The Brain, Emotion, and Depression

The Brain, Emotion, and Depression

Edmund T. Rolls
Oxford Centre for Computational Neuroscience, Oxford, England

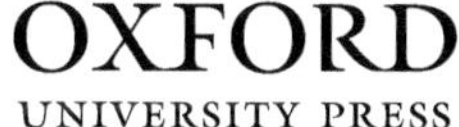

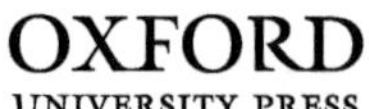

Great Clarendon Street, Oxford, OX2 6DP,
United Kingdom

Oxford University Press is a department of the University of Oxford. It furthers the University's objective of excellence in research, scholarship, and education by publishing worldwide. Oxford is a registered trade mark of Oxford University Press in the UK and in certain other countries

First Edition published in 2018
Impression: 1

Published in the United States of America by Oxford University Press
198 Madison Avenue, New York, NY 10016, United States of America

British Library Cataloguing in Publication Data
Data available

Library of Congress Control Number: 2018942778

ISBN 978–0–19–883224–9

Printed and bound by
CPI Group (UK) Ltd, Croydon, CR0 4YY

Preface

This book describes the brain mechanisms of emotion, and how they are leading to new approaches to understanding and treating depression.

The book is aimed at a non-specialist readership, including those with depression or those with friends or relatives with depression, and medical staff treating depression, as well as those interested in the science of emotion and decision-making, and how they are implemented in our brains. Indeed, **a key aim of the book is to describe research on understanding emotion and its underlying brain mechanisms, and to build an approach to understanding and treating depression that is based on this modern understanding of emotion and its brain mechanisms.**

The book has an innovative format, to help it to appeal to both non-specialist readers, and also to scientists interested in this research area. The sections in blue in this book are intended to be suitable for non-specialist readers, that is, for those who are not trained in neuroscience. But in addition, the sections not in blue consider some of the science in more detail, for the reader who either is a scientist, or wishes to start to delve into the science in more detail. This format has the promise to be very educational, in showing readers how to move from general understanding to the scientific evidence. It will enable the non-specialist reader, who may wish to read at first only the sections of the book in blue, to understand by delving into the other parts of the book, how scientists weigh the evidence to build an understanding based on how the evidence was obtained, which is a step beyond summarizing the main scientific conclusions. As an undergraduate reading medicine at the University of Cambridge, I was very impressed by how we were taught to look at the experimental evidence, to see how the science was performed, and what conclusions can be made from it. I believe that the approach taken in this book will provide the non-specialist reader with an understanding of the scientific approach, by looking into the non-blue sections. And I hope that the book as a whole will be useful to scientists and clinicians interested in emotion, its evolutionary functions, and its disorders, by providing a summary of the scientific evidence on these issues, and by providing a foundation for further research.

Non-specialist readers will notice that I provide citations to original published studies, usually citing the author(s) and year. The paper cited is listed in the reference section at the end of the book. The reason for this is that it must always be possible to go back to the original experiment or theoretical study, so that the evidence can be carefully examined, and evaluated. This is a very important part of the scientific method: that it must always be possible to go back to assess the original evidence. It does not mean that one has to go to read every paper cited: but the citations are provided, in case the reader wishes to check. The abstract of the original study can usually be found using Google Scholar (which may also lead one to a .pdf of the whole paper), or by using PubMed (https://www.ncbi.nlm.nih.gov/pubmed). (I note in parentheses that this is a rigorous and effective way to make progress in science, and that brief summaries on social media that do not cite their evidence have the risk of misleading rather than informing scientifically.) The references that I do cite focus on some of the key ground-breaking discoveries that are providing a framework for understanding emotion and its brain mechanisms and disorders such as depression, and there are therefore many follow-up studies that are not cited. However, many of these other studies can be found cited in *Emotion and Decision-Making Explained* (Rolls 2014b), and in the papers available as .pdfs on my website http://www.oxcns.org.

In addition, a glossary is provided in Appendix 1 on page 274.

Some of the key issues treated are: What produces emotions? Why do we have emotions? How do we have emotions? Why do emotional states feel like something? How do we take decisions? What happens in emotional disorders, including depression, and what are the new ideas that are emerging in these disorders, and possible new ways to treat them? This book seeks explanations of emotion and decision-making by considering these questions.

This book evolved from my earlier books *The Brain and Emotion* (Rolls 1999a), *Emotion Explained* (Rolls 2005) and *Emotion and Decision-Making Explained* (Rolls 2014b) as follows:

The Brain, Emotion and Depression (2018) is aimed at a wider readership, and aims to provide a new account of depression and its underlying brain mechanisms, which have implications for treatments. In addition, *The Brain, Emotion and Depression* updates some of the research described in *Emotion and Decision-Making Explained.* The present book, *The Brain, Emotion and Depression*, has the strength that a firm foundation is provided in *Emotion and Decision-Making Explained*, which those who find the present book of interest can turn to in order to find out in much more depth about what is considered here, and also about closely related topics such as neuroeconomics and the neuronal network mechanisms that implement many of the processes involved in emotion and decision-making. A unique aspect of the present book is its parts devoted to depression, which have been much less covered in *Emotion and Decision-Making Explained* (Rolls 2014b) and *Cerebral Cortex: Principles of Operation* (Rolls 2016c).

The Brain, Emotion and Depression goes beyond the brain mechanisms of emotion, in that it seeks to explain emotions in terms of the following: What produces emotions? (The general answer I propose is rewards and punishers, but with other factors too.) Why do we have emotions? (The overall answer I propose is that emotions are evolutionarily adaptive as they provide an efficient way for genes to influence our behaviour to increase their success.) How do we have emotions? (I answer this by describing what is known about the brain mechanisms of emotion.) Why do emotional states feel like something? This is part of the large problem of consciousness, which I address in Chapter 10.

Another way in which this book goes beyond brain mechanisms of emotion is to propose in Chapter 3 a Darwinian account of why animals (including humans) have emotions. The theory will I believe stand the test of time, in the same way as Darwin's theory of evolution by natural selection, and argues that emotions have the important evolutionary role of enabling genes to specify the goals (i.e. the rewards etc. that produce emotions) for actions, rather than the actions themselves. The advantage of this Darwinian design is that although the genes specify the goals, the actual actions are not prespecified by the genes, so that there is great flexibility of the actions themselves. This provides a new approach to the nature vs nurture debate in animal behaviour, for it shows how genes can influence behaviour without specifying a fixed, instinctive, behavioural response[1]. I hope that this will make the book of interest to a wide audience, including many interested in evolution and evolutionary biology.

Although in evolution Darwinian processes lead to gene-defined goals, it is also the case that in humans, goals may be influenced by other processes, including cultural processes. Indeed, some goals are defined within a culture, for example writing a novel like one by Tolstoy vs one by Virginia Woolf. But it is argued that it is primary reinforcers specified by genes of the general type shown in Table 2.1 on page 20 that make us want to be recognized

[1]There are some cases where genes do specify fixed responses, with one example that of a baby who feels the mother's breast on one cheek, and reflexively turns the head in the correct direction to suckle and obtain milk.

in society because of the advantages this can bring, to solve difficult problems, etc., and therefore to perform actions such as writing novels (see further Ridley (2003) Chapter 8, Ridley (1993b) pp. 310 ff, Laland & Brown (2002) pp. 271 ff, and Dawkins (1982)). Indeed, culture is influenced by human genetic propensities, and it follows that human cognitive, affective, and moral capacities are the product of a unique dynamic known as *gene-culture coevolution* (Gintis 2011, Gintis 2007).

We may also note that the theory that genes set many goals for action does not mean that our behaviour is determined by genes. Modern evolutionary theory has led to the understanding that many traits, particularly behavioural ones, may have some genetic basis but that does not mean that they will inevitably appear, because much depends on the environment (Dawkins 1995, Ridley 2003). Further, part of the power of the theory of emotion described here is that in evolution some genes specify rewards and punishers that are goals for action, but do not specify the actions themselves, which are flexible and can be learned. Further, it is shown in Chapter 10 that in humans (and other animals) with a reasoning capability, the reasoning can over-ride the gene-specified rewards to produce behaviour that is in the interests of the individual, the phenotype, and not the genes, and such behaviour is therefore even much less influenced (not 'determined') by genes.

Our understanding of emotion, decision-making, and the mechanisms of brain function, described in this book have wider implications, to for example aesthetics, ethics, and the philosophy of mind, and these wider implications are developed in *Neuroculture: On the Implications of Brain Science* (Rolls 2012d).

My book *Cerebral Cortex: Principles of Operation* (Rolls 2016c) shows how some of the neural mechanisms described in this book, and a number of others, provide a unifying computational neuroscience approach to understanding many aspects of brain function, including short-term memory, long-term memory, top-down attention, visual object recognition, and information representation in the brain, as well as decision-making. *Cerebral Cortex: Principles of Operation* (Rolls 2016c) includes Appendices that may be useful for those wishing an introduction to the computational neuroscience mechanisms involved in many aspects of brain function.

The Noisy Brain: Stochastic Dynamics as a Principle of Brain Function (Rolls & Deco 2010) describes in detail stochastic dynamics in the brain, how it can be understood with the techniques of theoretical physics, how it contributes to many aspects of brain function and behaviour, and how it provides new approaches to the cognitive changes that occur with aging, and to psychiatric disorders such as schizophrenia and obsessive-compulsive disorder.

It is hoped that this book will be of interest to all those interested in what emotions are, why we have them, how we have them, their disorders including especially depression, and how we take decisions based on emotions, as well as on rational thinking, and even how we choose between these types of decision-making.

The material in this text is the copyright of Edmund T. Rolls. Part of the material described in the book reflects research performed over many years in collaboration with many colleagues, whose tremendous contributions are warmly appreciated. The contributions of many will be evident from the references cited in the text. In addition, I have benefited enormously from the discussions I have had with a large number of colleagues and friends, many of whom I hope will see areas of the text that they have been able to illuminate. For example, discussions with Professor Jonathan Downar (University of Toronto) about depression were very much appreciated. Also, I pay tribute with this book and in a recent article (Rolls 2017d) to Larry Weiskrantz, who was a pioneering scientific thinker in the area of neuropsychology, an inspirational teacher when I was an undergraduate at Cambridge for me, David Marr, and many others, and who was a colleague at Oxford, and committed supporter and friend. Much of the work described would not have been possible without financial support from a number of sources, particularly the Medical Research Council of the UK, the Human Frontier Science Program, the Wellcome Trust, the McDonnell-Pew Foundation, and the Commission of the European Communities.

The book was typeset by the author in LaTeX using the WinEdt editor.

The cover shows part of the picture *Ulysses and the Sirens* painted in 1891 by John William Waterhouse. The metaphor relevant to understanding emotion is the rational conscious brain system in Ulysses resisting the gene-based emotion-related attractors, the sirens, by asking to be tied to the mast; and of Ulysses the explorer (the Greek Odysseus of Homer), always and indefatigably (like the author) seeking new discoveries about the world (and how it works). The cover shows that one of the themes of this book, the relation between emotional and rational (reasoning) processing has been a theme for many centuries, as the painting on this 5th century BC Greek Stamnos at the British Museum also shows Odysseus acting rationally by being tied to the mast. The other images are from 'Adam and Eve' painted in c. 1528 by Lucas Cranach the Elder (Uffizi Gallery, Florence), which provides an early interpretation of early human emotions, and emotion-related decision-making. This book provides a more recent, scientific, approach to emotions, and to decision-making, and to some of their disorders.

Updates to the publications cited in this book and .pdf files of many papers are available at `http://www.oxcns.org`.

Edmund T. Rolls dedicates this work to the overlapping group: his family, friends, and colleagues: *in salutem praesentium, in memoriam absentium.*

Contents

1 Introduction: the issues

1.1 Introduction

What are emotions? Why do we have emotions? What is their adaptive value? What are the brain mechanisms of emotion, and how can disorders of emotion be understood? Why does it feel like something to have an emotion? Why do emotions sometimes feel so intense? This book aims to provide answers to all these questions.

When we know what emotions are, why we have them, how they are produced by our brains, and why it feels like something to have an emotion, we will have a broad-ranging explanation of emotion.

We can similarly ask what motivates us: What is motivation? How is motivation controlled? How is motivation produced and regulated by the brain? What goes wrong in motivational disorders, for example in appetite disorders which produce overeating and obesity? How do these motivational control systems operate to ensure that we eat approximately the correct amount of food to maintain our body weight, or drink just enough to replenish our thirst? What are some of the underlying reasons for the different patterns of sexual behaviour found in different animals and humans? Why (and how) do we like some types of touch (e.g. a caress), and what is the relation of this to motivation? What brain processes underlie addiction? What is the relation between emotion, and motivational states such as hunger, appetite, and sexual behaviour? It turns out that the explanations for motivational behaviour are in many ways similar to those for emotional behaviour, and therefore I also treat motivation in this book.

Some of the aims of the book are to explain emotions in terms of the following:

1. What produces emotions? The general answer I propose is reinforcing stimuli, that is rewards and punishers, as described in Chapter 2.
2. Why do we have emotions? The overall answer I propose is that emotions are evolutionarily adaptive as they provide an efficient way for genes to influence our behaviour to increase their reproductive fitness (Chapter 3).
3. How do we have emotions? I answer this by describing what is known about the brain mechanisms of emotion (Chapter 4).
4. What is motivation? Motivation is a state in which we want a goal (e.g. a food reward, or avoiding pain) and are willing to perform an action to obtain the goal.
5. What are moods? These are states in which the eliciting stimulus may not be clear, or may have disappeared some time ago. (A description of all these terms is provided in Section 2.7.)
6. How do we take decisions?
   One answer I provide is in terms of attractor networks, which are described in Chapter 8. They have the interesting property that they are influenced by randomness in the exact times at which neurons fire in the brain, which makes our decision-making a little non-deterministic and probabilistic. This randomness

(or stochasticity) is evolutionarily adaptive, and contributes in other brain areas to original thought and creativity.

Another answer is that humans, and perhaps closely related animals, have a second, reasoning, system for making decisions (Chapter 10). This can make long-term decisions, which can be for the good of the individual, and not primarily for the good of the genes. These two properties make the two decision-making systems have quite different aims or goals, and this can lead to internal conflict in decision-making. I argue that these two systems are, generally across a large population, in balance; and that there may be considerable differences between individuals in their relative important. I also argue that which system (the emotional or the rational) is used for any particular decision is influenced by the randomness (stochasticity) just introduced.

7. Why do emotional states feel like something? This is part of the large problem of consciousness, which I address in Chapter 10.
8. Why can emotions feel so strong in humans? I address this in Chapter 10.
9. How can we understand emotional disorders such as depression? How will this better understanding help individuals to deal better with depressed feelings? What are the possibilities for new types of treatment now that we are advancing towards a way of understanding depression in terms of the underlying computational processes that take place in our brains? I address these important issues in Chapter 9.

Emotion and motivation are linked by the property that both involve rewards and punishers. Emotions can be thought of as states elicited by rewards or punishers. A full definition of emotion, and theory of emotion, with a starting point as the relation to rewards and punishers is described in Chapter 2. Motivation can be thought of as a state in which a goal is being sought, such as reward, or avoidance of a punisher. An example of a reward might be the food obtained when one has performed an action to obtain the food. An example of a motivational state might be hunger, when one wants to perform an action in order to obtain a food reward. This is made clear in Chapters 2, 3, 5, and 7.

Because of the importance of reward and punishment for emotion and motivation, I define in Section 1.2 reward and punishment, and describe some of the types of learning that involve rewards and punishers. This is useful groundwork for what follows in the rest of this book. However, for those who wish in a first reading to skip the definitions in Section 1.2 (which are provided to ensure that there is a firm foundation for understanding emotion and motivation), it may be useful simply to think of a reward as something for which an animal (which includes humans) will work, and a punisher as something that an animal will work to escape from or avoid.

Some stimuli are innately rewarding or punishing and are called primary reinforcers (for example no learning is necessary to respond to pain as aversive), while other stimuli are learned or secondary reinforcers (for example the sight of a chocolate cake is not innately rewarding, but may become a learned reinforcer, for which we may work, by the process of association learning between the sight of the cake and its taste, where the taste is a primary reward or reinforcer). This type of learning, which is important in emotion and motivation, is called stimulus–reinforcement association learning. (A better term is stimulus–reinforcer association learning, where reinforcer is being used to mean a stimulus that might be a reward or a punisher.)

1.2 Rewards and punishers, and learning about rewards and punishers: instrumental learning and stimulus–reinforcer association learning

A reward is something for which an animal (including of course a human) will work. A punisher is something that an animal will work to escape or avoid (or that will decrease the probability of actions on which it is contingent). In order to exclude simple reflex-like behaviour, the concept invoked here by the term 'work' is to perform an arbitrary behaviour (called an operant response) in order to obtain the reward or avoid the punisher. An example of an operant response might be putting money in a vending machine to obtain food, or for a rat pressing a lever to obtain food. In these cases, the food is the reward. Another example of an operant response might be moving from one place to another in order to escape from or avoid an aversive (punishing) stimulus such as a cold draught. If the aversive stimulus starts and then the response is made, this is referred to as *escape* from the punisher. If a warning stimulus (such as a flashing light) indicates that the punisher will be delivered unless the operant response is made, then the animal may learn to perform the operant response when the warning stimulus is given in order to *avoid* the punisher.

Because the definitions of reward and punisher make it a requirement that it must be at least possible to demonstrate learning of an arbitrary operant response (made to obtain the reward or to escape from or avoid the punisher), we see that learning is implicit in the definition of reward and punisher. (Merely swimming up a chemical gradient towards a source of food as occurs in single cell organisms is called a taxis as described in Chapter 3; it does not require learning, and does not make the food qualify as a reward under the definition.) In that rewards and punishers do imply the ability to learn what to do to obtain the reward or escape from or avoid the punisher, we call rewards and punishers 'instrumental reinforcers', because they are reinforcers that are obtained when actions are instrumental when trying to obtain goals, the rewards.

This introduction leads to the definition of instrumental **reinforcers** as stimuli that if their occurrence, termination, or omission is made contingent upon the making of an action, alter the probability of the future emission of that action (as a result of the contingency (i.e. dependency) on the action). The alteration of the probability of an action (or behavioural response) is the measure that instrumental learning has taken place to obtain a goal. A positive reinforcer (such as food) increases the probability of emission of an action on which it is contingent; the process is termed **positive reinforcement**, and the outcome is a reward (such as food). A negative reinforcer (such as a painful stimulus) increases the probability of emission of an action which causes the negative reinforcer to be omitted (as in active avoidance) or terminated (as in escape), and the procedure is termed **negative reinforcement**. In contrast, **punishment** refers to procedures in which the probability of an action is decreased. Punishment thus describes procedures in which an action decreases in probability if it is followed by a painful stimulus, as in passive avoidance. Punishment can also be used to refer to a procedure involving the omission or termination of a reward ('extinction' and 'time out' respectively), both of which decrease the probability of actions (Gray 1975, Mackintosh 1983, Dickinson 1980, Lieberman 2000, Mazur 2012).

My argument is that an affectively positive or 'appetitive' stimulus (which produces a state of pleasure) acts operationally as a **reward**, which when delivered acts instrumentally as a positive reinforcer, or when not delivered (omitted or terminated) acts to decrease the probability of actions on which it is contingent. Conversely I argue that an affectively negative or aversive stimulus (which produces an unpleasant state) acts operationally as a **punisher**, which when delivered acts instrumentally to decrease the probability of actions on which it is contingent, or when not delivered (escaped from or avoided) acts as a negative reinforcer in that it then increases the probability of the action on which its non-delivery is contingent[2] (Rolls 2014b).

Reinforcers, that is rewards or punishers, may be unlearned or **primary reinforcers**, or learned or secondary reinforcers. An example of a primary reinforcer is pain, which is innately a punisher. The first time a painful stimulus is ever delivered, it will be escaped from, and no learning that it is aversive is needed. Similarly, the first time a sweet taste is delivered, it can act as a positive reinforcer, so it is a primary positive reinforcer or reward. Other stimuli become reinforcing by learning, because of their association with primary reinforcers, thereby becoming '**secondary reinforcers**'. For example, a (previously neutral) sound that regularly precedes an electric shock can become a secondary reinforcer. Animals will learn operant responses (actions) reinforced by the secondary reinforcer, for example jumping to a place where the secondary reinforcer is not present or terminates. Secondary reinforcers are thus important in enabling animals to avoid primary punishers such as pain.

There is a close relation of all these processes to emotion, for as we will see in Chapter 2, fear is an emotional state that might be produced by a sound that has previously been associated with an electric shock. Shock in this example is the primary punisher, and fear is the emotional state that occurs to the tone stimulus as a result of the learning of the stimulus (i.e. tone)–reinforcer (i.e. shock) association. Another example of a secondary reinforcer is a visual stimulus associated with the taste of a food. For example, the first time we see a new type of food we do not treat the sight of the new visual stimulus as reinforcing, but if the stimulus has a good taste, the sight of the object becomes a positive secondary reinforcer, and we may choose the food when we see it in future by virtue of its association with a primary reinforcer. This type of learning is thus called '**stimulus–reinforcer association learning**'. (The operation is often referred to as stimulus–reinforcement association learning.) This type of learning is very important in many emotions, because it is as a result of this type of learning that many previously neutral stimuli come to elicit emotional responses, as in the example of fear above.

Unconditioned reinforcing stimuli often elicit autonomic responses. (Autonomic responses are those mediated through the autonomic nervous system, via the vagus and sympathetic nerves, which affect smooth muscle.) Examples include alterations of heart rate and of blood pressure which might be produced by a painful stimulus; and salivation which might be produced by the taste of food. Many endocrine (hormonal) responses are also mediated through the autonomic nervous system and so are autonomic responses, for example the release of adrenaline (epinephrine) from the adrenal gland during emotional excitement. Previously neutral stimuli, such as the sound in our previous example, can by pairing with unconditioned stimuli, such as shock in the previous example, come by learning the association, to produce learned autonomic responses. In the example the tone might by pairing with shock come to elicit a change in heart rate, and sweating. This type of learning is called **classical conditioning**, and also **Pavlovian conditioning** after Ivan Pavlov who performed many of the original studies of this type of learning, including learned salivation to the sound of a bell that predicted the taste of food. It is a type of learning that is very similar to stimulus–reinforcer association learning, except that in the case of classical conditioning the responses involved are autonomic and endocrine responses.

A key difference between **instrumental learning** and classical conditioning apart from

[2]Note that my definition of a punisher, which is similar to that of an aversive stimulus, is of a stimulus or event that can either decrease the probability of actions on which it is contingent, or increase the probability of actions on which its non-delivery is contingent. The term punishment is restricted to situations where the probability of an action is being decreased.

the response systems involved lies in the contingencies that operate. In classical conditioning the animal has no control over whether the unconditioned stimulus is delivered (as in the experiments of Pavlov just described). In contrast, the whole notion of instrumental learning is that what the animal does is instrumental in determining whether the reinforcer (the goal) is obtained, or escaped from or avoided. Both types of learning are important in emotions because (as we will see in Chapter 2) instrumental reinforcers produce emotional responses, but also typically produce autonomic responses that therefore typically occur during emotional states, and indeed mediate important effects of emotions such as preparing the body for action by increasing heart rate etc.

A more detailed description of the nature of classical (Pavlovian) conditioning and instrumental learning, and how both are related to emotion, are provided by Rolls (2014b).

Motivation refers to the state an animal is in when it is willing to work for a reward or to escape from or avoid a punisher. So for example we say that an animal is motivated to work for the taste of food, and in this case the motivational state is called hunger. The definition of motivation thus implies the capacity to perform any, arbitrary, operant response in order to obtain the reward or escape from or avoid the punisher. By implying an operant response, we exclude simple behaviours such as reflexes and taxes (such as swimming up a chemical gradient), as described above and in Chapter 2. By implying learning of any response to obtain a reward (or avoid a punisher), motivation thus focuses on behaviours in which a goal is defined. Motivation is one of the states that are involved in understanding brain design, related to the fundamental issue of how goals for behaviour are defined, and how an appropriate behaviour is selected, as described in this book and brought together into a theory in Chapter 2.

1.3 The approaches taken to emotion and motivation: their causes, functions, adaptive value, and brain mechanisms

To explain emotion, and motivation, a number of different approaches are taken, and some of these need some introduction.

1.3.1 The causes of emotion

To examine the causes of emotion, the environmental stimuli and situations that elicit emotions are identified. This is part of the subject of Chapter 2. It is shown how the different environmental stimulus conditions that produce emotions provide the basis for a classification of different emotions. Understanding the functions of emotion also provides part of the explanation of why we have emotions, and many of the functions of emotion are described in Chapter 3. These functions of emotion explain in part the adaptive value of emotion, and give part of an explanation about why emotion has evolved. However, it turns out that emotions provide a fundamental solution to the issue of how genes design brains to produce behaviour that is advantageous to the genes, and this deep understanding of the adaptive value of emotion, and in a sense the cause of emotion, is elaborated in Chapter 3. When considering the adaptive value of emotion in the context of evolution, we must remember that animals are generally social, and that evolution may have led to the development of special reward and punishment systems to help to produce emotional behaviour that is adaptive in social situations. This area, of understanding and explaining aspects of social behaviour in terms of its evolutionary adaptive value, is the field of sociobiology and evolutionary psychology (Buss 2015), and this approach is introduced especially in the context of sexual behaviour in Chapter 7.

1.3.1.1 Explanation of emotion at the 'ultimate' level of causation

At the 'ultimate' level of causation, the level of adaptive value in evolution (Mayr 1961, Tinbergen 1963), emotion is explained as an efficient and simple way for genes to influence behaviour for their own 'selfish' reproductive success, by specifying the rewarding and punishing goals for instrumental action with the resulting states being emotional states (Chapters 2 and 3). This is simpler and more efficient in terms of evolutionary adaptive value than for genes to specify the actions, the behavioural responses, to be produced by stimuli (Chapter 3).

1.3.1.2 Explanation of emotion at the 'proximate' level of causation

Another major approach taken to explain emotion and motivation, and their underlying reward and punishment systems, is in terms of the brain mechanisms that implement them. Understanding the brain processing and mechanisms of behaviour is one way to ensure that we have the correct explanation for how the behaviour is produced. Another important reason for investigating the actual brain mechanisms that underlie emotion and motivation, and reward and punishment, is not only to understand how our own brains work, but also to have the basis for understanding and treating medical disorders of these systems. This type of explanation of behaviour is referred to as the 'proximate' level of causation (Mayr 1961, Tinbergen 1963), and for emotion involves understanding the neuronal mechanisms in the orbitofrontal cortex, anterior cingulate cortex, amygdala, and connected brain regions.

In terms of decision-making, the explanation at the 'proximate' level of causation is in terms of the attractor cortical neuronal network mechanisms described in Chapter 8 that implement decision-making. An attractive feature of this explanation is that it is essentially the same type of cortical mechanism that is used in other cortical areas for long-term memory (e.g. the hippocampus episodic memory and temporal lobe semantic memory systems (Rolls 2016c, Kesner & Rolls 2015, Treves & Rolls 1994)) and for short-term memory (Rolls 2016c, Rolls, Dempere-Marco & Deco 2013). Moreover, the mechanism described for decision-making is a neuronal mechanism that specifies how the decision is taken in terms of the neuronal and neuronal network mechanisms (Wang 2002, Rolls & Deco 2010, Deco, Rolls, Albantakis & Romo 2013, Rolls 2016c) (see Chapter 8), and is different in this respect from a mathematical model such as a drift diffusion model that does not specify the neuronal mechanisms and so sets up artificial constructs for the source of the noise, the threshold at which a decision may be said to have been reached, etc. (Ratcliff & Rouder 1998, Ratcliff, Zandt & McKoon 1999, Gold & Shadlen 2007).

Another advantage of an explanation at the proximate level of the biological mechanism rather than a mathematical model is that an explanation at the biological level facilitates insight into biological factors that may influence the mechanisms, such as drug treatments for neuropsychiatric states such as depression (Chapter 9), schizophrenia, and obsessive-compulsive disorder (Rolls & Deco 2010, Rolls, Loh, Deco & Winterer 2008d, Rolls, Loh & Deco 2008c, Rolls 2016c).

Decision-making is explained at the 'ultimate' level of explanation by the evolutionary adaptive value of having accurate continuously graded representations of the decision variables such as value so that they can be represented precisely, and then following this by a non-linear choice mechanism that falls into one of two or more possible and stable decision states, so that behaviour and even the agonist and antagonist muscles are not being pulled in different directions simultaneously. Part of the evolutionary adaptive value of the attractor network decision-making mechanism described in Chapter 8 is that it implements a short-term memory mechanism that enables the decision to be maintained for some time so that behaviour can be directed for some time towards implementing the decision. Another part of the evolutionary adaptive value of the attractor network decision-making mechanism described in Chapter 8 is that although it makes a choice that is stable and is maintained for some time, the actual choice made can be influenced by noise in the brain, which as shown in Chapter 8 and by Rolls & Deco (2010) can be advantageous, including avoidance of predators, and creative thought. Decisions can be made by other brain systems with different neuronal mechanisms, for example by the direct mutual inhibition between neurons that is implemented in the basal ganglia as described in Chapter 6. However, the mechanism using direct mutual inhibition by neurons does not have the evolutionary adaptive value of maintaining the decision on-line using a short-term memory implemented by the recurrent excitatory connections in cortical networks, and indeed that is part of the 'ultimate' explanation for the value of cortical attractor decision-making networks as described in Chapter 8.

Thus emotion, motivation, and decision-making are provided with explanations at the 'proximate' and 'ultimate' levels in this book.

1.3.2 The importance of understanding the primate, including human, brain

It is because of the intended relevance to understanding human emotion and its disorders that emphasis is placed in this book on findings from research in non-human primates, including monkeys, as well as in humans. This is important, for many of the brain systems that are involved in emotion and motivation have undergone considerable development in primates (e.g. monkeys and humans) compared to non-primates (for example rats and mice).

For example, the temporal lobe has undergone great development in primates, and several systems in the temporal lobe are either involved in emotion (e.g. the amygdala), or provide some of the main sensory inputs to brain systems involved in emotion and motivation. In particular, the amygdala and the orbitofrontal cortex, key brain structures in emotion, both receive inputs from the highly developed temporal lobe cortical areas, including those involved in invariant visual object recognition and face identity and expression processing.

Another example is that the prefrontal cortex has also undergone great development in primates, and one part of it, the orbitofrontal cortex, is very little developed in rodents, yet is one of the major brain areas involved in emotion and motivation in primates including humans. Indeed, it has been argued that the granular prefrontal cortex is a primate innovation, and the implication of the argument is that any areas that might be termed orbitofrontal cortex in rats (Schoenbaum, Roesch, Stalnaker & Takahashi 2009) are homologous only to the agranular parts of the primate orbitofrontal cortex (shaded mid grey in Fig. 1.1), that is to areas 13a, 14c, and the agranular insular areas labelled Ia in Fig. 1.1 (Wise 2008, Passingham & Wise 2012). It follows from that argument that for most areas of the orbitofrontal and medial prefrontal cortex in humans and macaques (those shaded light grey in Fig. 1.1), special consideration must be given to research in macaques and humans. As shown in Fig. 1.1, there may be no cortical area in rodents that is homologous to most of the primate including human orbitofrontal cortex (Preuss 1995, Wise 2008, Passingham & Wise 2012).

The development of some of these cortical areas has been so great in primates that even evolutionarily old systems such as the taste system appear to have been rewired, compared with that of rodents, to place much more emphasis on cortical processing, taking place in areas such as the orbitofrontal cortex (Rolls & Scott 2003, Scott & Small 2009, Small & Scott 2009, Rolls 2016b, Rolls 2016e) (Fig. 4.2). In primates, the reward value of the taste is represented in the orbitofrontal cortex in that the responses of orbitofrontal taste neurons are modulated by hunger in just the same way as is the reward value or palatability of a taste. In particular, it has been shown that orbitofrontal cortex taste neurons stop responding to the taste of a food with which a monkey is fed to satiety, and that this parallels the decline in

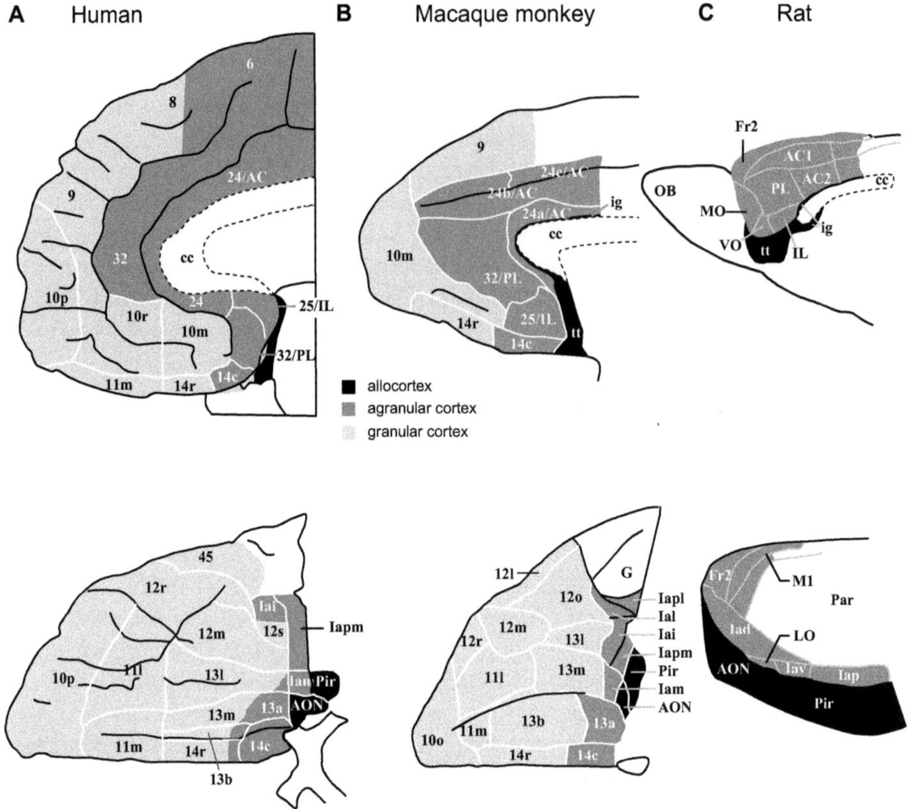

Fig. 1.1 Comparison of the orbitofrontal (below) and medial prefrontal (above) cortical areas in humans, macaque monkeys, and rats. (A) Medial (top) and orbital (bottom) areas of the human frontal codex (Ongur et al. 2003). (B) Medial (top) and orbital (bottom) areas of the macaque frontal cortex (Carmichael and Price 1994). (C) Medial (top) and lateral (bottom) areas of rat frontal cortex (Palomero-Gallagher and Zilles 2004). Rostral is to the left in all drawings. Top row: dorsal is up in all drawings. Bottom row: in (A) and (B), lateral is up; in (C), dorsal is up. Not to scale. Abbreviations: AC, anterior cingulate cortex; AON, anterior olfactory 'nucleus'; cc, corpus callosum; Fr2 second frontal area; la, agranular insular cortex; ig, induseum griseum; IL, infralimbic cortex; LO, lateral orbital cortex; MO, medial orbital cortex: OB, olfactory bulb; Pr, piriform (olfactory) cortex; PL, prelimbic cortex; tt, tenia tecta; VO, ventral orbital cortex; Subdivisions of areas are labelled caudal (c); inferior (i), lateral (l), medial (m); orbital (o), posterior or polar (p), rostral(r), or by arbitrary designation (a, b). (After Passingham and Wise (2012). (a) Adapted from Dost Ongur, Amon T. Ferry, and Joseph L. Price, Architectonic subdivision of the human orbital and medial prefrontal cortex, *Journal of Comparative Neurology*, 460 (3), pp. 425–49. doi.org/10.1002/cne.10609. Copyright © 2003 John Wiley and Sons. (b) Adapted from S. T. Carmichael and J. L. Price, Architectonic subdivision of the orbital and medial prefrontal cortex in the macaque monkey, *Journal of Comparative Neurology*, 346 (3), pp. 366–402 Copyright © 1994 John Wiley and Sons. (c) Adapted from Nicola Palomero-Gallagher and Karl Zilles, 'Isocortex', in Paxinos, George ed., *The Rat Nervous System*, 3e, pp. 729–757, doi.org/10.1016/B978-012547638-6/50024-9. Copyright © 2004 Elsevier Inc. All rights reserved.

the acceptability of the food (see Fig. 4.6) (Rolls, Sienkiewicz & Yaxley 1989b). In contrast, the representation of taste in the insular primary taste cortex of primates (Scott, Yaxley, Sienkiewicz & Rolls 1986, Yaxley, Rolls & Sienkiewicz 1990) is not modulated by hunger (Rolls, Scott, Sienkiewicz & Yaxley 1988, Yaxley, Rolls & Sienkiewicz 1988, Rolls 2016b). Thus in the primary taste cortex of primates (and at earlier stages of taste processing including the nucleus of the solitary tract), the reward value of taste is not represented, and instead the identity of the taste is represented (see Section 5.3.1). The importance of cortical processing of taste in primates, first for identity and intensity in the primary taste cortex, and then for reward value in the orbitofrontal cortex, is that both types of representation need to be interfaced to visual and other processing that requires cortical computation. For example, it may have adaptive value to be able to represent exactly what taste is present, and to link it by learning to the sight and location of the source of the taste, even when hunger and reward is not being produced, so that the source of that taste can be found in future, when it may have reward value. In line with cortical processing to dominate the processing of taste in primates, there is no modulation of taste responsiveness at or before the primary taste cortex, and the pathways for taste are directly from the nucleus of the solitary tract in the brainstem to the taste thalamus and then to the taste cortex (Fig. 4.2). In contrast, in rodents such as the rat, the nucleus of the solitary tract connects to a pontine taste area, the parabrachial nucleus, that is not present in primates (Rolls & Scott 2003, Scott & Small 2009, Small & Scott 2009, Rolls 2016b, Rolls 2016e). The rodent pontine taste area then not only has connections to the thalamus and thus to the cortex, but also has direct connections to many subcortical areas important in appetite control, including the amygdala and hypothalamus (Section 5.3.1.4). Moreover, in rodents, satiety reduces the responsiveness of neurons in the nucleus of the solitary tract to the taste of food by approximately 30%, so that taste processing in rodents is from the first synapse in the brain confounded by reward value, by hedonics. That makes the taste (and reward) system of rodents very difficult to understand functionally for different functions are not separated (taste identity and intensity vs hedonics), and makes the taste system of rodents a poor one with which to understand primate including human taste reward processing (Rolls 2016b, Rolls 2016e, Rolls 2016c). This evidence emphasizes the importance of understanding the evidence from primates including humans, even in a system such as the taste system that one might think is evolutionarily so old (Section 5.3.1.4).

Another reason for focusing interest on the primate brain is that there has been great development of the visual system in primates, and this itself has had important implications for the types of sensory stimuli that are processed by brain systems involved in emotion and motivation (Rolls 2014b, Rolls 2016c), and also in memory systems (Rolls & Wirth 2018). One example is the importance of face identity and face expression decoding, which are both important in primate emotional behaviour, and indeed provide an important part of the foundation for much primate social behaviour. These are among the reasons why emphasis is placed on brain systems in primates, including humans, in the approach taken here.

The overall medically relevant aim of the research described in this book is to provide a foundation for understanding in humans the brain mechanisms of emotion, motivation, and decision-making, and thus their disorders, including depression, anxiety, addiction, sociopathy, borderline personality disorder, schizophrenia, eating disorders, and decision-making disorders including pathological gambling.

1.3.3 Functional neuroimaging in humans, neuronal encoding, and understanding the brain computationally

When considering brain mechanisms involved in emotion and decision-making, findings with human brain imaging are described. These approaches include functional magnetic resonance imaging (fMRI) to measure changes in brain oxygenation level locally (using a signal from deoxyhaemoglobin) to provide an index of local brain activity, as well as positron emission tomography (PET) studies to estimate local regional cerebral blood flow, again to provide an index of local brain activity. It is, however, important to note that these functional neuroimaging approaches provide rather coarse approaches to brain function, in that the spatial resolution is seldom better than 3 mm, so that the picture given is one of 'blobs on the brain', which give some indication of what is happening where in the brain, and what types of dissociation of functions are possible.

However, because there are millions of neurons in each of the areas that can be resolved with functional neuroimaging, such imaging techniques give rather little evidence on how the brain works. For this, one needs to know what information is represented in each brain area at the level at which information is exchanged between the computing elements of the brain, the neurons (brain cells). One also needs to know how the representation of information (for example about stimuli or events in the world) changes from stage to stage of the processing in the brain, to understand how the brain works as a system. It turns out that one can 'read' this information from the brain by recording the activity of single neurons, or groups of single neurons (Rolls & Treves 2011). The reason that this is an effective procedure for understanding what is represented is that each neuron has one information output channel, the firing of its action potentials, so that one can measure the full richness of the information being represented in a region by measuring the firing of its neurons. This can reveal fundamental evidence crucial for understanding how the brain operates (Rolls 2016c). For example, neuronal recording can reveal all the information represented in an area even if parts of it are encoded by relatively small numbers, perhaps a few percent, of its neurons. (This is impossible with brain-imaging techniques, which also are susceptible to the interpretation problem that whatever causes the largest activation is interpreted as 'what' is being encoded in a region.)

Neuronal recording also provides evidence for the level at which it is appropriate to build computational models of brain function, the neuronal network level. Such neuronal network computational models consider how populations of neurons with the connections found in a given brain area, and with biologically plausible properties such as learning rules for altering the strengths of synaptic connections between neurons, actually could perform useful computation to implement the functions being performed by that brain area (Rolls 2016c). This approach should not really be considered as a metaphor for brain operation, but as a theory of how each part of the brain operates. The neuronal network computational theory, and any model or simulation based on it, may of course be simplified to some extent to make it tractable, but nevertheless the point is that the neuron-level approach, coupled with neuronal network models that analyse the functions of populations of neurons, together provide some of the fundamental elements for understanding how the brain actually works. For this reason, emphasis is also placed in this book on what is known about what is being processed in each brain area as shown by recordings from neurons. Such evidence, in terms of building theories and models of how the brain functions, can never be replaced by brain imaging evidence, although these approaches do complement each other very effectively.

The approach to brain function in terms of computations performed by neuronal networks in different brain areas is the subject of the books *Neural Networks and Brain Function* by Rolls & Treves (1998), *Computational Neuroscience of Vision* by Rolls & Deco (2002), *Memory, Attention, and Decision-Making: A Unifying Computational Neuroscience Approach* by Rolls (2016c), *The Noisy Brain: Stochastic Dynamics as a Principle of Brain Function* by Rolls & Deco (2010), and *Cerebral Cortex: Principles of Operation* by Rolls (2016c). The reader is referred to these books for more comprehensive accounts of this biologically plausible approach to brain function. It can be described as a mechanistic approach to understanding brain function, in that the underlying computational processes that underlie behaviour and thought must be explicitly understood (and are the 'proximate' causes of behaviour), and must be placed in the context of the evolutionary adaptive value of those mechanisms, the 'ultimate' causes of the behaviour. In this book, some of the neurophysiological evidence and its computational implications for understanding how our brains work to produce emotion and motivation, and the nature of their adaptive value, are described.

1.4 Emotion, motivation, and depression: the plan of the book

The plan of the book is that we consider in Chapters 2 and 3 the major issue of emotion, and its functions. These chapters address the explanation of emotion by defining emotion, and elucidating its functions. Another part of the explanation of emotion is how it actually works, that is how it is implemented in the brain, which is described in Chapter 4. By understanding its mechanisms, we not only understand better the different processes that contribute to emotion, but also we provide a fundamental basis for starting to understand many disorders of emotion, including for example depression, and how they can be treated.

Affective (emotional) states, and rewards, are involved in motivated behaviour such as eating, addiction, and sexual behaviour, and we consider these in Chapters 5, 6, and 7. These topics provide many clear examples of how the pleasantness or reward value of stimuli reflect a fundamental aspect of the design of both the brain and behaviour, and help to show the rewards, and punishers, that actually influence many aspects of our behaviour.

In Chapter 8 I consider how the brain takes decisions, and how confidence in our decisions is reflected by the machinery of the brain.

Building on what is in the rest of this book, Chapter 9 considers depression: its causes, brain mechanisms, and treatments.

In Chapter 10 the issue of emotional feelings, which is part of the large issue of consciousness, is considered, together with the brain processing involved in conscious feelings.

2 The nature of emotion

2.1 Introduction

In this Chapter, I describe emotion in terms of the events that cause emotions. Once we have an operational definition, this provides a basis for systematic research on emotion. I start with what is becoming a standard approach to understanding emotion. Then I compare this with some other approaches to emotion. The issues of emotional feelings, and more generally consciousness, are left to Chapter 10, for we can make great progress even before we fully understand what consciousness is. I provide a short version of the approach in this Chapter, with a much fuller description in *Emotion and Decision-Making Explained* (Rolls 2014b).

2.2 The outline of a theory of emotion

I will first introduce the essence of the definition of emotion that I propose:
Emotions are states elicited by rewards and punishers, that is, by instrumental reinforcers.

As described in Section 1.2, a reward is anything for which an animal will work. A punisher is anything that an animal will work to escape or avoid, or that will suppress actions on which it is contingent. I note that any change in the regular delivery of a reward or a punisher acts as an instrumental reinforcer. The force of 'instrumental' in this definition is that the emotional states are seen as defining the goals for arbitrary behavioural actions, made to obtain the instrumental reinforcer. This is very different from classical conditioning, in which a response, typically autonomic, may be elicited to a stimulus, without any need for an intervening state (see further Section 4.6.2). The relevant states elicited by the instrumental reinforcers are those with the particular functions described in Chapter 3.

An example of an emotion might thus be happiness produced by being given a reward, such as a hug, a pleasant touch, praise, winning a large sum of money, or being with someone whom one loves. All these things are rewards, in that we will work to obtain them. Another example of an emotion might be fear produced by the sound of a rapidly approaching bus when we are cycling, or the sight of an angry expression on someone's face. We will work to avoid such stimuli, which are punishers. Another example might be frustration, anger, or sadness produced by the omission of an expected reward such as a prize, or the termination of a reward such as the death of a loved one. Another example might be relief, produced by the omission or termination of a punishing stimulus, for example the removal of a painful stimulus, or sailing out of danger. These examples indicate how emotions can be produced by the delivery, omission, or termination of rewarding or punishing stimuli, and go some way to indicate how different emotions could be produced and classified in terms of the rewards and punishers received, omitted, or terminated.

Before accepting this proposal, we should consider whether there are any exceptions to the proposed rule. Indeed, at first this may appear to be a rather reductionist hypothesis about what produces emotions. However, one way to test the suggested definition of the events that cause emotions is to ask whether there are any rewards or punishers that do not produce emotions. Conversely, we should ask whether there are any emotions that are produced by stimuli, events, or remembered events that are not rewarding or punishing. As major exceptions to the overall principle are difficult to identify (see Rolls (2014b)), then we should accept the suggestion as a useful identification, summary, and operational definition of the conditions that produce emotions. The full theory of emotion must also take into account the issue of emotional feelings, which is part of the large issue of consciousness, and this is considered in Chapter 10.

The idea that rewards and punishers, that is instrumental reinforcers, are the stimuli that produce emotions has a considerable history, with origins that can be traced back to Watson (1930), Harlow & Stagner (1933), and Amsel (1962). More recently, the approach was developed by Millenson (1967), Larry Weiskrantz (1968), and Jeffrey Gray (1975, 1981).

The classification of emotions in terms of reinforcement contingencies is developed further in Section 2.3, and more formal definitions of rewards and punishers, and how they are related to learning theory concepts such as reinforcement, instrumental learning, and punishment are provided next, and are elaborated further in Sections 1.2 and 4.6.2.

Instrumental reinforcers are stimuli that, if their occurrence, termination, or omission is made contingent upon the making of an action, alter the probability of the future emission of that action (Gray 1975, Mackintosh 1983, Dickinson 1980, Lieberman 2000, Mazur 2012). Rewards and punishers are instrumental reinforcing stimuli. The notion of an action here is that an arbitrary action, e.g. turning right vs turning left, will be performed in order to obtain the reward or avoid the punisher, so that there is no pre-wired connection between the response and the reinforcing stimulus. Some stimuli are primary (unlearned) reinforcers (e.g., the taste of food if the animal is hungry, or pain); while others may become reinforcing by learning, because of their association with such primary reinforcers, thereby becoming 'secondary reinforcers'. This type of learning may thus be called 'stimulus–reinforcer association', and occurs via an associative learning process. A positive reinforcer (such as food) increases the probability of emission of a response on which it is contingent, the process is termed **positive reinforcement**, and the *outcome* is a reward (such as food). A negative reinforcer (such as a painful stimulus) increases the probability of emission of a response that causes the negative reinforcer to be omitted (as in active avoidance) or terminated (as in escape), and the procedure is termed **negative reinforcement**. In contrast, **punishment** refers to procedures in which the probability of an action is decreased. Punishment thus describes procedures in which an action decreases in probability if it is followed by a painful stimulus, as in passive avoidance. Punishment can also be used to refer to a procedure involving the omission or termination of a reward ('extinction' and 'time out' respectively), both of which decrease the probability of responses (Gray 1975, Mackintosh 1983, Dickinson 1980, Lieberman 2000, Mazur 2012). The learning of which action to perform to achieve the goal is 'action–outcome' learning. My argument is that an affectively positive or 'appetitive' stimulus (which produces a state of pleasure) acts operationally as a **reward**, which when delivered acts instrumentally as a positive reinforcer, or when not delivered (omitted or terminated) acts to decrease the probability of actions on which it is contingent. Conversely I argue that an affectively negative or aversive stimulus (which produces an unpleasant state) acts operationally as a **punisher**, which when delivered acts instrumentally to decrease the probability of responses on which it is contingent, or when not delivered (escaped from or avoided) acts as a negative reinforcer in that it then increases the probability of the action on which its non-delivery is contingent.

The link between emotion and instrumental reinforcers being made is partly an operational link. But the link is deeper than this, as we will see, in that the theory has been developed that genes specify primary reinforcers in order to encourage the animal to perform arbitrary actions to seek particular goals, thus increasing the probability of the genes' survival into the next generation (Rolls 1999a, Rolls 2014b). The emotional states elicited by the reinforcers have a number of functions, described in Chapter 3, related to these processes. The presence of an intervening state produced by the stimulus associated with a primary reinforcer (e.g. the sight of food, or a tone associated with shock) in instrumental learning that provides a goal for an action is a key concept in my theory of emotion (Rolls 2014b), for the intervening state is an affective or emotional state (Rolls 2013d).

Further, motivation can now be understood as a state in which the goal (i.e. the instrumental reinforcer) is being sought. We should reserve the term 'motivation' for states in which an instrumental reinforcer or goal is being sought. If in contrast the behaviour is a reflex such as protruding a proboscis when short of food, then we would not call this motivated behaviour, and the term 'drive' may be used.

Before considering how different emotions are related to different reinforcement contingencies in Section 2.3, I clarify a matter of terminology about *moods vs emotions*. A useful convention to distinguish between emotion and a mood state is as follows. An emotion consists of cognitive processing that results in a decoded signal that an environmental event (or remembered event) is reinforcing, together with the mood or affective or emotional state produced as a result. If the mood state is produced in the absence of the external sensory input and the cognitive decoding (for example by direct electrical stimulation of the brain (Rolls 2005)), then this is described only as a mood state, and is different from an emotion in that there is no object in the environment towards which the mood state is directed. (In that emotions are produced by stimuli or objects, and thus emotions 'take or have an object', emotional states are examples of what philosophers call intentional states.) It is useful to emphasize that there is great opportunity for cognitive processing (whether conscious or not) in emotions, for cognitive processes will very often be required to determine whether an environmental stimulus or event is an instrumental reinforcer.

2.3 Different emotions

As introduced in Section 2.2, the different emotions can in part be described and classified according to whether the instrumental reinforcer is positive or negative, and by the reinforcement contingency. An outline of such a classification scheme, elaborated by Rolls (1990a, 1999a, 2000a, 2005, 2014b) is shown in Fig. 2.1.

Movement away from the centre of the diagram represents increasing intensity of emotion, on a continuous scale. The diagram shows that emotions associated with the delivery of a reward (S+) include pleasure, elation and ecstasy. Of course, other emotional labels can be included along the same axis. Emotions associated with the delivery of a punisher (S–) include apprehension, fear, and terror (see Fig. 2.1). Emotions associated with the omission of a reward (S+) or the termination of a reward (S+!) include frustration, anger and rage. Emotions associated with the omission of a punisher (S–) or the termination of a punisher (S–!) include relief. Although the classification of emotions presented here (and by Rolls (1986a, 1986b, 1990a, 1999a, 2005, 2014b)) differs from earlier theories, the approach adopted here of defining and classifying emotions by instrumentally reinforcing effects is one that has been developed in a number of earlier analyses (e.g. Millenson (1967), and

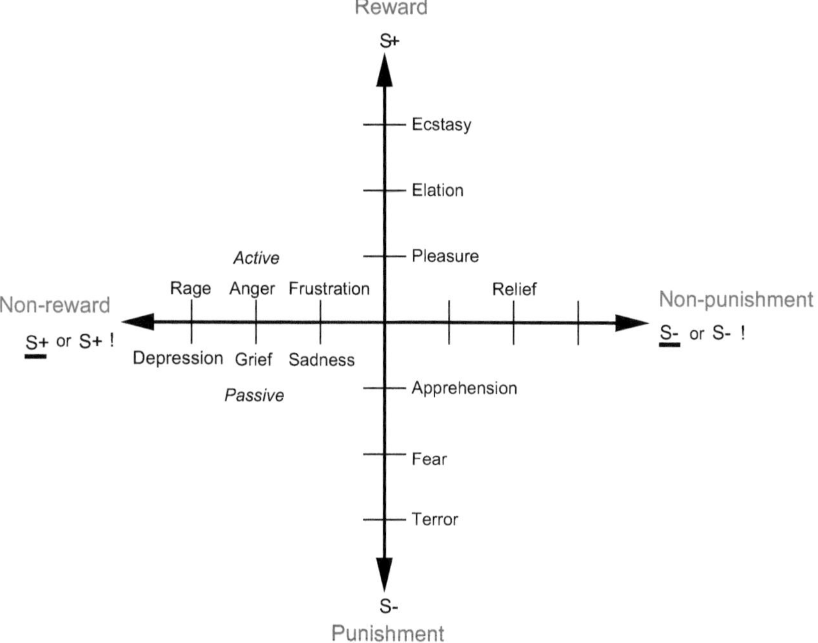

Fig. 2.1 Some of the emotions associated with different reinforcement contingencies are indicated. Intensity increases away from the centre of the diagram, on a continuous scale. The classification scheme created by the different reinforcement contingencies consists with respect to the action of (1) the delivery of a reward (S+), (2) the delivery of a punisher (S–), (3) the omission of a reward (S+) (extinction) or the termination of a reward (S+!) (time out), and (4) the omission of a punisher (S–) (avoidance) or the termination of a punisher (S–!) (escape). Note that the vertical axis describes emotions associated with the delivery of a reward (up) or punisher (down). The horizontal axis describes emotions associated with the non-delivery of an expected reward (left) or the non-delivery of an expected punisher (right). For the contingency of non-reward (horizontal axis, left) different emotions can arise depending on whether an active action is possible to respond to the non-reward, or whether no action is possible, which is labelled as the passive condition. The diagram summarizes emotions that might result for one reinforcer as a result of different contingencies. Every separate reinforcer has the potential to operate according to contingencies such as these. This diagram does not imply a dimensional theory of emotion, but shows the types of emotional state that might be produced by a specific reinforcer. Each different reinforcer will produce different emotional states, but the contingencies will operate as shown to produce different specific emotional states for each different reinforcer.

Gray(1975, 1981); see Strongman (2003)).

I should make it clear that the scheme shown in Fig. 2.1 is not intended to be a dimensional scheme. [A dimensional scheme is one in which independent factors or dimensions have been identified that account for the major and independent sources of variation in a data set. Some investigators work to show that these dimensions can be interpreted both biologically (for example as differing in autonomic, endocrine, or arousal-related ways) and psychologically (e.g. as representing anger vs fear), as described in Section 2.4.3.] However, the import of what is shown in Fig. 2.1 is to set out a set of logical possibilities of ways in which reinforcement contingencies can vary, and to show how they may be related to some different types of emotion. I emphasize that there are many different types of instrumental reinforcer, as will be shown with Table 2.1, and that each reinforcer is capable of acting by many of the types of contingency summarized in Fig. 2.1, with each reinforcer producing its own specific and different type of emotion.

It is actually a possibility that the four directions shown in Fig. 2.1 are at least partly independent from each other, and that a four-dimensional space is spanned by what is shown in Fig. 2.1. For example, sensitivity to (that is the ability to respond to) reward (S+) could be at least partly independent from sensitivity to punishers (S–), sensitivity to non-reward ($\underline{S+}$ and S+!), and sensitivity to non-delivery of a punisher ($\underline{S-}$ and S–!). The dimensions or independent ways in which emotions may differ from each other could thus span 4 dimensions even with what is shown in Fig. 2.1, and these ways are expanded greatly as shown by the following further effects that make different emotions different to each other.

One important point about Fig. 2.1 is that there are a large number of different primary reinforcers, and that for example the reward label S+ shows states that might be elicited by just one type of reward, such as a pleasant touch. There will be a different reward axis (S+) and non-reward axis ($\underline{S+}$ and S+!) for each type of reward (e.g. pleasant touch vs sweet taste); and, correspondingly, a different punisher axis (S–) and non-punisher axis ($\underline{S-}$ and S–!) for each type of punisher (e.g. pain vs bitter taste).

Different reinforcement contingencies can thus be used to classify a wide range of emotions. However, some of my tutorial pupils at Oxford sometimes expressed the view that reinforcement contingencies alone might not be able to account for the full range of human emotions. I therefore set out for them ways in which a system based on reinforcement contingencies could be developed in a number of different ways to give an account of most emotions. This extended set of ways of accounting for different emotions was published in 1986 (Rolls 1986a, Rolls 1986b), and developed a little in later publications (e.g. Rolls (1995, 1999a, 2005, 2014b)). It is described, and elaborated further next. If the reader can think of any emotions that cannot be accounted for by a combination of the ways described next, then it would be interesting to consider what further extensions might be needed.

1. **Reinforcement contingency**

The first way in which different classes of emotion could arise is because of different reinforcement contingencies, as described above and indicated in Fig. 2.1.

2. **Intensity**

Second, different intensities within these classes can produce different degrees of emotion (see above and Millenson (1967)). For example, as the strength of a positive reinforcer being presented increases, emotions might be labelled as pleasure, elation, and ecstasy. Similarly, as the strength of a negative reinforcer being presented increases, emotions might be labelled as apprehension, fear, and terror (see Fig. 2.1). It may be noted here that anxiety can refer to the state produced by stimuli associated with the non-delivery of a reward; or with the delivery of a punisher (Gray 1987).

3. **Multiple reinforcement associations**

Third, any environmental stimulus might have a number of different reinforcement associations. For example, a stimulus might be associated with both reward and punishment, allowing states such as conflict and guilt to arise. The different possible combinations greatly increase the number of possible emotions.

4. **Different primary reinforcers**

Fourth, emotions elicited by stimuli associated with different primary reinforcers will be different even within a reinforcement category (i.e. with the same reinforcement contingency), because the original reinforcers are different. Thus, for example, the state elicited by a stimulus associated with a reward such as the taste of food will be different from that elicited by a reward such as being groomed. Indeed, it is an important feature of the association memory mechanisms described here that when a stimulus is applied, it acts as a key which 'looks up' or recalls the original primary reinforcer with which it was associated (Rolls 2016c). Thus emotional stimuli will differ from each other in terms of the original primary reinforcers with which they were associated.

A summary of many different primary reinforcers is provided in Table 2.1, and inspection of this will help to show how some different emotions are produced by different primary reinforcers. For example, from Table 2.1 it might be surmised that one of the biological origins of the emotion of jealousy might be the state elicited in a male when his partner is courted by another male, because this threatens his parental investment in the offspring he raises with his partner, as described in Chapter 7. Jealousy in females would arise in a corresponding way, especially if her resources were threatened. Examples of how further emotions including guilt, shame, anger, forgiveness, envy and love may arise in relation to particular primary reinforcers are provided later in this section, throughout this chapter, in Chapters 3 and 7, and in many other places in this book.

5. **Different secondary reinforcers**

A fifth way in which emotions can be different from each other is in terms of the particular (conditioned) stimulus that elicits the emotion, and the situation in which it occurs. Thus, even though the reinforcement contingency and even the unconditioned reinforcer may be identical, emotions will still be different cognitively, if the conditioned stimuli that give rise to the emotions are different (that is, if the objects of the emotion are different). For example, the emotional state elicited by the sight of one person may be different from that elicited by the sight of another person because the people, and thus the cognitive evaluations associated with the perception of the stimuli, are different. In another example, not obtaining a monetary reward in a gambling task might lead to frustration, but being blocked by another person from obtaining a reward might lead to anger directed at the person.

Thus evolution may have shaped different reinforcers to contribute in different ways and depending on the environmental circumstances to the exact emotion produced. For example, some emotions may be related to social reinforcers (e.g. love, anger, envy, and breaking rules of society so that shame is produced, see further Section 11.3 and Rolls (2012d)), others to non-social reinforcers (such as fear of a painful stimulus), and others to solving difficult problems. By taking into account the nature of the primary reinforcer, the nature of the secondary reinforcer, and the environmental circumstances in which these apply, many different emotions can thus be accounted for, and cognitive factors taken into account. The common underlying basis of emotion remains however that it is related to goals/instrumental reinforcers, and the reinforcement contingencies that operate. The variety of different goals, and the contingencies and environmental situations in which they occur, combine to contribute to the richness in the variety of emotional states.

6. **The behavioural responses that are available**

A sixth possible way in which emotions can vary arises when the environment constrains the types of behavioural response that can be made. For example, if an active behavioural response can occur to the omission of an expected reward, then anger might be produced and directed at the person who prevented the reward being obtained, but if only passive behaviour is possible, then sadness, depression or grief might occur (see Fig. 2.1).

By realizing that these six possibilities can occur in different combinations, it can be seen that it is possible to account for a very wide range of emotions, and this is believed to be one of the strengths of the approach described here. It is also the case that the extent to which a stimulus is reinforcing on a particular occasion (and thus an emotion is produced) depends on the prior history of reinforcements (both recently through processes that include sensory-specific satiety, and in the longer term), and that the current mood state can affect the degree to which a stimulus (a term that includes cognitively decoded events and remembered events) is reinforcing (see Section 4.9).

If we wish to consider the number of independent ways in which emotions may differ from each other (for comparison with the 'dimensional' theories described in Section 2.4.3) we see immediately that a vast subtlety of emotions can be systematically described using the approach described here. For example, based on the four different reinforcement contingencies shown in Fig. 2.1 we have four at least potentially independent 'dimensions', which are combined with perhaps another 100–500 independently varying (in that they are gene-specified) primary reinforcers, some of which are included in Table 2.1. These are combined with constraints to the actions that may be possible when a reinforcer is received (the 'coping potential' of appraisal theorists), which potentially at least doubles the number of emotions that can be described. We add further combinatorial possibilities by noting (point 3 above) that a given stimulus in the world may have many different reinforcement associations producing states such as conflict. The possible number of different emotions can be further multiplied by the fact that each primary reinforcer may have associated with it almost any neutral stimulus to produce a secondary reinforcer.

The resulting number of emotional states that can be described and categorized is clearly enormous, even if we do not assume that each of the above factors operates strictly independently. For example, it is likely that if a gene were to specify a particular reward as being particularly intense in an individual, for example the pleasantness of touch, then omitting ($\underline{S+}$) or terminating (S+!) this reward might also be expected to be particularly intense, so the contributions of reinforcement contingency and identity of the primary reinforcer might combine additively rather than multiplicatively. Even if there is only partial independence of the different processes 1–6 above, and of variation within each process, then nevertheless many different emotions can be systematically classified and described. It does of course remain an interesting issue of how the processes described above do combine, and of the extent to which a few factors actually do account for a great deal in the variation between different emotions. For example, if in an individual's sensitivity to non-reward is generally much more intense than the individual's sensitivity to reward, then this will shape the emotions in that individual, and account for quite a deal of the character of that individual's emotional states. Such a factor might also account for quite an amount of the variation in emotions and personality between individuals (see Section 2.5).

Some examples of how different emotions might be classified using the above criteria now follow. **Fear** is a state that might be produced by a stimulus that has become a secondary reinforcer by virtue of its learned association with a primary negative reinforcer such as pain (see Fig. 2.1). **Anger** is a state that might be produced by the omission of an expected reward, frustrative non-reward, when an active behavioural response is possible (see Fig. 2.1). (In particular, anger may occur if another individual prevents an expected reward from being obtained.) **Guilt** may arise when there is a conflict between an available reward and a rule or law of society. **Jealousy** is an emotion that might be aroused in a male if the faithfulness of his partner seems to be threatened by her liaison (e.g. flirting) with another male. In this case the reinforcement contingency that is operating is produced by a punisher, and it may be that males are specified genetically to find this punishing because it indicates a potential threat to their paternity and paternal investment, as described in Chapters 7 and 3. Similarly, a female may become jealous if her partner has a liaison with another female, because the resources available to the 'wife' useful to bring up her children are threatened. Again, the punisher here may be gene-specified, as described in Chapter 3. **Envy** or **disappointment** might be produced if a prize is obtained by a competitor. In this case, part of the way in which the frustrative non-reward is produced is by the cognitive understanding that this is a competition in which there will be a winner, and that the person has set himself or herself the goal of obtaining it.

The partial list of primary reinforcers provided in Table 2.1 should provide readers with a foundation for starting to understand the rich categorisation scheme for different types of emotion that can be understood in this way.

Many other similar examples can be surmised from the area of evolutionary psychology (Ridley 1993a, Buss 2015, Buss 2016, Barrett, Dunbar & Lycett 2002). For example, there may be a set of reinforcers that are genetically specified to help promote social cooperation and even reciprocal altruism. Such genes might specify that emotion should be elicited, and behavioural changes should occur, if a cooperating partner defects or 'cheats' (Cosmides & Tooby 1999). Moreover, the genes may build brains with genetically specified rules that are useful heuristics for social cooperation, such as acting with a strategy of 'generous tit-for tat', which can be more adaptive than strict 'tit-for-tat', in that being generous occasionally is a good strategy to help promote further cooperation that has failed when both partners defect in a strict 'tit-for-tat' scenario (Ridley 1996). Genes that specify good heuristics to promote social cooperation may thus underlie such complex emotional states as feeling forgiving.

It is suggested that many apparently complex emotional states have their origins in designing animals to perform well in such sociobiological and socioeconomic situations (Ridley 1996, Glimcher 2004, Glimcher 2011a, Glimcher & Fehr 2013, Rolls 2014b). Indeed, many principles that humans accept as ethical may be closely related to strategies that are useful heuristics for promoting social cooperation, and emotional feelings associated with ethical behaviour may be at least partly related to the adaptive value of such gene-specified strategies. These ideas are developed in Section 11.3 and by Rolls (2012d).

These examples indicate that an emotional state can be systematically specified and classified using the six principles described above in this Section. The similarity between particular emotions will depend on how close they are in the space defined by the above principles. Refinements of Rolls' theory of emotion are described in *Emotion and Decision-Making Explained* (Rolls 2014b).

Table 2.1 Some primary reinforcers, and the dimensions of the environment to which they are tuned

Taste	
Salt taste	reward in salt deficiency
Sweet	reward in energy deficiency
Bitter	punisher, indicator of possible poison
Sour	punisher
Umami	reward, indicator of protein; produced by monosodium glutamate and inosine monophosphate
Tannic acid	punisher; it prevents absorption of protein; found in old leaves; probably somatosensory not gustatory (Critchley and Rolls 1996a)
Odour	
Putrefying odour	punisher; hazard to health
Pheromones	reward (depending on hormonal state)
Somatosensory	
Pain	punisher
Touch	reward
Grooming	reward; to give grooming may also be a primary reinforcer.
Washing	reward
Temperature	reward if tends to help maintain normal body temperature; otherwise punisher
Texture of food	reward (e.g. pleasant mouth feel) or punisher
Visual	
Snakes, etc.	punisher for, e.g., primates
Youthfulness	reward, associated with mate choice
Beauty, e.g. symmetry	reward
Secondary sexual characteristics	rewards
Face expression	reward (e.g. smile) or punisher (e.g. threat)
Blue sky, cover, open space	reward, indicator of safety
Flowers	reward (indicator of fruit later in the season?)
Auditory	
Warning call	punisher
Aggressive vocalization	punisher
Soothing vocalization	reward (part of the evolutionary history of music, which at least in its origins taps into the channels used for the communication of emotions)

Table 2.1 continued **Some primary reinforcers, and the dimensions of the environment to which they are tuned**

Reproduction	
Courtship	reward
Sexual behaviour	reward (different reinforcers, including a low waist-to-hip ratio, and attractiveness influenced by symmetry and being found attractive by members of the other sex, are discussed in Chapter 7).
Mate guarding	reward for a male to protect his parental investment. Jealousy results if his mate is courted by another male, because this may ruin his parental investment
Nest building	reward (when expecting young)
Parental attachment (love)	reward (good for the parent's genes both when the attachment is to the other parent or an infant)
Infant attachment to parents (love)	reward (good for the infant's genes)
Crying of infant	punisher to parents; produced to promote successful development
Power, status, wealth, resources	Attractive to females, who may benefit from resources for their offspring. Attractive to males as they make males attractive to females.
Body size	Large in males may be attractive to females as a signal for the provision of protection and of the ability of her male offspring to compete for a mate. Small in females may be attractive to males as a neotenous sign of youth, and therefore fertility
Other	
Novel stimuli	rewards (encourage animals to investigate the full possibilities of the multidimensional space in which their genes are operating)
Sleep	reward; minimizes nutritional requirements and protects from danger
Altruism to genetic kin	reward (kin altruism)
Altruism to other individuals	reward while the altruism is reciprocated in a 'tit-for-tat' reciprocation (reciprocal altruism). Forgiveness, honesty, and altruistic punishment are some associated heuristics. May provide underpinning for some aspects of what is felt to be moral.
Altruism to other individuals	punisher when the altruism is not reciprocated
Group acceptance, reputation	reward (social greeting might indicate this). These goals can account for why some cultural goals are pursued
Control over actions	reward
Play	reward
Danger, stimulation, excitement	reward if not too extreme (adaptive because of practice?)
Exercise	reward (keeps the body fit for action)
Mind reading	reward; practice in reading others' minds, which might be adaptive
Solving an intellectual problem	reward (practice in which might be adaptive)
Storing, collecting	reward (e.g. food)
Habitat preference, home, territory	reward
Some responses	reward (e.g. pecking in chickens, pigeons; adaptive because it is a simple way in which eating grain can be programmed for a relatively fixed type of environmental stimulus)
Breathing	reward

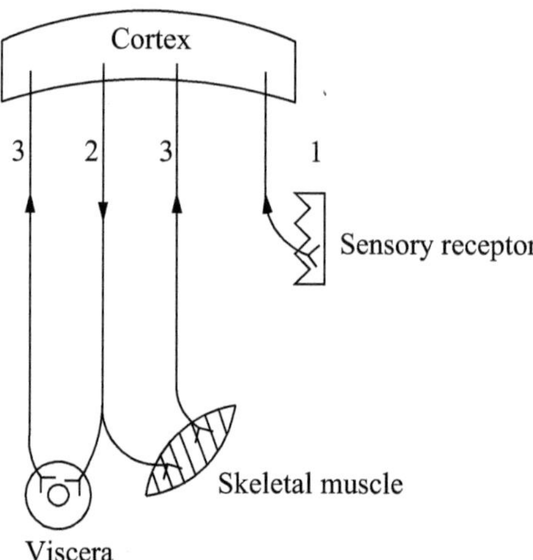

Fig. 2.2 The James–Lange theory of emotion proposes that there are three steps in producing emotional feelings. The first step is elicitation by the emotion-provoking stimulus (received by the cortex via pathway 1 in the Figure) of peripheral changes, such as skeleto-muscular activity to run away, and autonomic changes, such as alteration of heart rate (via pathways labelled 2 in the Figure). The second step is the sensing of the peripheral responses (e.g. altered heart rate, and somatosensory effects produced by running away) (via pathways labelled 3 in the Figure). The third step is elicitation of the emotional feeling in response to the sensed feedback from the periphery.

2.4 Other theories of emotion

In the following subsections, I outline some other theories of emotion, and compare them with the above (Rolls') theory of emotion. Surveys of some of the approaches to emotion that have been taken in the past are provided by Strongman (2003) and Oatley, Keltner & Jenkins (2018).

2.4.1 The James–Lange and other bodily theories of emotion including Damasio's theory

James (1884) believed that emotional experiences were produced by sensing bodily changes, such as changes in heart rate or in skeletal muscles. Lange (1885) had a similar view, although he emphasized the role of autonomic feedback (for example from the heart) in producing the experience of emotion. The theory, which became known as the James–Lange theory, suggested that there are three steps in producing emotional feelings (see Fig. 2.2). The first step is elicitation by the emotion-provoking stimulus of peripheral changes, such as skeleto-muscular activity to produce running away, and autonomic changes, such as alteration of heart rate. But, as pointed out above, the theory leaves unanswered perhaps the most important issue in any theory of emotion: Why do some events make us run away (and then feel emotional), whereas others do not? This is a major weakness of this type of theory. The second step is the sensing of the peripheral responses (e.g. running away, and altered heart rate). The third step is elicitation of the emotional feeling in response to the sensed feedback from the periphery.

The history of research into peripheral theories of emotion starts with the fatal flaw that step one (the question of which stimuli elicit emotion-related responses in the first place) leaves unanswered this most important question. The history continues with the accumulation of empirical evidence that has gradually weakened more and more the hypothesis that peripheral responses made during emotional behaviour have anything to do with producing the emotional behaviour (which has largely already been produced anyway according to the James–Lange theory), or the emotional feeling. Some of the landmarks in this history are described by Rolls (2014b).

2.4.2 Appraisal theory

Appraisal theory, (Frijda 1986, Scherer 2009, Moors, Ellsworth, Scherer & Frijda 2013, Oatley et al. 2018) generally holds that two types of appraisal are involved in emotion. Primary appraisal holds that "an emotion is usually caused by a person consciously or unconsciously evaluating an event as relevant to a concern (a goal) that is important; the emotion is felt as positive when a concern is advanced and negative when a concern is impeded" (from Oatley & Jenkins (1996), p. 96). The concept of appraisal presumably involves assessment of whether something is a reward or punisher, that is whether it will be worked for or avoided. The description in terms of rewards and punishers adopted here (and by Rolls (2014b)) simply seems much more precisely and operationally specified. If primary appraisal is defined with respect to goals, it might be helpful to note that goals may just be the reinforcers specified in Rolls' theory of emotion (Rolls 1999a, Rolls 2005, Rolls 2014b), and if so the reinforcer/punisher approach provides clear definitions of goals.

Secondary appraisal is concerned with coping potential, that is with whether for example a plan can be constructed, and how successful it is likely to be.

Scherer (2009) summarizes his approach as follows. He suggests that there are four major appraisal objectives to adaptively react to a salient event:
(a) Relevance: How relevant is this event for me? Does it directly affect me or my social reference group?
(b) Implications: What are the implications or consequences of this event and how do they affect my well-being and my immediate or long-term goals?
(c) Coping Potential: How well can I cope with or adjust to these consequences?
(d) Normative Significance: What is the significance of this event for my self-concept and for social norms and values?
To attain these objectives, the organism evaluates the event and its consequences on a number of criteria or stimulus evaluation checks, with the results reflecting the organism's subjective assessment (which may well be unrealistic or biased) of consequences and implications on a background of personal needs, goals, and values. He states that an important feature of the model is that it does not include overt instrumental behaviour. Instead he sees emotion as a reaction to significant events that prepares action readiness and different types of alternative, possibly conflicting, action tendencies but not as a sufficient cause for their execution. This is a clear difference from my theory, in that my theory is that emotions are states that have a key role in brain design by providing a way for stimuli to produce states that are the goals for instrumental actions (Chapter 3). Of course stimuli that are instrumental reinforcers, goals for action, can also produce adaptive autonomic and skeletomotor reflexes (such as freezing), but these are responses, and can be classically conditioned, but do not require intervening goal-related representations or states, which are emotional and motivational states.

I note that appraisal theory is in many ways quite close to the theory that I outline here and elsewhere (Rolls 1999a, Rolls 2005, Rolls 2014b), and I do not see them as rivals. Instead, I hope that those who have an appraisal theory of emotion will consider whether much of what is encompassed by primary appraisal is not actually rather close to assessing whether stimuli or events are instrumental reinforcers; and whether much of what is encompassed by secondary appraisal is rather close to taking into account the actions that are possible in particular circumstances, as described above in Section 2.2.

An aspect of some flavours of appraisal theory with which I do not agree is that emotions have as one of their functions releasing particular actions, which seems to make a link with species-specific action tendencies or responses, or 'fixed action patterns' (Tomkins 1995, Panksepp 1998) or more 'open motor programs' (Ekman 2003). I argue in Chapter 3 that rarely are behavioural responses programmed by genes (see Table 2.1), but instead genes optimize their effects on behaviour if they specify the goals for (flexible) actions, that is if they specify rewards and punishers. The difference is quite considerable, in that specifying goals is much more economical in terms of the information that must be encoded in the genome; and in that specifying goals for actions allows much more flexibility in the actual actions that are produced. Of course I acknowledge that there is some preparedness to learn associations between particular types of secondary and primary reinforcers (Seligman 1970), and see this just as an economy of sensory–sensory convergence in the brain, whereby for example it does not convey much advantage to be able to learn that flashing lights (as contrasted with the taste of a food just eaten) are followed by sickness.

2.4.3 Dimensional and categorical theories of emotion

Dimensional and categorical theories of emotion suggest that there are a number of fundamental or basic emotions. Charles Darwin for example in his book *The Expression of the Emotions in Man and Animals* (1872) showed that some basic expressions of emotion are similar in animals and humans. Some of the examples he gave are shown in Table 2.1. His focus was on the continuity between animals and humans of how emotion is expressed.

In a development of this approach, Ekman (1992, 2003) has suggested that humans categorize face expressions into a number of basic categories that are similar across cultures. These face expression categories include happy, fear, anger, surprise, grief and sadness.

A related approach is to identify a few clusters of variables or factors that result from multidimensional analysis of questionnaires, and to identify these factors as basic emotions. (Multidimensional analyses such as factor analysis seek to identify a few underlying sources of variance to which a large number of data values such as answers to questions are related.)

One potential problem with some of these approaches is that they risk finding seven plus or minus two categories, which is the maximal number of categories with which humans normally operate, as described in a famous paper by George Miller (1956). A second problem is that there is no special reason why the first few factors (which account for most of the variance) in a factor analysis should provide a complete or principled classification of different emotions, or of their functions. In contrast, the theory described here does produce a principled classification of different emotions based on reinforcement contingencies, the nature of the primary and secondary reinforcers, etc., as set out in Sections 2.2 and 2.3. Moreover, the present theory links the functions of emotions to the classification produced, by showing how the functions of emotion can be understood in terms of the gene-specified reinforcers that produce different emotions (see Chapter 3).

An opposite approach to the dimensional or categorical approach is to attempt to describe the richness of every emotion (e.g. Ben-Ze'ev (2000)). Although it is important to understand the richness of every emotion, I believe that this is better performed with a set of underlying principles of the type set out above (in Section 2.2), rather than without any obvious principles to approach the subtlety of emotions.

2.4.4 Other approaches to emotion

LeDoux (1992, 1995, 1996, 2012) has described a theory of the neural basis of emotion that is probably conceptually similar to that of Rolls (1975, 1986a, 1986b, 1990a, 1995, 1999a,

2000a, 2005, 2014b), except that he focuses mostly on the role of the amygdala in emotion (and not on other brain regions such as the orbitofrontal cortex, which are poorly developed in the rat); except that he focuses mainly on fear (based on his studies of the role of the amygdala and related structures in fear conditioning in the rat); and except that he suggests from his neurophysiological findings that an important route for conditioned emotional stimuli to influence behaviour is via the subcortical inputs (especially auditory from the medial part of the medial geniculate nucleus of the thalamus) to the amygdala. In contrast, I suggest that cortical processing to the object representation level before the representation is then sent to areas such as the amygdala and orbitofrontal cortex is normally involved in emotion, as emotions normally occur to objects, faces, etc. and not to spots of light or pure tones, which is what are represented precortically. Further, LeDoux (2012) has emphasized especially reflexes and classically conditioned reflexes such as autonomic responses and freezing, which I argue have adaptive value or in LeDoux's words 'survival value', whereas Rolls' theory is that emotional and motivational states are important intervening states in relation to instrumental actions. The way in which the rodent and amygdala literature has focussed on conditioned responses and not on emotional feelings is described by LeDoux and colleagues (LeDoux 2012, LeDoux & Pine 2016, LeDoux & Daw 2018).

Panksepp's approach to emotion had its origins in neuroethological investigations of brainstem systems that when activated lead to behaviours like fixed action patterns, including escape, flight and fear behaviour (Panksepp 1998, Panksepp 2011). Using evidence from brain stimulation that elicits behaviours, he has postulated that there are a set of basic emotions, including for example Seeking, Rage, Fear, Lust, Care, Panic/Grief and Play. He argued that these are 'natural kinds', things that exist in nature as opposed to being inventions (constructions) of the human mind. My view is that there are not a few basic emotions, that emotions do not involve fixed action patterns as these do not require intervening emotional states to support goal-directed instrumental actions, and that emotions can be classified based on the specific reinforcer, the specific reinforcement contingency, the actions that are available, etc. as described earlier in this chapter in Rolls' theory of emotion.

Other approaches to emotion are summarized by Strongman (2003) and Oatley et al. (2018).

2.5 Individual differences in emotion, personality, and emotional intelligence

Sensitivity to rewards and punishers, and the ability to learn and be influenced by rewards and punishers, may be important in personality, and are thus closely involved in emotion according to the theory developed here. An extreme example might be that if humans were insensitive to social punishers following orbitofrontal cortex damage, we might expect social problems and impulsive behaviour, and indeed Tranel, Bechara & Denburg (2002) have used the term 'acquired sociopathy' to describe some of these patients.

We might expect sensitivity to different types of reinforcer (including social reinforcers) to vary between individuals both as a result of gene variation and as a result of learning, and this, operating over a large number of different social reinforcers, might produce many different variations of personality based on the sensitivity to a large number of different reinforcers. Further, insofar as the functions of particular brain regions may be related to particular processes involved in emotion [with evidence for example that the human orbitofrontal cortex is involved in face expression decoding, and in impulsiveness, but not in some other aspects of personality (see Section

4.5.4)], then it may be possible in future to understand different particular modules for inter-relations between reward/punishment and personality systems.

The concept of the relation between differential sensitivity to different types of reward and punisher might produce individuals showing many types of conditional evolutionarily stable strategies, where the conditionality of the strategy might be influenced in different individuals by differential sensitivity to different rewards and punishers. Examples of behaviours that might be produced in this way are included in Chapter 7.

Hans J. Eysenck developed the theory that personality might be related to different aspects of conditioning. He analysed the factors that accounted for the variance in the differences between the personality of different humans (using, for example, questionnaires), and suggested that the first two factors in personality (those which accounted for most of the variance) were introversion vs extraversion, and neuroticism (related to a tendency to be anxious). He performed studies of classical conditioning on groups of subjects, and also obtained measures of what he termed arousal. Based on the correlations of these measures with the dimensions identified in the factor analysis, he suggested that introverts showed greater conditionability (to weak stimuli) and are more readily aroused by external stimulation than extraverts; and that neuroticism raises the general intensity of emotional reactions (Eysenck & Eysenck 1985).

Jeffrey A. Gray (1970) reinterpreted the findings, suggesting that introverts are more sensitive to punishment and frustrative non-reward than are extraverts; and that neuroticism reflects the extent of sensitivity to both reward and punishment (see Matthews & Gilliland (1999)). A related hypothesis is that extraverts may show enhanced learning in reward conditions, and may show enhanced processing of positively valent stimuli (Rusting & Larsen 1998). Matthews & Gilliland (1999), reviewing the evidence, show that there is some support for both hypotheses about introversion vs extraversion, namely that introverts may in general condition readily, and that extraverts may be relatively more responsive to reward stimuli (and correspondingly, introverts to punishers). However, Matthews & Gilliland (1999) go on to show that extraverts may perform less well at vigilance tasks (in which the subject must detect stimuli that occur with low probability); may tend to be more impulsive; and perform better when arousal is high (e.g. later in the day), and when rapid responses rather than reflective thought is needed (see also Matthews, Zeidner & Roberts (2002)). With respect to neuroticism and trait anxiety, anxious individuals tend to focus attention on potentially threatening information (punishers) at the cost of neglecting neutral or positive information sources; and may make more negative judgements, especially in evaluating self-worth and personal competence (Matthews, Zeidner & Roberts 2002).

More recent evidence comes from functional neuroimaging studies. For example, Canli, Sivers, Whitfield, Gotlib & Gabrieli (2002) have found that happy face expressions are more likely to activate the human amygdala in extraverts than in introverts. In addition, positively affective pictures interact with extraversion, and negatively affective pictures with neuroticism to produce activation of the amygdala (Canli, Zhao, Desmond, Kang, Gross & Gabrieli 2001, Hamann & Canli 2004). This supports the conceptually important point made above that part of the basis of personality may be differential sensitivity to different rewards and punishers, and omission and termination of different rewards and punishers.

The observations just described are consistent with the hypothesis that part of the basis of extraversion is increased reactivity to positively affective (as compared to negatively affective) face expressions and other positively affective stimuli including pictures. The exact mechanisms involved may be revealed in the future by genetic studies, and these might potentially address for example whether genes control responses to positively affective stimuli, or whether some more general personality trait by altering perhaps mood produces differential top-down biasing of face expression decoding systems in the way outlined in Section 4.9.

In one update of this approach, links have been made to behavioural economics by relating loss aversion to greater negative valuation sensitivity compared to positive valuation sensitivity; by suggesting that tendencies to approach or avoid have distinct sensitivities to those of the valuation systems; that approach-avoidance conflict is distinct process from the basic approach and avoidance systems; and linking these to a reinforcer sensitivity theory of personality (Corr & McNaughton 2012).

Another example is the impulsive behaviour that is a part of Borderline Personality Disorder (BPD), which could reflect factors such as less sensitivity to the punishers associated with waiting for rational processing to lead to a satisfactory solution, or changes in internal timing processes that lead to a faster perception of time (Berlin, Rolls & Kischka 2004, Berlin & Rolls 2004) (see Section 4.5.4). It was of considerable interest that the BPD group (mainly self-harming patients), as well as a group of patients with damage to the orbitofrontal cortex, scored highly on a Frontal Behaviour Questionnaire that assessed inappropriate behaviours typical of orbitofrontal cortex patients including disinhibition, social inappropriateness, perseveration, and uncooperativeness. In terms of measures of personality, using the Big Five personality measure (which identifies five major components of personality (Trull & Widiger 2013)), both groups were also less open to experience (i.e. less open-minded). In terms of other personality measures and characteristics, the orbitofrontal and BPD patients performed differently: BPD patients were less extraverted and conscientious and more neurotic and emotional than the orbitofrontal group (Berlin, Rolls & Kischka 2004, Berlin & Rolls 2004, Berlin, Rolls & Iversen 2005). Thus some aspects of personality, such as impulsiveness and being less open to experience, but not other aspects, such as extraversion, neuroticism and conscientiousness, were differentially related to orbitofrontal cortex function.

Daniel Goleman (1995) has popularized the concept of *emotional intelligence*. The rather sweeping definition given was "Emotional intelligence [includes] abilities such as being able to motivate oneself and persist in the face of frustrations, to control impulse and delay gratification; to regulate one's moods and keep distress from swamping the ability to think; to empathize and to hope" (Goleman (1995), p. 34).

One potential problem with this definition of emotional intelligence as an ability is that different aspects within this definition (such as impulse control and hope) may be unrelated, so a unitary ability described in this way seems unlikely. An excellent critical evaluation of the concept has been produced by Matthews, Zeidner & Roberts (2002). They note (p. 368) that in a rough and ready way, one might identify personality traits of emotional stability (low neuroticism), extraversion, agreeableness, and conscientiousness/self-control as dispositions that tend to facilitate everyday social interaction and to promote more positive emotion. (Indeed, one measure of emotional intelligence, the EQ-i (Bar-On 1997), has high correlations with some of the Big Five personality traits, especially, negatively, with neuroticism, and the EQ-i may reflect three constructs, self-esteem, empathy, and impulse control (Matthews et al. 2002).) But these personality traits are supposed to be independent, so linking them to a single ability of emotional intelligence is inconsistent. Moreover, this combination of personality traits might well not be adaptive in many circumstances, so the concept of this combination as an 'ability' is inappropriate.

2.6 Cognition and emotion

It may be noted that while the definition of emotions as states elicited by instrumental reinforcers (with particular functions) is operational, it should not be criticized (Katz 2000) as behaviourist. For example, the definition has nothing to do with stimulus–response (habit) associations, but instead with a two-stage type of learning, in which a first stage is learning which environmental stimuli or events are associated with instrumental reinforcers (goals) to represent value, which potentially is a very rapid and flexible process; and a second stage produces appropriate instrumental and arbitrary actions performed in order to achieve the goal (which might be to obtain a reward or avoid a punisher). In the instrumental stage, animals learn about the outcomes of their actions (Dickinson 1994, Pearce 2008, Cardinal, Parkinson, Hall & Everitt 2002, Mazur 2012, Rolls 2014b)).

To determine what is a goal for an action, every type of cognitive operation may be involved. The proposal is that whatever cognitive operations are involved, then if the outcome is that a certain event, stimulus, thought (or any one of these remembered) leads to the evaluation that the event is a reward or punisher, then an emotion will be produced. So cognition is very much included.

Indeed, cognitive operations may produce emotions when operating at three levels of the architecture, as described more fully in Chapter 3. The first is the implicit level (see Fig. 4.3), where a primary reinforcer, or a stimulus or event associated with a primary reinforcer, may lead to emotions. The second level is where a (first-order) syntactic symbol processing system performing "what ... if" computations to implement planning results in identification of a rewarding or punishing outcome. The third level is the higher-order linguistic thought level described in Chapter 10, where thinking about and evaluating the operations of a first-order linguistic processor may result in a reinforcing outcome such as "I should not spend further time thinking about that set of plans, as it would be better now to devote my linguistic resources (which are limited and serial) to this other set of plans".

Another way in which cognition influences emotion is that cognitive states, even at the level of language, can modulate subjective and brain responses to the reward value of affective stimuli, as analysed in Section 4.5.3.6. There an experiment is described in which a word label ('cheese' vs 'body odour') influences the subjective pleasantness ratings, and the activations in olfactory stages at least as early as the secondary olfactory cortex in the orbitofrontal cortex, to a standard test odour (De Araujo, Rolls, Velazco, Margot & Cayeux 2005). An implication of these findings is that language-based cognitive states can influence even relatively early cortical representations of rewards and punishers, and thus potentially modulate how much emotion is felt subjectively to an emotion-provoking stimulus.

I suggest that this top-down modulation of affective representations by cognition occurs in a way that is analogous to top-down attentional effects, which are believed to be implemented by a top-down biased competition mechanism (Rolls & Deco 2002, Deco & Rolls 2003, Deco & Rolls 2005b, Rolls & Stringer 2001, Rolls 2016c, Rolls 2013a). In this case, the semantic, language-based, representation is the source of the biased competition, and the effect could be not only to bias the early cortical representation of a reward or punisher in one direction or another, but also by providing much or little top-down modulation, to influence how much emotion is felt (see Chapter 10), by modulating the processing of emotion-related stimuli (including remembered stimuli or events) at relatively early processing stages. This could be a mechanism by which cognition can influence how much emotion is felt under conditions in which emotions such as empathy and pity may occur, and when for example reading a novel, attending a play, listening to music, etc. (see Section 11.4). Analysis of the mechanisms by which the top-down biased competition operates are becoming detailed (Desimone & Duncan 1995, Rolls & Deco 2002, Deco & Rolls 2003, Deco & Rolls 2004, Deco & Rolls 2005b, Rolls 2016c, Rolls 2013a), and are included in a model in which a rule module exerts a top-down influence on neurons that represent stimulus–reward and stimulus–punisher combinations to influence which stimulus should currently be interpreted as reward-related (Deco & Rolls 2005a).

Another way in which cognitive factors are related to emotion is that mood can affect cognitive processing, and one of the effects of this is to promote continuity of behaviour (see Chapter 3). One of the mechanisms described (in Section 4.9) utilizes backprojections to cortical areas from the amygdala and orbitofrontal cortex, so that reciprocal interactions between cognition and emotion are made possible.

2.7 Emotion, motivation, reward, and mood

It is useful to be clear about the difference between motivation, emotion, reward, and mood (Rolls 2000a, Rolls 2005). **Motivation** makes one work to obtain a reward, or work to escape from or avoid a punisher. One example of motivation is hunger, and another thirst, which in these cases are states set largely by internal homeostatically-related variables such as plasma glucose concentration and plasma osmolality (Chapter 5, Rolls (2005)). A **reward** is a stimulus or event that one works to obtain, such as food, and a punisher is what one works to escape from or avoid (or which suppresses an action on which its delivery is contingent), such as a painful stimulus or the sight of an object associated with a painful stimulus. Obtaining the reward or avoiding the punisher is the goal for the instrumental action. An **instrumental action** is an arbitrary action performed to obtain a goal, for example, raising one's arm, or lowering one's arm. A motivational state is one in which a goal is *desired*. An **emotion** is a state elicited when a goal is obtained, that is by an instrumental reinforcer (i.e. a reward or punisher, or omission or termination of a reward or punisher), for example fear produced by the sight of the object associated with pain. This makes it clear that emotions are states elicited by rewards or punishers that have particular functions. Another term used for an emotional state is an **affective state**.

Of course, one of the functions of emotions is that they are motivating, as exemplified by the case of the fear produced by the sight of the object that can produce pain, which motivates one to avoid receiving the painful stimulus, which is the goal for the action. In that emotion-provoking stimuli or events produce motivation, then arousal is likely to occur, especially for reinforcers that lead to the active initiation of actions. However, arousal alone is not sufficient to define motivation or emotion, in that the motivational state must specify the particular type of goal that is the object of the motivational state, such as water if we are thirsty, food if we are hungry, and avoidance of the painful unconditioned stimulus signalled by a fear-inducing conditioned stimulus.

A **mood** is a continuing state normally elicited by a reinforcer, and is thus part of what is an emotion. The other part of an emotion is the decoding of the stimulus in terms of whether it is a reward or punisher, that is, of what causes the emotion, or in philosophical terminology of what the emotion is about or the object of the emotion. Mood states help to implement some of the persistence-related functions of emotion, can continue when the originating stimulus may be forgotten (by the explicit system described in Chapter 10), and may occur spontaneously not because such spontaneous mood swings may have been selected for, but because of the difficulty of maintaining stability of the neuronal firing that implements mood (or affective) state (see *The Brain and Emotion*, Rolls (1999a), pp. 62, 66; and Rolls (2016c)). Mood states are thus not necessarily about an object.

Thus, motivation may be seen as a state in which one is working for a goal, and emotion as a state that occurs when the goal, a reinforcer, is obtained, and that may persist afterwards. The concept of gene-defined reinforcers providing the goals for action helps to understand the relation between motivational states (or desires) and emotion, as the organism must be built to be motivated to obtain the goals, and to be placed in a different state (emotion) when the goal is or is not achieved by the action. The close but clear relation between motivation and emotion is that both are states related to goals, for example motivational states such as feeling hungry (wanting to obtain the goal of food reward), and emotional or affective states such as liking the taste of a food, and feeling happy because a social reinforcer has been received. However, we should note that emotional states may be motivating, as in frustrative non-reward which may motivate us to try again to obtain the reward (Section 3.4.3). The Darwinian theory of the functions of emotion developed in Chapter 3 which shows how emotion is adaptive because it reflects the operation of a process by which genes define goals for action applies just as much to motivation (see further Section 3.6), in that emotion can be thought of as states elicited by goals (rewards and punishers), and motivation can be thought of as states elicited when goals are being sought.

By specifying goals, the genes must specify both that we must be motivated to obtain those goals, and that when the goals are obtained, further states, emotional states with further functions, are produced. In this sense, my Darwinian approach to the functions of gene-specified instrumental reinforcers provides a fundamental and unifying approach to emotion and motivation.

2.8 Advantages of the approach to emotion described here (Rolls' theory of emotion)

I now evaluate the advantages of, and justifications for, starting with the concept that emotions are states elicited by instrumental reinforcers, even though one proposes that a full definition requires the principles summarized in Section 2.2, and incorporating a statement of the functions elicited by those states (Chapter 3).

One advantage is that this definition in terms of rewards and punishers may provide a concise operational definition of the environmental stimuli or events that actually lead to emotions. If we can agree that the environmental conditions that lead to emotions are those that can be described as rewarding or punishing, and that those that are not rewards or punishers do not lead to states that are described as emotional, then we are a long way forward in producing a conceptualization of what emotions may be. No commentators on the *Précis of The Brain and Emotion* (Rolls 2000a) actually produced clear exceptions to this correspondence. If we accept this operational definition, it provides us with a powerful way forward to start to examine emotions (because we accept that they are states elicited by rewards or punishers, and have a useful delimitation of what events produce emotion). This leads directly to an analysis of the brain mechanisms that implement emotions as those brain mechanisms that decode environmental stimuli as primary reinforcers, those brain mechanisms that implement stimulus–reinforcer association learning, and the brain mechanisms that link the resulting emotional states to actions.

A second advantage of this definition is that it enables us to see emotions in the context of what I propose is their most important function, namely as a way to provide a mechanism for the genes to influence behaviour in a brain that evolves by gene selection. It is argued in Chapter 3 that the genes do this by specifying the stimuli or events that the animal is built to find rewarding or punishing, i.e. to find reinforcing, so that the genes specify the goals for action, not the actions themselves. The definition of emotions as states elicited by reinforcers thus links directly to the Darwinian theory I propose for why we have emotions, which is that some genes specify reinforcers, that is goals for action, that will increase the fitness of these genes. It is these particular genes that specify reinforcers that provide the foundation I propose for emotional states. The definition of emotion in terms of states elicited by reinforcers should not be seen thus as behaviourist, but instead as part of a much broader theory that takes an adaptive, Darwinian, approach to the functions of emotion, and how they are important in brain design (see Section 3.5).

A third advantage is that the definition offers a principled way to approach emotion. Different emotions can be classified and understood in terms of different reinforcement contingencies and different reinforcers, and hence directly in terms of their functions. This is recommended as being more advantageous than categorizing emotions based on clusters of variables or factors that result from multidimensional analysis of questionnaires etc., or by correlation with autonomic or face expression measures, which do not lead directly to an understanding of the different functions of different emotions (and run the risk of producing seven plus or minus two categories, which is the typical number of categories that humans form (Miller 1956)), as described in Section 2.4.3. This definition of emotion also leads to an operational, and thus clearly specified, approach to emotions, whereas approaches such as appraisal theory may suffer from the disadvantage that they quickly become somewhat under-specified and intractable, as described in Section 2.4.2. Moreover, this principled way of understanding emotions provides a systematic and fundamental way to approach the brain mechanisms involved in emotion, in that brain regions involved in decoding primary reinforcers, and brain regions involved in learning associations of events to primary reinforcers, can be seen to have a clear information-processing role in emotion. Analysing the information processing performed by each connected stage in the brain provides a fruitful approach to understanding neural computation (Rolls & Treves 1998, Rolls & Deco 2002, Rolls 2016c).

A fourth advantage of conceptualizing emotions as states elicited by instrumental reinforcers is that this provides an immediate way into understanding the relation between emotion and personality (see Section 2.5).

A complex issue related to one's definition of emotion is where the boundaries for emotional states should be set. Should our definition result in emotions being states that occur in invertebrates such as Aplysia, as suggested by Kupferman (2000)? My own answer to this is to set off from emotions those behaviours that are performed with fixed responses, that is without the possibility for selecting arbitrary types of behaviour as the goals for actions (see Chapter 3). Such fixed-response behaviours include taxes, such as might be performed by a single cell organism swimming up a chemical gradient towards a source of nutrient. Other examples include fixed action patterns, and autonomic and even skeletomotor responses such as freezing, even when conditioned. One reason why these types of behaviour with fixed responses are excluded from emotion (though they may be forerunners to it) is that the behaviour does not occur by elicitation of a persistent or continuing state to a reinforcing stimulus that provides the motivation for (arbitrary) instrumental responses to obtain the goal. (That an instrumental (or operant) response is being made is demonstrated most precisely by the bidirectional criterion that either a response, or its opposite, may be performed as an action to obtain a goal.) It is the intervening persistent state elicited by reinforcing stimuli and the ability to allow stimuli to be interfaced to arbitrary instrumental actions that is one of the prime functions of emotion described here (see Chapter 3), and is therefore incorporated into the definition of emotion. The definition thus provides a clear way of dividing states into emotional or not, as it includes only those states that allow instrumental learning, that is arbitrary actions to be performed to obtain reinforcing outcomes (such as obtaining rewards and avoiding punishers).

Although animals that do not perform instrumental learning may not qualify according to this criterion as having emotions, they may of course have states that are precursors to emotions. This discussion thus leads to one possible way to separate animals that have emotions from those that do not, a way that is related to one of the fundamental functions of emotion, but it is realized that the separation made at this point should be seen as a useful separating point with a clear principle underlying it, but not a separating point that need be thought of as more than a useful convention in this context.

3 The functions of emotion: reward, punishment, and emotion in brain design

3.1 Introduction

We now confront the fundamental issue of why we, and other animals, are built to have emotions, as well as motivational states. Biologists would describe this as an 'ultimate' explanation for emotion and motivation. I will propose that we are built to have emotions, and motivational states, because we (and many other animals) use rewards and punishers to guide our behaviour, and that this is a good design for a system that is built by genes where some of the genes are increasing their survival (reproductive success) by specifying the goals for behaviour.

The emotions arise and are an inherent part of such a system because they are the states, typically persisting, that are elicited by rewards and punishers and stimuli associated with them, and that are the goals for instrumental actions. I will show that this is a very adaptive way for evolution to design complex animals without having to specify the details of the behavioural responses, the actions, as it is much more flexible in an uncertain environment for responses and actions to be learned.

What results from this analysis is thus a thoroughly Darwinian theory (though not anticipated by Darwin, and operating at the level of individual genes) that places emotion at the heart of brain design because it reflects the way in which genes build our brains in such a way that our genes can specify the goals of our actions, and thus what we do. There is thus a close conceptual link between instrumental learning and emotion, for primary reinforcers (primary rewards and punishers) are the gene-specified goals for our actions, and we use instrumental learning to learn any actions during our life-times that will lead to the gene-specified goals.

In Section 3.2, I outline several types of brain design, with differing degrees of complexity, and suggest that evolution can operate much better with only some of these types of design.

3.2 Brain design and the functions of emotion

3.2.1 Taxes, rewards, and punishers: gene-specified goals for actions, and the flexibility of actions

3.2.1.1 Taxes

A simple design principle is to incorporate mechanisms for taxes into the design of organisms. Taxes consist at their simplest of orientation towards stimuli in the environment, for example the bending of a plant towards light that results in maximum light collection by its photosynthetic surfaces. (When just turning rather than locomotion is possible, such responses are called tropisms.) With locomotion possible, as in animals, taxes include movements towards sources of nutrient, and movements away from hazards such as very high temperatures. The design principle here is that animals have, through a process of natural selection, built receptors for certain dimensions of the wide range of stimuli in the environment, and have linked these receptors to response mechanisms in such a way that the stimuli are approached or escaped from.

3.2.1.2 Rewards and punishers

As soon as we have approach to stimuli at one end of a dimension (e.g. a source of nutrient) and away from stimuli at the other end of the dimension (in this case lack of nutrient), we can start to wonder when it is appropriate to introduce the terms 'rewards' and 'punishers' for the stimuli at the different ends of the dimension. By convention, if the response consists of a fixed response to obtain the stimulus (e.g. locomotion up a chemical gradient), we shall call this a taxis not a reward-related instrumental action.

If a fixed behavioural response or 'action pattern' such as skeletomotor freezing and autonomic responses are elicited by a stimulus, they may be adaptive, but are essentially stimulus-response reflexes, with no need for an intervening state such as a goal to be reached. An example is the baby being stimulated by the touch of the mother's breast to turn the head and thus find the source of milk. These types of fixed response pattern can be useful, as they can operate without the need to learn an appropriate action, and can be useful for example in early life.

On the other hand, if an arbitrary instrumental (or operant) action can be performed by the animal in order to obtain the stimulus, then we will call this rewarded behaviour, and the stimulus that the animal works to obtain, the reward, is the goal for the action. (The arbitrary operant action can be thought of as any arbitrary action that the animal will perform to obtain the stimulus, such as either raising, or lowering, the arm to obtain a reward. That is a definition of an instrumental action.)

This criterion, of an arbitrary operant action, is often tested by bidirectionality. For example, if a rat can be trained to either raise its tail, or lower its tail, in order to obtain a piece of food, then we can be sure that there is no fixed relationship between the stimulus (e.g. the sight of food) and the response, as there is in a taxis. Some authors, including me, reserve the term '**motivated behaviour**' for that in which an arbitrary operant action will be performed to obtain a reward or to escape from or avoid a punisher. If this criterion is not met, and only a fixed response can be performed, then the term '**drive**' can be used to describe the state of the animal when it will work to obtain or escape from the stimulus.

We can thus distinguish a first level of approach/avoidance mechanism complexity in a taxis, with a fixed response available for the stimulus, from a second level of complexity in which any arbitrary response (or action) can be performed, in which case we use the term reward when a stimulus is being approached, and punisher when the action is to escape from or avoid the stimulus.

The role of natural selection in this process is to guide animals to build sensory systems that will respond to dimensions of stimuli in the natural environment along which actions of the animals can lead to better survival to enable genes to be passed on to the next generation, which is what we mean by fitness. (Fitness refers to the fitness of genes, but this must be measured by the effects that the genes have on the organism.) The animals must be built by such natural selection to perform actions that will enable them to obtain more rewards, that is to work to obtain stimuli that will increase their fitness. Correspondingly, animals must be built to perform actions that will enable them to escape from, or avoid when learning mechanisms are introduced, stimuli that will reduce their fitness. There are likely to be many dimensions of environmental stimuli along which actions of the animal can alter fitness. Each of these dimensions may be a separate reward–punisher dimension. An example of one of these dimensions might be food reward. It increases fitness to be able to sense nutrient need, to have sensors that respond to the taste of food, and to perform behavioural responses to obtain such reward stimuli when in that need or motivational state. Similarly, another dimension is water reward, in which the taste of water becomes rewarding when there is body-fluid depletion (Rolls & Rolls 1982a, Rolls 1999a, Rolls 2005).

One aspect of the operation of these reward–punisher systems that these examples illustrate is that with very many reward–punisher dimensions for which actions may be performed, there is a need for a selection mechanism for actions performed to these different dimensions. In this sense, rewards and punishers provide a common currency that provides one set of inputs to action selection mechanisms. Evolution must set the magnitudes of each of the different reward systems so that each will be chosen for action in such a way as to maximize overall fitness. Food reward must be chosen as the aim for action if some nutrient depletion is present, but water reward as a target for action must be selected if current water depletion poses a greater threat to fitness than does the current degree of food depletion. This indicates that for a competitive selection process for rewards, each reward must be carefully calibrated in evolution to have the right value on a common scale for the selection process (but not converted into a common currency (Rolls 2014b). Other types of behaviour, such as sexual behaviour, must be performed sometimes, but probably less frequently, in order to maximize fitness (as measured by gene transmission into the next generation).

There are many processes that contribute to increasing the chances that a wide set of different environmental rewards will be chosen over a period of time, including not only need-related satiety mechanisms that reduce the rewards within a dimension, but also sensory-specific satiety mechanisms, which facilitate switching to another reward stimulus (sometimes within and sometimes outside the same main dimension), and attraction to novel stimuli. (As noted in Sections 3.4.6 and 4.6.6, attraction to novel stimuli, i.e. finding them rewarding, is one way that organisms are encouraged to explore the multidimensional space within which their genes are operating. The suggestion is that animals should be built to find somewhat novel stimuli rewarding, for this encourages them to explore new parts of the environment in which their genes might do better than others' genes. Unless animals are built to find novelty somewhat rewarding, the multidimensional genetic space being explored by genes in the course of evolution might not find the appropriate environment in which they might do better than others' genes.)

3.2.1.3 Stimulus–response (habit) learning reinforced by rewards and punishers

In this second level of complexity, involving reward or punishment, learning may occur. If an organism performs trial-and-error responses, and as the result of performing one particular response is more likely to obtain a reward, then the response may become linked by a learning process to that stimulus as a result of the reward received. The reward is said to reinforce the response to that stimulus, and we have what is described as stimulus–response or habit learning. The reward acts as a positive reinforcer in that it increases the probability of a response on which it is made contingent. A punisher reduces the probability of a response on which it is made contingent. (It should be noted that this is an operational definition, and that there is no implication that the punisher feels like anything – the punisher just has in the learning mechanism to reduce the probability of responses followed by the punisher.) Stimulus–response or habit learning is typically evident after over-training, and once habits are being executed, the behaviour becomes somewhat independent of the reward value of the goal, as shown in experiments in which the reward is devalued. This is described in more detail in Section 4.6.2 on page 96.

3.2.1.4 Stimulus–reinforcer association learning, and two-factor learning theory for instrumental actions

Two-process learning introduces a third level of complexity and capability into the ways in which behaviour can be guided. Rewards and punishers still provide the basis for guiding behaviour within a dimension, and for selecting the dimension towards which action should be directed.

The first stage of the learning is stimulus–reinforcer association learning, in which the reinforcing value of a previously neutral, e.g. visual or auditory, stimulus is learned because of its association with a primary reinforcer, such as a sweet taste or a painful touch. This learning is of an association between one stimulus, the conditioned or secondary reinforcer, and the primary reinforcer, and is thus stimulus–stimulus association learning. This stimulus–reinforcer learning can be very fast, in as little as one trial. For example, if a new visual stimulus is placed in the mouth and a sweet taste is obtained, a simple approach response such as reaching for the object will be made on the next trial. Moreover, this stimulus–reinforcer association learning can be reversed very rapidly. For example, if subsequently the object is made to taste of salt, then approach no longer occurs to the stimulus, and the stimulus is even likely to be actively pushed away. This process leads to representations of expected value in the orbitofrontal cortex (Chapter 4).

The second process or stage in this type of learning is instrumental learning of an action (or 'operant response') made in order to obtain the stimulus now associated with reward (or avoid a stimulus associated by learning with the punisher). This is action–outcome learning (implemented in brain regions such as the cingulate cortex). The outcome could be a primary reinforcer, but often involves a secondary reinforcer learned by stimulus–reinforcer association learning. The action–outcome learning may be much slower, for it may involve trial-and-error learning of which action is successful in enabling the animal to obtain the stimulus now associated with reward or avoid the stimulus now associated with a punisher. However, this second stage may be greatly speeded if an operant response or strategy that has been learned previously to obtain a different type of reward (or avoid a different punisher) can be used to obtain (or avoid) the new stimulus now known to be associated with reinforcement. It is in this flexibility of the response that two-factor learning has a great advantage over stimulus–response learning. The advantage is that any action can be performed once an association has been learned between a stimulus and a primary reinforcer. This flexibility in the response is much more adaptive (and could provide the difference between survival or not) than no learning, as in taxes, or stimulus–response learning.

The different processes that are involved in instrumental learning are described in more detail in Section 4.6.2.

Another key advantage of this type of two-stage learning is that after the first stage the different rewards and punishers available in an environment can be compared in a selection mechanism, using the common scale of different rewards and punishers for the comparison and selection process. In this type of system, the many dimensions of rewards and punishers are again the basis on which the selection of a behaviour to perform is made.

Part of the process of evolution can be seen as identifying the factors or dimensions that affect the fitness of an animal, and providing the animal with sensors that lead to rewards and punishers that are tuned to the environmental dimensions that influence fitness. The example of sweet taste receptors being set up by evolution to provide reward when physiological nutrient need is present has been given above.

To help specify the way in which stimulus–reinforcer association learning operates, a list of what may be in at least some species primary reinforcers is provided in Table 2.1 on page 20. The reader will doubtless be able to add to this list, and it may be that some of the reinforcers in the list are actually secondary reinforcers. The reinforcers are categorized where possible by modality, to help the list to be systematic. Possible dimensions to which each reinforcer is tuned are suggested.

3.2.2 Explicit systems, language, and reinforcement

A fourth level of complexity to the way in which behaviour is guided is by processing that includes syntactic operations on semantically grounded symbols (see Section 10). This allows multistep one-off plans to be formulated. Such a plan might be: if I do this, then B is likely to do this, C will probably do this, and then X will be the outcome. Such a process cannot be performed by an animal that only performs instrumental actions to obtain a gene-specified reward, or secondary reinforcers. The process may enable an available reward to be deferred for another reward that a particular multistep strategy could lead to. What are the roles of rewards and punishers in such a system?

The language system can still be considered to operate to obtain rewards and avoid punishers. This is not merely a matter of definition, for many of the rewards and punishers will be the same as those described above, those that have been tuned by evolution to the dimensions of the environment that can enable an animal to increase fitness. The processing afforded by language can be seen as providing a new type of strategy to obtain such gene-specified rewards or avoid such punishers. If this were not generally the case, then the use of the language system would not be adaptive: it would not increase fitness.

However, once a language system has evolved, a consequence may be that certain new types of reward become possible. These may be related to primary reinforcers already present, but may develop beyond them. For example, music may have evolved from the system of non-verbal communication that enables emotional states to be communicated to others. An example might be that lullabies could be related to emotional messages that can be sent from parents to offspring to soothe them. Music with a more military character might be related to the sounds given as social signals to each other in situations in which fighting (or co-operation in fighting) might occur. The prosodic quality of voice expression may be part of the same emotion communication system, and brain systems that are activated by prosody may be strongly engaged in women even in tasks that do not require prosody to be analysed (Schirmer, Zysset, Kotz & von Cramon 2004). Then on top of this, the intellectualization afforded by linguistic (syntactic) processing would contribute further aspects to music. Another example here is that solving problems by intellectual means should itself be a primary reinforcer as a result of evolution, for this would encourage the use of intellectual abilities that have potential advantage if used. A further set of examples of how, when a language system is present, there is the possibility for further types of reinforcer, comes from the possibility that the evolution of some mental abilities may have been influenced by sexual selection (see Section 7.7.2).

An additional principle enabled by language is that the rewards and punishers need not be defined only in the interests of the genes, but can be instead in the interests of the individual, the phenotype, as shown in Section 10.1.4.

3.2.3 Special-purpose design by an external agent vs evolution by natural selection

The above mechanisms, which operate in an evolutionary context to enable animals' behaviour to be tuned to increase fitness by evolving reward–punisher systems tuned to dimensions in the environment that increase fitness, may be contrasted with typical engineering design. In the latter, we may want to design a robot to work on an assembly line. Here there is an external designer, the engineer, who defines the function to be performed by the robot (e.g. picking a nut from a box, and attaching it to a particular bolt in the object being assembled). The engineer then produces special-purpose design features that enable the robot to perform this task, by for example providing it with sensors and an arm to enable it to select a nut, and to place the nut in the correct position in the 3D space of the object to enable the nut to be placed on the bolt and tightened.

In the case of the animal, there is a multidimensional space within which many optimizations to increase fitness must be performed. The solution to this is to evolve multiple reward–punisher systems tuned to each dimension in the environment that can lead to an increased fitness if the animal performs the appropriate actions. Natural selection guides evolution to find these dimensions. In contrast, in the robot arm, there is an externally defined movement to be performed, of placing the nut on the bolt, and the robot does not need to tune itself to find the goal to be performed. The contrast is between design by evolution that is 'blind' to the purpose of the animal, and design by a designer who specifies the job to be performed (cf. Dawkins (1986b)).

The implication of this comparison is that operation by animals using reward and punisher systems tuned to dimensions of the environment that increase fitness provides a mode of operation that can work in organisms that evolve by natural selection. It is clearly a natural outcome of Darwinian evolution to operate using reward and punisher systems tuned to fitness-related dimensions of the environment, if arbitrary actions are to be made by the animals rather than just preprogrammed movements such as are involved in tropisms and taxes. This may be the reason why we are built to work for rewards, avoid punishers, have emotions, and feel needs (motivational states). These concepts do not appear to have been developed within selfish gene theory (Dawkins 1976, Dawkins 1982, Dawkins 1986b), and bear on developments in the field of artificial life (see, e.g. Boden (1996)).

3.3 Selection of behaviour: cost–benefit 'analysis' of net value

One advantage of a design based on rewards and punishers is that the decoding of stimuli to a reward or punisher value can provide a common scale of value as inputs to the mechanism that selects which behavioural action should be performed. Thus, for example, a moderately sweet taste when little hunger is present would have a smaller reward value than the taste of water when thirst is present. A reward-selection mechanism could thus include in its specification competition between the different rewards, all represented on a common scale of value, with the most active specific reward or value representation indicating the stimulus most likely to be selected for action. As described above, to make sure that different types of reward are selected when appropriate, natural selection would need to ensure that different types of reward would operate on similar scales (from minimum to maximum), so that each type of reward would be selected if it reaches a high value on the common scale (Rolls 2014b). Mechanisms such as sensory-specific satiety can be seen as contributing usefully to this mechanism which ensures that different types of reward will be selected for action.

However, the action selection mechanisms must take into account not only the relative value of each type of reward, but also the cost of obtaining each type of reward. If there is a very high cost of obtaining a particular reward, it may be better, at least temporarily, until the situation changes, to select an action that leads to a smaller reward, but is less costly. It appears that animals do operate according to such a cost–benefit analysis, in that if there is a high cost for an action, that action is less likely to be performed. One example of this comes from the fighting of deer. A male deer is less likely to fight another if he is clearly inferior in size or signalled prowess (Clutton-Brock & Albon 1979, Dawkins 1995). Thus the value of a stimulus or course of action, that is its intrinsic value minus the cost of the actions needed to obtain it and any resulting consequences of obtaining it, needs to be produced in a system that represents net value. Decisions can then be taken between these net value representations, and then actions can be selected as a separate process to obtain the winning stimulus or goal for action.

There may also be a cost to switching behaviour. If the sources of food and water are very distant, it would be costly to switch behaviour (and perhaps walk a mile) every time a mouthful of food or a mouthful of water was swallowed. This may be part of the adaptive value of incentive motivation or the 'salted nut' phenomenon – that after one reward is given early on in working for that reward the incentive value of that reward may increase. This may be expressed in the gradually increasing rate of working for food early on in a meal. By increasing the reward value of a stimulus for the first minute or two of working for it, hysteresis may be built into the behaviour selection mechanism, to make behaviour 'stick' to one reward for at least a short time once it is started.

Reward and punisher signals provide a common scale of value for different sensory inputs, and can be seen as important in the selection of which actions are performed. Evolution ensures that the different reward and punisher signals are made potent to the extent that each will be chosen when appropriate. For example, food will be rewarding when hungry, but as hunger falls, the current level of thirst may soon become sufficient to make the reward produced by the taste of water greater than that produced by food, so that water is ingested. If however a painful input occurs or is signalled at any time during the feeding or drinking, this may be a stronger signal in the common scale of value, so that behaviour switches to that appropriate to reduce or avoid the pain. After the painful stimulus or threat is removed, the next most rewarding stimulus in the common value scale might be the taste of water, and drinking would therefore be selected.

An implication is that a decision process must be implemented in the brain between options each represented by their net value. An option is an action that might be chosen, and these decision processes are examined in Chapter 8.

The overall aim of the cost–benefit analysis in animals is to maximize *fitness*. By fitness we mean the probability that an animal's genes will be passed on into the next generation. To maximize this, there may be many ways in which different stimuli have been selected during evolution to be rewards and punishers (and among punishers we could include costs). All these rewards and punishers should operate together to ensure that over the lifetime of the animal there is a high probability of passing on genes to the next generation; but in doing this, and maximizing fitness in a complex and changing environment, all these rewards and punishers may be expected to lead to a wide variety of behaviour.

Once language enables rewards and punishers to be intellectualized, so that, for example, solving complex problems in language, mathematics, or music becomes rewarding, behaviour might be less obviously seen as adapted for reproductive fitness. Indeed, it is argued in Chapter 10 that language enables humans to takes decision based on reasoning, which enables human behaviour to be less dependent on gene-specified reinforcers and the associated emotions, and made instead on the basis of reasoning, which can enable humans to make decisions that might be against what gene-specified reinforcers might favour, as for example when we choose to select a nutritionally good food what may not be especially delicious. This makes human decision-making particularly interesting, as shown in Chapter 10.

3.4 Further functions of emotion

The fundamental function of emotion, to enable an efficient way for the goals for actions to be defined by genes during evolution and to be implemented in the brain, has been described in Sections 3.2 and 3.3. The simple brain implementation provided as a result of evolution allows the different goals to be selected and compared by using reward and punisher evaluation or appraisal of stimuli, and of the stimuli that may be obtained by different courses of action. This function allows flexibility of the behavioural responses that will be performed to obtain gene-specified goals.

Next we consider some further functions and properties of emotion, and also highlight some particularly interesting examples of the types of emotional behaviour that result from the fundamental operation of emotional systems described above.

3.4.1 Autonomic and endocrine responses

An additional function of emotion is the elicitation of autonomic responses (e.g. a change in heart rate) and endocrine responses (e.g. the release of adrenaline). It is of clear survival value to prepare the body, for example by increasing the heart rate, so that actions such as running which may be performed as a consequence of the reinforcing stimulus can be performed more efficiently. The neural connections from the amygdala and orbitofrontal cortex via the visceral insula (its antero-ventral part) and the hypothalamus as well as directly towards the brainstem autonomic motor nuclei may be particularly involved in this function (see Chapter 4).

3.4.2 Flexibility of behavioural actions, because emotions are related to the rewards and punishers that specify the goals for action

A function of emotion inherent in the gene-based theory described above is providing flexibility of behavioural responses, and this function of emotion is elaborated now. The thesis here is that when a rewarding or punishing stimulus in the environment elicits an emotional state, we can perform any appropriate and arbitrary action to obtain the reward, or avoid the punisher. That is, the reward or punisher defines the goal for the action, but does not specify the action itself. The action itself can be selected by the animal as appropriate in the current circumstances as that most appropriate for obtaining the reward or avoiding or escaping from the punisher. This is more flexible than simply learning a fixed behavioural response to a stimulus, which is what was implied by the stimulus–response (S–R) or habit learning theories of the 1930s.

This flexibility of behavioural responses is made very clear when we consider the learning processes that typically occur when emotion-provoking stimuli occur. Let us consider as an example avoidance learning. An example of this might be learning an action to perform when a tone sounds in order to avoid an electrical shock. The learning would take place in two stages, with different processes involved in each stage. In the first stage, stimulus–reinforcer association learning would produce an emotional state such as fear to a tone associated with the shock. This learning stage may be very rapid, and may occur in one trial. (We will see in Chapter 4 that the orbitofrontal cortex and amygdala are especially involved in this type of learning.) The second stage of the avoidance learning would be instrumental learning of an operant response (i.e. an action), motivated by and performed in order to terminate the fear-inducing stimulus. Finding an appropriate action to remove the fear-inducing stimulus may occur by trial-and-error, and may take many trials.

The suggestion made here is that this general type of two-stage learning process is closely related to the design of animals for many types of behaviour, including emotional behaviour. It simplifies the interface of sensory systems to motor systems. Instead of having to learn a particular response or habit to a particular stimulus by slow, trial-and-error, learning, two-stage learning allows very fast (often one trial) learning of an emotional state to a rewarding or punishing stimulus. Then the action system can operate in a quite general way, sometimes using new trial-and-error learning, but often using many previously learned strategies, to approach the reward or avoid the punisher, which act as goals.

It may be emphasized that emotions are thus an important part of brain design by enabling actions to be selected on the basis of goals, in allowing flexibility of the action performed, but also, and extremely importantly, by enabling a very simple type of one-trial learning, stimulus–reinforcer association learning, which is also very fast, to enable animals to respond to new attractive or dangerous stimuli with learning that may take as little as one trial.

3.4.3 Emotional states are motivating

Another function of emotion is that it is motivating. For example, fear learned by stimulus–reinforcer association formation provides the motivation for actions performed to avoid noxious stimuli. Similarly, positive reinforcers elicit incentive motivation, so that we will work harder to obtain the rewards. Another example where emotion affects motivation is when a reward becomes no longer available, that is frustrative non-reward (see Fig. 2.1). If an action is possible, then increased motivation facilitates behaviour to produce harder working to obtain that reinforcer again or another reinforcer. If no action is possible to obtain again that reward (e.g. after a death in the family), then as described in Chapter 2, grief or sadness may result. This may be adaptive, by preventing continuing motivated attempts to regain the positive reinforcer that is no longer available, and helping the animal in due course to therefore be sensitive to other potential reinforcers to which it might be adaptive to switch. As described in Chapter 2, if such frustrative non-reward occurs in humans when no action is possible, depression may occur.

A depressed state that lasts for a short time may be seen as being adaptive for the reason just given. However, the depression may last for a very long time perhaps because long-term explicit (conscious) knowledge in humans enables the long-term consequences of loss of the positive reinforcer to be evaluated and repeatedly brought to mind as described in Chapters 9 and 10, and this may make long-term (psychological) depression maladaptive. Thus a discrepancy between the evolutionary and current environment caused by the rapid development of an explicit system may contribute to some emotional states that are no longer adaptive.

In an interesting evolutionary approach to depression, Nesse (2000) has argued that humans may set long-term goals for themselves that are difficult to attain, and may spend years trying to attain these goals. An example of such a goal might be obtaining a particular position in one's career, or professional qualification, which may take years of a person's life. If the goal is not attained, then the lack of the reinforcer may lead to prolonged depression. Humans may find it difficult to reorganize their long-term aims to identify other, replacement and more attainable, goals, and without facility at this reorganization of long-term goals, the depression may be prolonged. The evolutionary aspect of this is that with our long-term explicit planning system (described in Chapter 10) and the value that society places on long-term goals and the status that attaining these may confer, humans find themselves in an environmental situation in which their explicit long-term planning system did not evolve, so that it is not well adapted to identifying goals that are realistic. The explicit system then provides a long-lasting non-reward signal to the emotion system (which in addition did not evolve to deal with such long-lasting non-reward inputs), and this contributes to long-lasting depression. A therapeutic solution would be to help depressed people identify possible precipitating factors such as unachieved long-term goals, and readjust their life aims so that positive reinforcers start to be obtained again, helping to lift the person out of the depression.

In addition to these motivating effects of emotion-provoking stimuli, I also emphasize that my Darwinian view that some genes specify the goals for actions leads not only to an account of emotion, but also to an account of motivation. As described in Chapter 2, motivation does not require an inherently different mechanism to emotion, in that if genes are specifying the reward value of some stimuli ('primary reinforcers'), then the behavioural system must be built to seek to obtain these stimuli (i.e. be motivated to treat them as goals), for otherwise the stimuli would not be operationally describable as rewards. A simple way to think about this is that *motivation is a state in which we are performing instrumental actions to obtain gene-defined goals; and emotions are states that are elicited when those goals are obtained, or are not obtained.*

3.4.4 Communication

Because of its survival value, the ability to decode signals from other animals as being rewarding or punishing is important. The reward or punisher value may in some cases be innate, and in other cases learned. It may also be adaptive to send such signals, and in some cases the sending of such signals may be 'honest' and in other cases 'deceptive'. These communicated signals may indicate for example the extent to which animals are willing to compete for resources, and they may influence the behaviour of other animals (Hauser 1996). Communicating emotional states may have survival value, for example by reducing fighting.

Darwin (1872), in his book entitled *The Expression of the Emotions in Man and Animals* had as a goal emphasizing the similarity, and therefore the possible phylogenetic closeness, of the expressions of man and his closest living relatives, but nevertheless noted the communicative value of such expressions.

The observation that expressions can evoke a response in the receiver underlies the idea that expressions can also be communicative rather than simply outward signs of affect (Chevalier-Skolnikoff 1973). Expression can be seen as a way of inviting/inducing certain responses in the receiver, much as a smile can appease, a laugh can invite participation, and fear could enlist assistance. In non-human primates, expression is used as a tool with which to regulate and maintain social relations. For example, in the macaque if a subordinate grimaces in an aggressive encounter with a dominant, this signals submission. However, the use of expression is not necessarily so straightforward, for if the same expression were to be given by a dominant individual approaching a subordinate, it no longer signals submission but the positive intention of the dominant. In this way, the communicative effect of expression can be said to be context-dependent, and it depends on the age, sex, dominance and kinship of the senders and receivers (Chevalier-Skolnikoff 1973).

To argue that the expression of emotion is utilized in social communication, then the ability to decode these signals must be demonstrated. We will see in Chapter 4 that brain systems have evolved in primates to identify the expression on a face, and the identity of the face, for both are very important to deciding what action to take to a face expression.

3.4.5 Social attachment

Another area in which emotion is important is in social bonding. Examples of this are the emotions associated with the attachment of the parents to their young, with the attachment of the young to their parents, and with the attachment of the parents to each other (see Section 7.2). In the theory of the ways in which the genes affect behaviour ('selfish gene' theory, see Dawkins (1989), Ridley (2003)), it is held that (because, e.g., of the advantages of parental care) all these forms of emotional attachment have the effect that genes for such attachment are more likely to survive into the next generation. Kin-altruism can also be considered in these terms (see e.g. Dawkins (1989) and Section 7.7.2). In these examples, social bonding is related to primary (gene-specified) reinforcers. In other cases, the emotions involved in social interactions may arise from reinforcers involved in reciprocal altruism, utilizing for example 'tit-for-tat' strategies. In these cases it is crucial to remember which reinforcers are exchanged with particular individuals, so that cheating does not lead to disadvantages for some of those involved. This type of social bonding can be stable when there is a net advantage to both parties in cooperating (see Section 11.3).

Some investigators have argued that the main functions of emotion are in social situations (see Strongman (2003)). While it is certainly the case that many emotions are related to social situations (as can be inferred from Table 2.1), many are not, including for example the fear of snakes by primates, or the fear that is produced by the sight of an object that has produced pain previously.

3.4.6 Separate functions for each different primary reinforcer

It is useful to highlight that each primary (gene-specified) reinforcer (of which a large number are suggested in Table 2.1) not only leads to a different set of emotions, but also implements a different function. A few examples of these functions are elaborated here. This should make it possible for the reader to complete the elaboration for the other primary reinforcers in Table 2.1.

Before considering these examples, let us remember that each function is related to the survival value or sexually selected value being provided by the specifying gene by increasing reproductive success for the gene; and that in so far as emotional states are associated with feelings (see Chapter 10), anything that feels pleasant or unpleasant to the organism, and is instrumentally reinforcing, is likely to have survival value, and to implement another function of emotion.

One example of a primary reinforcer taken from Table 2.1 is slight novelty, which may feel good and be positively reinforcing because it may lead to the discovery of better opportunities for survival in the environment (e.g. a new food).

Another example from Table 2.1 is gregariousness, which may assist the identification of new social partners, which could provide advantage.

Probably related to the effects of novelty is sensory-specific satiety, the phenomenon whereby pleasant tastes during a meal gradually become less pleasant as satiety approaches (see Chapter 5). This may be an aspect of a more general adaptation to ensure that behaviour does eventually switch from one reinforcer to another.

Of course the genes may be misled sometimes and lead to behaviour that does not have survival value, as when for example the non-nutritive sweetener saccharin is eaten by animals. This does not disprove the theory, but only points out that the genes cannot specify correctly for every possible stimulus or event in the environment, but must only on average lead to behaviour feeling pleasant that increases reproductive fitness, i.e. is appropriate for gene survival.

3.4.7 The mood state can influence the cognitive evaluation of moods or memories

Another property of emotion is that the current mood state can affect the cognitive evaluation of events or memories (Blaney 1986, Robinson, Watkins & Harmon-Jones 2013), and this may have the function of facilitating continuity in the interpretation of the reinforcing value of events in the environment. A theory of how this occurs is presented in Section 4.9 'Effects of emotion on cognitive processing and memory'.

3.4.8 Facilitation of memory storage

An eighth function of emotion is that it may facilitate the storage of memories. One way in which this occurs is that episodic memory (i.e. one's memory of particular episodes) is facilitated by emotional states. This may be advantageous in that storage of as many details as possible of the prevailing situation when a strong reinforcer is delivered may be useful in generating appropriate behaviour in situations with some similarities in the future. This function may be implemented in the brain by the relatively non-specific projecting systems to the cerebral cortex and hippocampus, including the cholinergic pathways in the basal forebrain and medial septum, and the ascending noradrenergic pathways (Rolls 2016c, Rolls 2014b, Rolls & Treves 1998, Rolls 1999a, Wilson & Rolls 1990a, Wilson & Rolls 1990b, Wilson & Rolls 1990c).

A second way in which emotion may affect the storage of memories is that the current emotional state may be stored with episodic memories, providing a mechanism for the current emotional state to affect which memories are recalled. In this sense, emotion acts as a contextual retrieval cue, that as with other contextual effects influences the retrieval of episodic memories (Rolls 2016c, Rolls & Treves 1998, Kesner & Rolls 2015).

A third way in which emotion may affect the storage of memories is by guiding the cerebral cortex in the representations of the world that are set up. For example, in the visual system, it may be useful to build perceptual representations or analysers that are different from each other if they are associated with different reinforcers, and to be less likely to build them if they have no association with reinforcers. Ways in which backprojections from parts of the brain important in emotion (such as the amygdala) to parts of the cerebral cortex could perform this function are discussed in Section 4.9 'Effects of emotion on cognitive processing and memory'; and by Rolls (2016c).

3.4.9 Emotional and mood states are persistent, and help to produce persistent motivation

A ninth function of emotion is that by enduring for minutes or longer after a reinforcing stimulus has occurred, it may help to produce persistent motivation and direction of behaviour. For example, if an expected reward is not obtained, the persisting state of frustrative non-reward may usefully keep behaviour directed for some time at trying to obtain the reward again.

3.4.10 Emotions may trigger memory recall and influence cognitive processing

A tenth function of emotion is that it may trigger recall of memories stored in neocortical representations. Amygdala and orbitofrontal cortex backprojections to cortical areas could perform this for emotion in a way analogous to that in which the hippocampus could implement the retrieval in the neocortex of recent memories of particular events or episodes (Rolls 2016c, Kesner & Rolls 2015, Rolls 2015d). This is thought to operate as follows. When a memory is stored in a neocortical area or the hippocampus, any mood state that is present and reflected in the firing of neurons in the orbitofrontal cortex or amygdala will become associated with that memory by virtue of the associatively modifiable synaptic connections from the backprojecting neurons onto the neocortical or hippocampal system neurons. Then later, a particular mood state represented by the firing of neurons in the amygdala or orbitofrontal cortex will by the associatively modified backprojection connections enhance or produce the recall of memories stored when that mood state was present. These effects have been formally modelled by Rolls & Stringer (2001), and are described further in Section 4.9.

One consequence of these effects is that once in a particular mood state, memories associated with that mood state will tend to be recalled and incoming stimuli will be interpreted in the light of the current mood state. The result may be some continuity of emotional state and thus of behaviour. This continuity may sometimes be advantageous, by keeping behaviour directed towards a goal, and making behaviour interpretable by others, but it may become useful in human psychiatric conditions to break this self-perpetuating tendency.

3.5 The functions of emotion in an evolutionary, Darwinian, context

In this book (see for example Section 3.2), the question of why we have emotions is a fundamental issue that I answer in terms of a Darwinian, functional, approach, producing the answer that emotions are states elicited by the goals (rewards and punishers) for instrumental actions, and that this is part of an adaptive process by which genes can specify the behaviour of the animal by specifying goals for behaviour rather than fixed responses. The emotional states elicited with respect to the goals depend on the reinforcement contingencies, as illustrated in Fig. 2.1. The states themselves may be the goals for action, such as reducing fear, and additionally maintain behaviour by being persistent, and act in other ways as described in Section 3.4.

This theory of emotion provides I believe a powerful approach to understanding how genes influence behaviour. In much thinking in zoology, an approach has been to understand how genes may determine particular behaviours. For example, Niko Tinbergen (1963, 1951) considered that innate releasing stimuli might elicit fixed action patterns. An example is the herring gull chick's pecking response elicited as a fixed action pattern by the innate releasing stimulus of a red spot on its parent's bill. A successor in this approach in the context of emotion is Panksepp (1998), who specifies fixed action patterns.

The details of the stimulus, or the context in which it occurs, may be taken into account, to influence the instinctive response (Dawkins 1995), but there is still no arbitrary relation between the stimulus and the action, as in instrumental learning.

In contrast, the most important function of emotion that I propose is for genes to specify the stimuli that are the goals for actions. This means that the genetic specification can be kept relatively simple, in that it is stimuli that are specified by the genes, such as a taste or touch, and this is generally simpler than specifying the details of a response (such as climbing a tree, running along a branch, picking an apple, and placing it into the mouth). It also means that relatively few genetic specifications are needed, for instead of having to encode many relations between particular stimuli and particular behavioural responses, the genes need to span the dimensionality of the stimulus space of primary reinforcers. Examples of some of these primary, gene-encoded, reinforcers are shown in Table 2.1.

Another way in which the genetic specification required can be kept low is that stimulus–reinforcer association learning can then be used to enable quite arbitrary stimuli occurring in the lifetime of an animal to become associated with primary reinforcers by stimulus–reinforcer association learning, and thus to lead to actions.

But the most important advantage conferred by emotion is that the behaviour required need not be genetically specified, for arbitrary actions can be learned in the lifetime of the animal by instrumental, action–outcome, learning to obtain or avoid the goals specified by the genes. The actions are arbitrary operants, in that any action may be made to obtain the goal (Rolls 2014b). Thus the genetic specification of the behaviour that emotion allows is one in which the behaviour is not pre-programmed with respect to the stimulus (as in instinctive behaviour such as fixed action patterns), but instead the action is not specified by the genes, and the goals to which actions are directed are specified by the genes. Of course this does not deny that some behavioural responses are genetically specified as responses, and examples might include pecking to particular stimuli in birds, orientation to and suckling of the nipple in mammals, and some examples of preparedness to learn (Rolls 2014b).

Darwinian natural selection of genes that encode the goals for action (i.e. encode reinforcers) rather than the actions themselves, and thus allows great flexibility of the resulting behaviour, can be thought of as liberating 'The Selfish Gene' (Dawkins 1976, Dawkins 1989). When Richard Dawkins wrote *The Selfish Gene* (Dawkins 1976), he was careful to make it clear that the concept that selection and competition operate at the level of genes (Hamilton 1964, Hamilton 1996) does not lead inevitably to genetic determinism of behaviour. Nevertheless the concept was criticized on these grounds, and Dawkins devoted a whole chapter of *The Extended Phenotype* to addressing this further (Dawkins 1982). The concepts developed in *Emotion and Decision-Making Explained* help to resolve this further, for I argue that an important way in which genes influence behaviour (and in doing so produce emotion), is by specifying the reinforcers, the goals for actions, rather than particular behaviours (Rolls 1999a, Rolls 2014b). This helps to avoid the charge that selfish genes 'determine' the behaviour. Instead, many of the genes that influence behaviour operate by competing with each other in a world of reinforcing stimuli or goals for actions, and thus there is great flexibility in the behaviour that results. We are led to think not of behaviours being inherited or 'determined by selfish genes', but instead of genes exploring by natural selection reinforcers that may guide behaviour successfully so that the fitness of the genes is increased. In this sense, the selfish gene (in particular, those involved in specifying reinforcers) is liberated from directly 'determining' behaviour, to providing goals for (instrumental) actions that can involve completely flexible behaviour made to obtain the goal. In these cases, the heritability of behaviour is best understood as the heritability of reinforcers in a stimulus space not in a behavioural or response space.

An interesting consequence of this fundamental adaptive value of emotion that I propose is that the genetic specification does need to include specification for several synapses through the nervous system from the sensory input to the brain region where the reward or punishment value of the goal stimulus is made explicit in the representation. It is thus a prediction that genes specify the connectivity to the stage of processing in the brain where goals and rewards are specified, so that appropriate actions can be learned to the goals. Evidence is described in Chapters 4 and 5 that the goals may not be made explicit, that is related to neuronal firing, until stages of information processing such as the orbitofrontal cortex and amygdala. An example of this specification is that sweet taste receptors on the tongue must be connected to neurons that specify food reward, and whose responses are modulated by hunger signals (see Chapter 5).

The definition I provide of emotions, that they are states (with particular functions) elicited by instrumental reinforcers (see Chapter 2), thus is consistent with what I see as the most important function of emotion, that of being part of a design by which genes can specify (some) goals or reinforcers of our actions. This means that the theory of emotion that I propose should not be seen as behaviourist, but instead as part of a much broader theory that takes an adaptive, Darwinian, approach to the functions of emotion, and how they are important in brain design. Further, the theory shows how cognitive states can produce and modulate emotion (see Sections 2.6 and 4.5.3.6), and in turn how emotional states can influence cognition (see Section 4.9).

I believe that this approach leads to a fundamental understanding of why we have emotions that is likely to stand the test of time, in the same way that Darwinian thinking itself provides a fundamental way of understanding biology and many 'why' questions about life. This is thus intended to be a thoroughly Darwinian theory of the adaptive value of emotion in the design of organisms.

3.6 The functions of motivation in an evolutionary, Darwinian, context

Motivation may be seen as a state in which one is working for a goal, and emotion as a state that occurs when the goal, a reinforcer, is obtained, and that may persist afterwards. The concept of gene-specified reinforcers providing the goals for action helps the understanding of the relation between motivational states and emotion, as the organism must be built to be motivated to obtain the goals, and to be placed in a different state (emotion) when the goal is or is not achieved by the action. The close but clear relation between motivation and emotion is that both involve what humans describe as affective states (e.g. feeling hungry, liking the taste of a food, feeling happy because of a social reinforcer), and both are about goals. The Darwinian theory of the functions of emotion developed in this chapter, which shows how emotion is adaptive because it reflects the operation of a process by which genes define goals for action, applies just as much to motivation. By specifying goals, the genes must specify both that we must be motivated to obtain those goals, and that when the goals are obtained, further states, emotional states with further functions, are produced.

In motivated behaviour, many factors influence how rewarding or punishing the goal is. In terms of motivated states relevant to internal homeostatic needs, the reward or goal value of a sensory stimulus such as the taste of food or water is set up genetically to be influenced by the relevant internal signals, such as plasma glucose concentration or plasma osmolality in the cases of hunger and thirst, as described in Chapter 5 and for thirst in Rolls (2005). If a gene-specified goal such as the taste of expected food is not obtained, then we are left in a state of frustrative non-reward in which the original goal remains rewarding, which will leave us motivated to still obtain it if it may still be available, or will lead to a learned change in its reward value, and to extinction of that behaviour, if we learn that no action will obtain the goal (see Section 3.4.3).

3.7 Are all goals for action gene-specified?

Finally in this chapter, we can ask whether all goals are gene-specified. An important concept of this chapter has been that part of the adaptive value of emotion is that it is part of the process that results from the way in which genes specify reinforcers, that is the goals for action. Emotions may thus be elicited by primary reinforcers, or by stimuli that become associated by learning with primary reinforcers, i.e. secondary reinforcers. But are there goals related to emotional and motivational states that are not related to goals defined in this way by gene-specified reinforcers?

I think it is likely that most reinforcers can be traced back to a gene-specified goal, even if they are in some cases rather general goals. Some examples of these types of reinforcer (and there are likely to be many others) are included in Table 2.1, such as goals for social cooperation and group acceptance, mind reading, and solving an intellectual problem. However, when an explicit, rational, reasoning system capable of syntactic operations on symbols (as described in Chapter 10) evolves, it is possible that goals that are not very directly related to gene specifications become accepted. This may be seen in some of the effects of culture. Indeed, some goals are defined within a culture, for example writing a novel. But it is argued that it is primary reinforcers specified by genes of the general type shown in Table 2.1 that make us want to be recognized in society because of the advantages this can bring, to solve difficult problems, etc., and therefore to perform actions such as writing novels (see further Chapters 7 and 10, Ridley (2003) Chapter 8, Ridley (1993b) pp. 310 ff, Laland & Brown (2002) pp. 271 ff, Dawkins (1982), and *Neuroculture* Rolls (2012d)). Indeed, culture is influenced by human genetic propensities, and it follows that human cognitive, affective, and moral capacities are the product of a unique dynamic known as *gene-culture coevolution* (Gintis 2007, Bowles & Gintis 2005, Gintis 2003, Boyd, Gintis, Bowles & Richerson 2003).

Nevertheless, there may be cases where the explicit, reasoning, system might specify a goal, and thus lead to emotions, that could not be related to any genetic adaptive value, whether current or specified in evolutionary history. In these cases I would argue that although emotion has evolved and is generally adaptive in relation to gene-specified reinforcers, when the explicit, reasoning, system evolves, this can set up alternative goals that tap into and utilize the existing emotional system for facilitating actions, but with respect to which the goals might be genetically unspecified and even non-adaptive. Indeed, it is argued in Chapters 10 and 11 that much implicit emotion acts in the interests of the genes, whereas reasoning in the explicit system can allow gene-specified rewards to be rejected, in the long-term interests of the individual person, for example to stay alive for a long time (which may not be in the interests of the genes). Thus there can be some goals for action that are not in the interests of the genes.

4 The brain mechanisms underlying emotion

4.1 Introduction

Part of the explanation provided in this book of emotions is the way in which emotions are implemented in our brains. What happens in our brains during emotions? What processes taking place in our brains make us have emotions, and behave the way we do? We start with diagrams to show some of the brain regions we will be discussing. Then there is a short summary of the general principles involved in the brain mechanisms underlying emotion.

Given that emotions can be considered as states elicited by reinforcers (Chapter 2), a principled approach to the brain processes involved in emotion is to consider where primary reinforcers are represented in the brain (by neuronal firing) (Section 4.3), where and how potential secondary (learned) reinforcers are represented (Section 4.4), then the brain regions that implement stimulus–reinforcer, i.e. emotional, learning, considering in turn the orbitofrontal cortex (Section 4.5), and amygdala (Section 4.6). Then we consider a brain system involved in learning actions to obtain reward outcomes, the anterior cingulate cortex (Section 4.7). Then we consider other output systems for emotions.

Some of the main brain regions implicated in emotion will now be considered in the light of the introduction given in Chapters 2 and 3 on the nature and functions of emotion. These brain regions include the orbitofrontal cortex, amygdala, cingulate cortex, and basal forebrain areas including the hypothalamus, which are shown in Figs. 4.1 and 4.2. Particular emphasis is placed on investigations of the functions of these regions in primates (usually monkeys and humans), because the ways in which the brain is organized for emotion in rodents is rather different, as described in Section 1.3.2 and more fully elsewhere (Rolls 2014b).

4.2 Overview of brain systems involved in emotion

The way in which recent studies in primates including humans indicate that the neural processing of emotion is organized is as follows (see Fig. 4.2).

1. In Tier 1 (Fig. 4.2), information is processed to a level at which the neurons represent 'what' the stimulus is, independently of the reward or punishment and hence emotional value of the stimulus.
   For example, neurons in the primary taste cortex represent what the taste is, and its intensity; but not its reward value (including how pleasant or unpleasant the taste is).

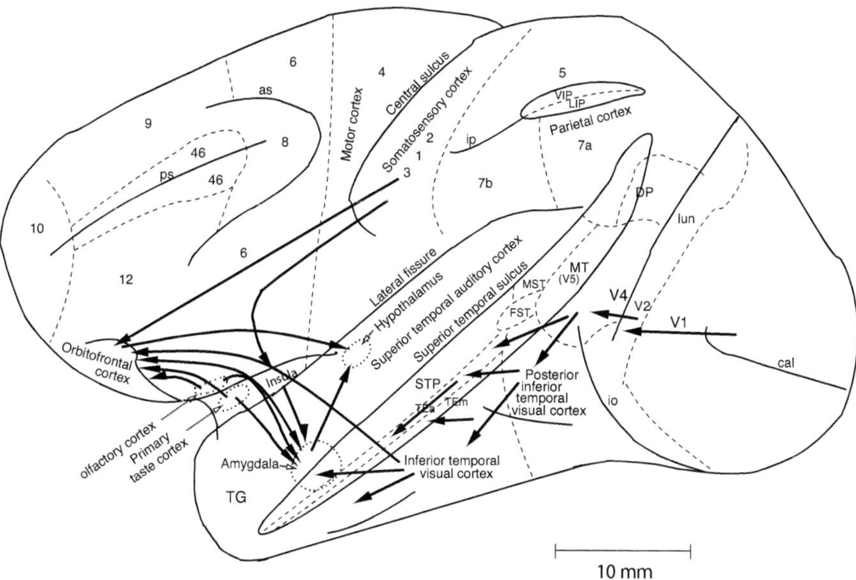

Fig. 4.1 Some of the pathways involved in emotion described in the text are shown on this lateral view of the brain of the macaque monkey. Connections from the primary taste and olfactory cortices to the orbitofrontal cortex and amygdala are shown. Connections are also shown in the 'ventral visual system' from V1 to V2, V4, the inferior temporal visual cortex, etc., with some connections reaching the amygdala and orbitofrontal cortex. In addition, connections from the somatosensory cortical areas 1, 2, and 3 that reach the orbitofrontal cortex directly and via the insular cortex, and that reach the amygdala via the insular cortex, are shown. as, arcuate sulcus; cal, calcarine sulcus; cs, central sulcus; lf, lateral (or Sylvian) fissure; lun, lunate sulcus; ps, principal sulcus; io, inferior occipital sulcus; ip, intraparietal sulcus (which has been opened to reveal some of the areas it contains); sts, superior temporal sulcus (which has been opened to reveal some of the areas it contains). AIT, anterior inferior temporal cortex; FST, visual motion processing area; LIP, lateral intraparietal area; MST, visual motion processing area; MT, visual motion processing area (also called V5); PIT, posterior inferior temporal cortex; STP, superior temporal plane; TA, architectonic area including auditory association cortex; TE, architectonic area including high order visual association cortex, and some of its subareas TEa and TEm; TG, architectonic area in the temporal pole; V1–V4, visual areas V1–V4; VIP, ventral intraparietal area; TEO, architectonic area including posterior visual association cortex. The numerals refer to architectonic areas, and have the following approximate functional equivalence: 1,2,3, somatosensory cortex (posterior to the central sulcus); 4, motor cortex; 5, superior parietal lobule; 7a, inferior parietal lobule, visual part; 7b, inferior parietal lobule, somatosensory part; 6, lateral premotor cortex; 8, frontal eye field; 12, part of orbitofrontal cortex; 46, dorsolateral prefrontal cortex.

In the inferior temporal visual cortex, the representation is of objects and faces, invariantly with respect to the exact position on the retina, size, and even view. Forming invariant representations involves a great deal of cortical computation in the hierarchy of visual cortical areas from the primary visual cortex V1 to the inferior temporal visual cortex (Rolls 2016c, Rolls 2012e). The fundamental advantage of this separation of 'what' processing in Tier 1 from reward value processing in Tier 2 is that any learning in Tier 2 of the value of an object or face seen in one location on the retina, size, and view will generalize to other views etc, because the representation provided by Tier 1 is invariant.

Evidence that there is no such clear separation of 'what' from 'value' representations in rodents, for example in the taste system, is described in Sections

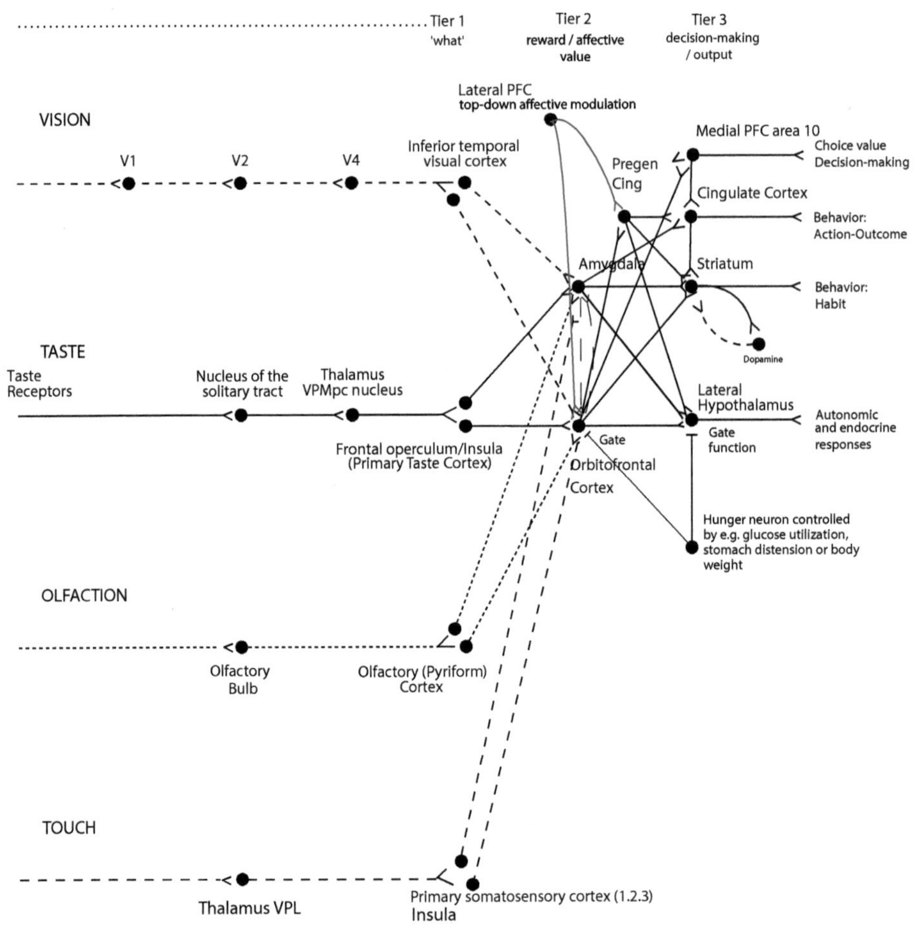

Fig. 4.2 Schematic diagram showing some of the connections of the taste, olfactory, somatosensory, and visual pathways in the brain. V1, primary visual (striate) cortex; V2 and V4, further cortical visual areas. PFC, prefrontal cortex. The Medial PFC area 10 is part of the ventromedial prefrontal cortex (VMPFC). VPL, ventro-postero-lateral nucleus of the thalamus, which conveys somatosensory information to the primary somatosensory cortex (areas 1, 2 and 3). VPMpc, ventro-postero-medial nucleus pars parvocellularis of the thalamus, which conveys taste information to the primary taste cortex. Pregen Cing, pregenual cingulate cortex. For purposes of description, the stages can be described as Tier 1, representing what object is present independently of reward value; Tier 2 in which reward value is represented; and Tier 3 in which decisions between stimuli of different value are taken, and in which value is interfaced to behavioural output systems. A pathway for top-down attentional and cognitive modulation of emotion is shown in red.

1.3.2 and 5.3.1.4, and this property makes the processing in rodents not only different from that in primates including humans, but also much more difficult to analyse.

2. There are brain mechanisms in Tier 2 that are involved in computing the reward value of primary (unlearned) reinforcers. Because reward value is represented in Tier 2, it becomes involved in emotional processing.

The primary reinforcers include taste, touch (both pleasant touch and pain), and to some extent smell, and perhaps certain visual stimuli, such as face expression. There is evidence that there is a representation of the (reward/punishment) value of many primary reinforcers in the orbitofrontal cortex, including taste, positive touch and pain, face expression, face beauty, and auditory consonance/dissonance.

3. Brain regions in Tier 2 are also concerned with learning associations between previously neutral stimuli (such as the sight of objects or of individuals' faces), and primary reinforcers. The representations thus include the 'expected value' of stimuli. An example might be the expected value produced when we see our favourite food being prepared, which may soon lead to the primary reward of the taste of the food.
   These expected value signals in Tier 2 are sent to Tier 3 where they provide the goals for action systems.
   Because reward-related signals are being represented by these expected value neurons, Tier 2 is further involved in emotions.
   These Tier 2 brain regions include the orbitofrontal cortex and amygdala.
4. In the orbitofrontal cortex in Tier 2, the representation is of the value of stimuli, and actions are not represented.
   The value of very many different types of stimuli, events or goals are represented separately at the neuronal level, providing the basis for choice between stimuli, and the selection at later stages of processing of appropriate actions to obtain the chosen goal.
5. Rewards and subjective pleasure tend to be reflected in neural activity in the medial (towards the midline) and middle orbitofrontal cortex, areas BA 13 and 11 (which are shown in Fig. 1.1), as shown in Fig. 4.14.
   Not obtaining rewards, punishers, and subjective unpleasantness tend to be reflected in neural activity in the lateral orbitofrontal cortex, areas BA 12/47 and the adjacent part of the inferior frontal gyrus (which are shown in Fig. 1.1), as shown in Fig. 4.14. It is the lateral orbitofrontal cortex that therefore may be related directly to depression, which can be produced by no longer receiving expected or hoped-for rewards.
6. Whereas the orbitofrontal cortex in Tier 2 represents the value of stimuli (potential goals for action) on a continuous scale, an area anterior to this, medial prefrontal cortex area 10 (sometimes called ventromedial prefrontal cortex, VMPFC) (in Tier 3), is implicated in decision-making between stimuli, in which a selection must be made, moving beyond representation of value on a continuous scale towards a decision between goods based on their value.
7. The brain regions in which the reinforcing, and hence emotional, value of stimuli are represented interface to four main types of output system (Fig. 4.3): The first is the autonomic and endocrine system, for producing such changes as increased heart rate and release of adrenaline (the Greek form is epinephrine), which prepare the body for action.
   The second type of output is to brain systems concerned with performing habit-related responses. Such a brain system is the basal ganglia, which include the striatum (caudate, putamen, and ventral striatum), and globus pallidus and substantia nigra. These are for 'stimulus-response' behaviour, which can occur

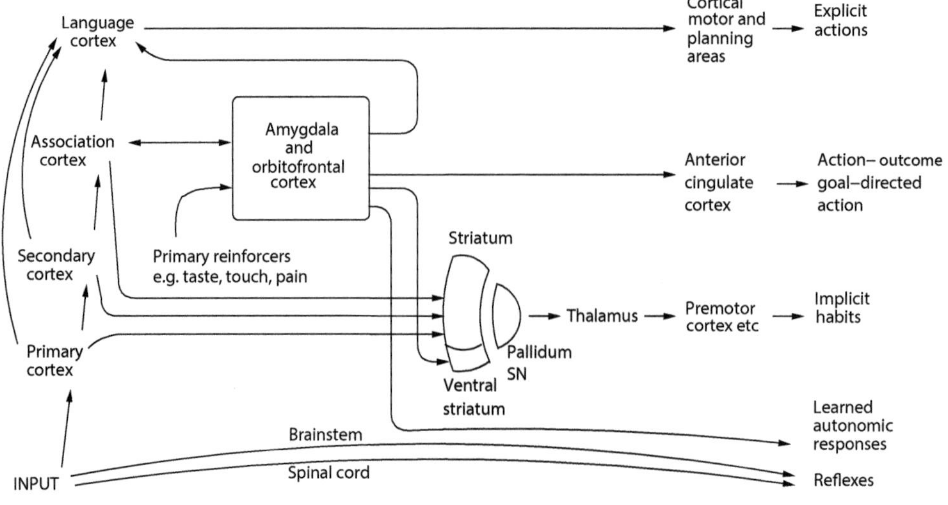

Fig. 4.3 Multiple routes to the initiation of actions and responses to rewarding and punishing stimuli. The inputs from different sensory systems to brain structures such as the orbitofrontal cortex and amygdala allow these brain structures to evaluate the reward- or punishment-related value of incoming stimuli, or of remembered stimuli. One type of route is via the language systems of the brain, which allow explicit (verbalizable) decisions involving multistep syntactic planning to be implemented. The other type of route may be implicit, and includes the anterior cingulate cortex for action–outcome, goal-dependent, learning; and the striatum and rest of the basal ganglia for stimulus–response habits. Pallidum / SN – the globus pallidus and substantia nigra. Outputs for autonomic responses can also be produced using outputs from the orbitofrontal cortex and anterior cingulate cortex (some of which are routed via the ventral, visceral, part of the anterior insular cortex) and amygdala.

when a behaviour has been overlearned, and which may not be associated with much emotion when the behaviour is highly learned and automatic.

The third type of output is to brain systems concerned with performing actions in order to obtain the goals of rewards or of avoiding punishers. These brain systems include the anterior cingulate cortex for action–outcome, that is, goal-directed, learning. (The 'outcome' is the reward or punisher that is or is not obtained when the action is performed.) The learning of the correct action typically occurs by trial and error.

The fourth type of output is to a system capable of planning many steps ahead, and for example deferring short-term rewards in order to execute a multiple-step long-term plan. This system may use syntactic processing to perform the multiple-step planning, and is therefore part of a linguistic system. Such a system can perform explicit (conscious) processing and reasoning, as described more fully in Chapter 10.

4.3 Representations of primary reinforcers, i.e. of unlearned value

Emotions can be produced by primary reinforcers. (Primary reinforcers are unlearned reinforcers, that is they are innately reinforcing.) Other, previously neutral, stimuli, such as the sight of an object, can by association learning with a primary reinforcer come to be a secondary (or learned) reinforcer, which can also produce an emotional response. For these reasons, in order to understand the neural basis of emotion it is necessary to know where in the processing systems in the brain a sensory input comes to be represented in terms of its reward value by neuronal activity, and examples of some of the evidence for primary reinforcers is provided next, with much fuller evidence available elsewhere (Rolls 2014b).

4.3.1 Taste

In primates, the evidence that the representation of taste is independent of its rewarding properties as far as and including the primary taste cortex is described in Chapter 5. In the secondary taste cortex, which is part of the orbitofrontal cortex, the representation is of the food reward value of the taste, in that the taste responses of neurons are modulated by hunger in devaluation experiments, and decrease to zero when the animal is satiated, and the taste is no longer rewarding (see Section 4.5.3.1 and Chapter 5). Water also has reward value when thirsty, and this value representation reflects neural activity in the primate including human orbitofrontal cortex (Rolls 2005, De Araujo, Kringelbach, Rolls & McGlone 2003b, Rolls, Sienkiewicz & Yaxley 1989b, Rolls, Yaxley & Sienkiewicz 1990).

4.3.2 Smell

For olfaction, it is known that some orbitofrontal cortex olfactory neurons respond to the smell of food only when a monkey has an appetite for that food (Critchley & Rolls 1996c), and consistent results have been found in humans with functional neuroimaging (O'Doherty, Rolls, Francis, Bowtell, McGlone, Kobal, Renner & Ahne 2000, Gottfried, O'Doherty & Dolan 2003). The responses of these neurons thus reflect the reward value of these food-related olfactory stimuli.

Consistently, the reward value of odours is represented in the human medial orbitofrontal cortex, in that activation here is correlated with the pleasantness but not intensity ratings of six odours (Rolls, Kringelbach & De Araujo 2003c), and is increased by paying attention to pleasantness but not intensity (Rolls, Grabenhorst, Margot, da Silva & Velazco 2008a). Further, there is evidence in humans that the primary olfactory cortical areas (including the pyriform cortex and cortico-medial amygdala region) represent the identity and intensity of olfactory stimuli but not the reward value, in that in a functional magnetic resonance imaging (fMRI) investigation, activation of these regions was correlated with the subjective intensity ratings but not the subjective pleasantness ratings of six odours (Rolls, Kringelbach & De Araujo 2003c).

In humans there is some evidence that pheromone-like odours can influence behaviour, though probably not through the vomero-nasal olfactory system, which appears to be vestigial in humans (see Section 7.8). In rodents and many mammals (but

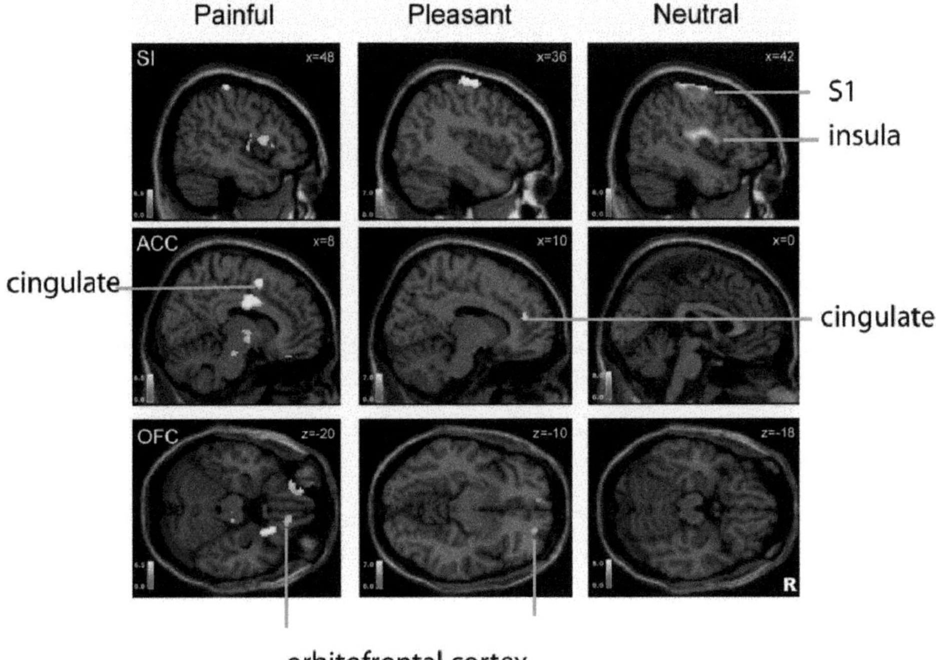

Fig. 4.4 Brain activation to painful, pleasant and neutral touch of the human brain. The top row shows strongest activation of the somatosensory cortex S1/insula by the neutral touch, on sagittal sections (parallel to the midline). The middle row shows activation of the most anterior part of the anterior cingulate cortex by the pleasant touch, and of a more posterior part by the painful touch, on sagittal sections. The bottom row shows activation of the orbitofrontal cortex by the pleasant and by the painful touch, in axial slices (in the horizontal plane). The activations were thresholded at $p<0.0001$ to show the extent of the activations. (This material was originally published in *Cerebral Cortex* 13 (3) Representations of Pleasant and Painful Touch in the Human Orbitofrontal and Cingulate Cortices, pp. 308–17 by E.T. Rolls, J. O'Doherty, M.L. Kringelbach, S. Francis, R. Bowtell and F. McGlone, and has been reproduced by permission of Oxford University Press http://cercor.oxfordjournals.org/content/13/3/308.full.)

not humans and Old World monkeys), signals in an accessory olfactory system which includes the vomeronasal organ and the accessory olfactory bulb could act as primary reinforcers which affect attractiveness and aggression, and act as primary reinforcers (see Section 7.8 and Wyatt (2014)).

4.3.3 Pleasant and painful touch

Experiments have been performed to investigate where in the human touch-processing system (see Figs. 4.1 and 4.2) tactile stimuli are decoded and represented in terms of their rewarding value or the pleasure they produce. In order to investigate this, Rolls, O'Doherty, Kringelbach, Francis, Bowtell & McGlone (2003d) performed functional magnetic resonance imaging (fMRI) of humans who were receiving pleasant, neutral, and painful tactile stimuli. They found that a weak but very pleasant touch of the hand with velvet produced much stronger activation of the orbitofrontal cortex than a more intense but affectively neutral touch of the hand with wood. In contrast, the pleasant stimuli produced much less activation of the primary somatosensory cortex S1 than the neutral stimuli (see Fig. 4.4). It was concluded that part of the orbitofrontal cortex is concerned with representing the positively affective aspects of somatosensory stimuli.

It was also notable that the pleasant touch activated the most anterior (pregenual) part of the anterior cingulate cortex, which receives inputs from the orbitofrontal cortex (see Fig. 4.4). In another study, it was found that pleasant, light, slow, rubbing touch to the forearm, which activates C tactile afferent fibres, produces activation in the human orbitofrontal cortex (McCabe, Rolls, Bilderbeck & McGlone 2008, Rolls 2010c, Rolls 2016a).

Warm touch can be pleasant, and cold touch can be unpleasant. In an fMRI investigation we showed that the mid-orbitofrontal and pregenual cingulate cortex have activations that are correlated with the subjective pleasantness ratings made to warm (41°C) and cold (12°C) stimuli, and combinations of warm and cold stimuli, applied to the hand (Rolls, Grabenhorst & Parris 2008b) (Fig. 4.31 on page 115). Activations in the lateral and some more anterior parts of the orbitofrontal cortex were correlated with the unpleasantness of the stimuli.

Oral texture can also be pleasant and rewarding. For example, the pleasantness of the fat texture of ice cream, and of cream with strawberries, can be pleasant, with the evolutionary foundation that fat is a source of high energy. Neurons in the primate orbitofrontal cortex respond selectively to the slick oily texture of fat, and represent its reward value in that feeding to satiety with cream selectively reduces to zero the neuronal response to fat (Rolls, Critchley, Browning, Hernadi & Lenard 1999a, Verhagen, Rolls & Kadohisa 2003, Rolls 2011e, Rolls, Mills, Norton, Lazidis & Norton 2018c) (see Fig. 5.5). In humans, fMRI investigations show that fat texture is represented in areas such as the taste insula and orbitofrontal cortex (De Araujo & Rolls 2004), and that the subjective pleasantness of oral fat texture reflects activations in the orbitofrontal and anterior cingulate cortex (Grabenhorst, Rolls, Parris & D'Souza 2010b).

The issue of where the reinforcing and affective properties of activation of the pain pathways is decoded is complex (Melzack & Wall 1996, Perl & Kruger 1996, Kobayashi 2012, Brodersen, Wiech, Lomakina, Lin, Buhmann, Bingel, Ploner, Stephan & Tracey 2012, Wiech & Tracey 2013), with some of the evidence as follows.

In the fMRI study of Rolls, O'Doherty, Kringelbach, Francis, Bowtell & McGlone (2003d) painful inputs (produced by a stylus) were also applied to the hand, and we found that the orbitofrontal cortex was more strongly activated by the painful touch than by the neutral touch, whereas the somatosensory cortex was relatively more activated by the physically heavier neutral touch (see Fig. 4.4). This provides evidence that negative as well as positive aspects of affective touch are especially represented in the orbitofrontal cortex. In our study, as in many studies (Vogt & Sikes 2000), a part of the anterior cingulate cortex in or near to the cingulate motor area was also activated by pain (see example in Fig. 4.4 and Section 4.7). Consistent with this, patients with lesions or disconnection of the orbitofrontal cortex may say that they can identify the input as painful, but that it does not produce the same affective feeling as previously (Freeman & Watts 1950, Melzack & Wall 1996). However, the perception of pain is complex, and the literature referred to above addresses some of the complexities.

4.3.4 Visual stimuli

Although most visual stimuli are not primary reinforcers, but may become secondary reinforcers as a result of stimulus–reinforcer association learning, it is possible that some visual stimuli, such as the sight of a beautiful face, of a smiling face, or of an angry face, could be primary reinforcers.

Indeed, we discovered a population of face-selective neurons in the orbitofrontal cortex (Rolls, Critchley, Browning & Inoue 2006) (see Section 4.5.3.4), and some of these neurons by being tuned to face expression could represent the primary reinforcing value of a face. Consistent with this, orbitofrontal and cingulate cortex lesions can impair humans' ability to identify the emotional expression in a face (Hornak, Rolls & Wade 1996, Rolls 1999c, Hornak, Bramham, Rolls, Morris, O'Doherty, Bullock & Polkey 2003) (see Section 4.5.4), and the sight of an angry face expression which signals that behaviour should be changed activates the lateral orbitofrontal cortex (Kringelbach & Rolls 2003).

Further, in humans, it has been found that activation of the orbitofrontal cortex is correlated with the attractiveness of the face being viewed (O'Doherty, Winston, Critchley, Perrett, Burt & Dolan 2003). This may be an example of a visual primary reinforcer being represented in the orbitofrontal cortex. Systems such as this may contribute to aesthetic appreciation (Rolls 2011d, Rolls 2012d, Ishizu & Zeki 2011, Ishizu & Zeki 2013, Rolls 2017a).

It is possible that some auditory stimuli can be primary reinforcers. Where the reinforcement value may be decoded is not yet known, though auditory neurons that respond to vocalization have been found in the orbitofrontal cortex (Rolls, Critchley, Browning & Inoue 2006) and may also be present in the cingulate cortex (Jurgens 2002, West & Larson 1995); and orbitofrontal and cingulate cortex lesions can impair humans' ability to identify the emotional expression in a voice (Hornak, Rolls & Wade 1996, Hornak, Bramham, Rolls, Morris, O'Doherty, Bullock & Polkey 2003) (see Section 4.5.4). Activations in the human orbitofrontal cortex have been related to consonant (pleasant) vs dissonant musical sounds (Blood, Zatorre, Bermudez & Evans 1999, Blood & Zatorre 2001), and to the resolution of harmony towards pleasant stability (Fujisawa & Cook 2011). A possible evolutionary foundation for dissonance being a primary reinforcer is that dissonant sounds may be produced by the non-linear distortion produced by overloaded vocal cords making shouting angry or warning sounds, in contrast to a soft soothing mother's lullaby.

As discussed in Chapter 3 and Section 4.6.6, novel stimuli are somewhat rewarding and in this sense act as primary reinforcers. The value of this type of reinforcer is that it encourages animals to explore new environments in which their genes might produce a fitness advantage. Neurons that respond to visual stimuli that are associated with rewards, and also to novel stimuli, have been discovered in the primate amygdala, and this evidence suggests that these neurons are involved in the primary reinforcing properties of novel stimuli (Wilson & Rolls 1993, Wilson & Rolls 2005). These neurons may provide inputs to the basal forebrain, probably cholinergic, neurons that project this information to the cerebral cortex, and probably influence arousal and synaptic modification to enhance learning when such stimuli are present (Rolls 2014b). We have also discovered that there is a population of neurons in the primate orbitofrontal cortex that responds to novel visual stimuli (Rolls, Browning, Inoue & Hernadi 2005a), and these may perform similar functions. Consistent evidence has been found for humans (Petrides 2007).

Further examples of visual primary reinforcers are given in Section 3.2.1.4 and Table 2.1.

Given that primary reinforcers are represented in the orbitofrontal cortex, and that the rewards and punishers provide the goals for action, we should expect that gene specifications of primary reinforcers such as sweet and bitter taste, pleasant and painful touch, etc. should have a genetically specified set of connections all the way to the orbitofrontal cortex. This needs to arrange that for example sweet taste receptors have a molecular recognition mechanism that ensures that sweet taste receptors end up making connections, after many synapses through the taste system, to the correct neurons in the orbitofrontal cortex that will represent the goals for actions that action systems will try to activate by learning the correct actions to activate the reward-specific orbitofrontal cortex neurons. A start has been made on such tracing that specifies which classes of neurons should connect to which other classes of neurons (Rolls & Stringer 2000) in the olfactory system (Mombaerts 2006).

4.4 Learning associations between stimuli and primary reinforcers: emotion-related learning

Many stimuli, such as the sight of an object, have no intrinsic emotional effect. They are not primary reinforcers. Yet they can come as a result of learning to have emotional significance. This type of learning is called stimulus–reinforcer association, and the association is between the sight of the neutral visual stimulus (the potential secondary reinforcer) and the primary reward or punisher (for example the taste of food, or a painful stimulus). In that the potential secondary reinforcer and the primary reinforcer are both stimuli, stimulus–reinforcer association learning is a type of stimulus–stimulus association learning.

We discovered that this type of learning is implemented in the orbitofrontal cortex. A brief summary of some of the key evidence follows in Section 4.4.1, and is considered in more detail elsewhere (Rolls 2014b, Rolls 2017d). Then in Section 4.4.2, the source of the visual inputs in the temporal lobe cortex is described. It is shown that the reward or emotional value of stimuli is not represented in the temporal cortical visual areas, but that they provide a representation of visual stimuli that is excellently adapted for the emotion-related learning that takes place in the next stages of processing, the orbitofrontal cortex and amygdala.

4.4.1 Emotion-related learning about visual stimuli in the orbitofrontal cortex

We have been able to show that there is a major visual input to many neurons in the orbitofrontal cortex, and that what is represented by these neurons is in many cases the reinforcer (reward or punisher) association of visual stimuli. Many of these neurons reflect the relative preference or reward value of different visual stimuli, in that their responses decrease to zero to the sight of one food on which the monkey is being fed to satiety, but remain unchanged to the sight of other food stimuli. In this sense the visual reinforcement-related neurons predict the reward value that is available from the primary reinforcer, the taste.

The fact that these neurons represent the reinforcer associations of visual stimuli

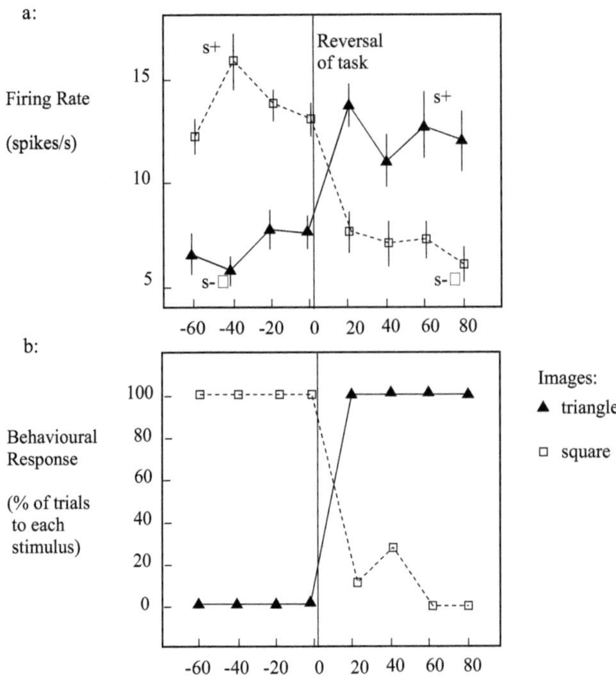

Fig. 4.5 Orbitofrontal cortex: visual discrimination reversal. The activity of an orbitofrontal visual neuron during performance of a visual discrimination task and its reversal. The stimuli were a triangle and a square presented on a video monitor. (a) Each point represents the mean poststimulus activity in a 500 ms period of the neuron based on approximately 10 trials of the different visual stimuli. The standard errors of these responses are shown. After 60 trials of the task the reward associations of the visual stimuli were reversed. s+ indicates that a lick response to that visual stimulus produces fruit juice reward; s– indicates that a lick response to that visual stimulus results in a small drop of aversive tasting saline. This neuron reversed its responses to the visual stimuli following the task reversal. (b) The behavioural response of the monkey to the task. It is shown that the monkey performs well, in that he rapidly learns to lick only to the visual stimulus associated with fruit juice reward. (Reproduced from *Journal of Neurophysiology*, 75 (5), Orbitofrontal cortex neurons: role in olfactory and visual association learning, E. T. Rolls, H. D. Critchley, R. Mason, and E. A. Wakeman, pp. 1970–1981, © 1996, The American Physiological Society.)

and hence the expected value has been shown to be the case in formal investigations of the activity of orbitofrontal cortex visual neurons, which in many cases reverse their responses to visual stimuli when the taste primary reinforcer with which the visual stimulus is associated is reversed by the experimenter (Thorpe, Rolls & Maddison 1983, Rolls, Critchley, Mason & Wakeman 1996a). An example of the responses of an orbitofrontal cortex neuron that reversed the visual stimulus to which it responded during reward-reversal is shown in Fig. 4.5. This reversal by orbitofrontal visual neurons can be very fast, in as little as one trial, that is a few seconds.

These neurons thus reflect the information about which stimulus is currently associated with reward during reversals of visual discrimination tasks – they are reward predicting neurons, that is, they represent *expected value*.

Another way in which it has been shown that the visual neurons in the orbitofrontal cortex reflect the expected value predicted by visual stimuli is by reducing the reward value by feeding to satiety in devaluation experiments. With this sensory-specific satiety (or reward devaluation) paradigm, it has been shown that the visual (as well as the olfactory and taste) responses of orbitofrontal cortex neurons in the macaque decrease to zero as the monkey is fed to satiety with one food, but remain unchanged to another food not eaten in the meal (Critchley & Rolls 1996c) (see example in Fig. 4.6). In that these neurons parallel the changing preference of the monkey for the food being eaten to satiety vs the food not being eaten to satiety, they reflect the relative preference for different visual stimuli, that is the expected value (Thorpe, Rolls & Maddison 1983, Rolls, Critchley, Mason & Wakeman 1996a) (as found also by Tremblay & Schultz (1999) and Wallis & Miller (2003)).

Further evidence that these orbitofrontal cortex neurons encode expected value is that they represent choices made when the 'offers' (the visual stimuli) are different qualities or different amounts of the 'goods' (for example the type of fruit juice that is the reward outcome of the choice, and different probabilities of obtaining reward) (Padoa-Schioppa & Assad 2006, Padoa-Schioppa 2011).

Consistent with these neurophysiological discoveries, damage to the caudal orbitofrontal cortex in the monkey produces emotional changes. These include reduced aggression to humans and to stimuli such as a snake and a doll, a reduced tendency to reject foods such as meat (Butter, Snyder & McDonald 1970, Butter & Snyder 1972, Butter, McDonald & Snyder 1969), and a failure to display the normal preference ranking for different foods (Baylis & Gaffan 1991). The visual discrimination reversal learning deficit shown by monkeys with orbitofrontal cortex damage (Jones & Mishkin 1972, Baylis & Gaffan 1991, Murray & Izquierdo 2007) may be due at least in part to the tendency of these monkeys not to withhold responses to non-rewarded stimuli (Jones & Mishkin 1972) including objects that were previously rewarded during reversal (Rudebeck & Murray 2011), and including foods that are not normally accepted (Butter et al. 1969, Baylis & Gaffan 1991). Consistently, orbitofrontal cortex (but not amygdala lesions) impaired instrumental extinction (in that the behaviour continued even when rewards were no longer available) (Murray & Izquierdo 2007). In a further investigation of possible dissociations, it was found that lesions of areas 11/13 (medial orbitofrontal cortex), disrupted the rapid updating of object value during selective satiation (Rudebeck & Murray 2011). (Selective satiation is a way of measuring reward value that relates to the discovery and much further evidence that reducing the value of a food stimulus by feeding to satiety decreases the responses of orbitofrontal cortex neurons (and activations in humans) selectively to the food with which satiety was produced, providing direct evidence for value representations in the orbitofrontal cortex (Rolls, Sienkiewicz & Yaxley 1989b, Critchley & Rolls 1996a, Kringelbach, O'Doherty, Rolls & Andrews 2003, Rolls & Grabenhorst 2008, Grabenhorst & Rolls 2011).) In relation to neuroeconomics, the estimation of predicted reward value as influenced by reward size, and delay to reward, or both, is impaired by orbitofrontal cortex lesions in macaques (Simmons, Minamimoto, Murray & Richmond 2010). Simpler measures, of emotional responses to an artificial snake, are impaired by both orbitofrontal cortex and amygdala lesions (Murray & Izquierdo 2007).

In the human, euphoria, irresponsibility, lack of affect, and impulsiveness can follow frontal lobe damage (Kolb & Whishaw 2015, Damasio 1994, Eslinger & Damasio 1985), particularly orbitofrontal cortex damage (Rolls, Hornak, Wade & McGrath 1994a, Hornak, Bramham, Rolls, Morris, O'Doherty, Bullock & Polkey 2003, Berlin, Rolls & Kischka 2004, Berlin, Rolls & Iversen 2005). The effects of damage to the orbitofrontal cortex in humans are described further in Section 4.5.4.

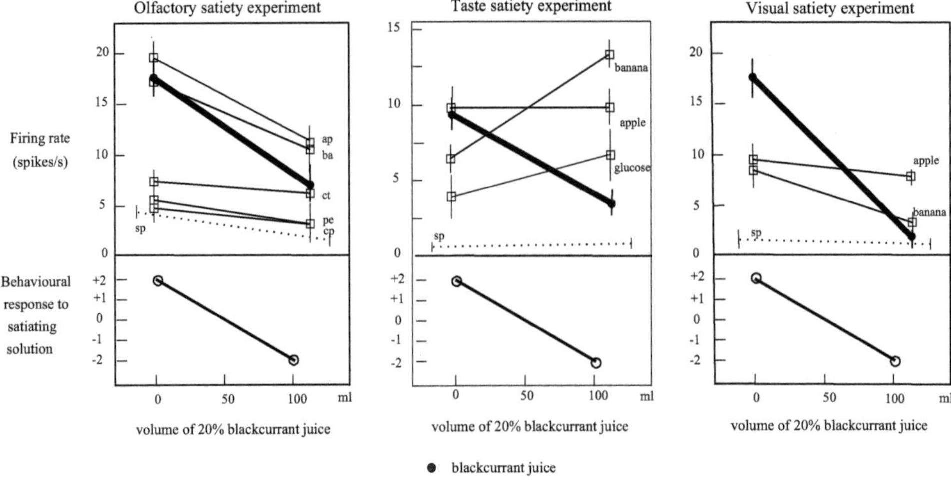

Fig. 4.6 Sensory-specific satiety. Orbitofrontal cortex neuron with visual, olfactory and taste responses, showing the responses before and after feeding to satiety with blackcurrant juice. The solid circles show the responses to blackcurrant juice. The olfactory stimuli included apple (ap), banana (ba), citral (ct), phenylethanol (pe), and caprylic acid (cp). The spontaneous firing rate of the neuron is shown (sp). (Reproduced from *Journal of Neurophysiology*, 75 (4), Hunger and satiety modify the responses of olfactory and visual neurons in the primate orbitofrontal cortex, H. D. Critchley and E. T. Rolls pp. 1673–1886, © 1996, The American Physiological Society.)

Reward reversal learning is also impaired in humans by damage to the orbitofrontal cortex (Rolls et al. 1994a, Hornak et al. 2003, Berlin et al. 2004, Berlin et al. 2005).

All this evidence provides strong support for the theory that the orbitofrontal cortex is a key brain region in emotion, and that part of its role in emotion is to rapidly learn associations between visual stimuli and primary reinforcers, and then to be able to reverse these very quickly when the rewards provided change (Rolls 2014b). This is very important in social as well as most types of emotional behaviour, and further evidence is described in Section 4.5 and elsewhere (Rolls 2014b).

4.4.2 The visual inputs from the temporal lobe cortex to the orbitofrontal cortex and amygdala for emotion-related learning

This reversal learning found in orbitofrontal cortex neurons probably is implemented in the orbitofrontal cortex, for it does not occur one synapse earlier in the visual inferior temporal cortex (IT) (Rolls, Judge & Sanghera 1977, Rolls, Aggelopoulos & Zheng 2003a) which provides the visual inputs to the orbitofrontal cortex. This is shown by the fact the IT neurons do not reverse their responses in a visual discrimination reversal task in which one visual stimulus is associated with reward and the other with punishment, that is, the valence of the stimulus is not represented in primates in the IT cortex nor at any earlier stage of processing (Rolls et al. 1977, Rolls et al. 2003a). (Of course, there could be non-specific effects if a stimulus is associated with reward vs neutral, or for that matter punishment vs neutral, but this is not encoding of valence,

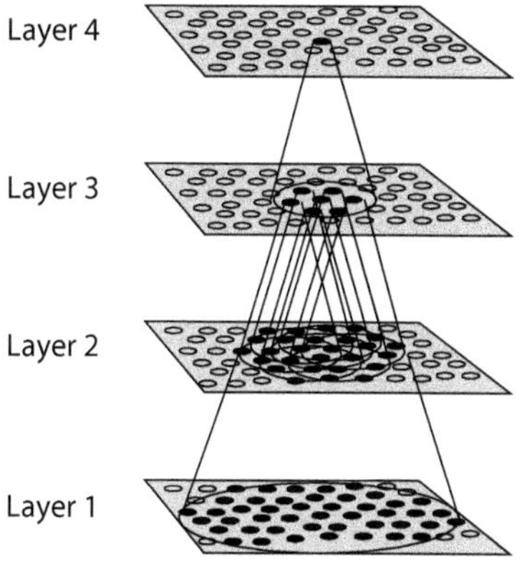

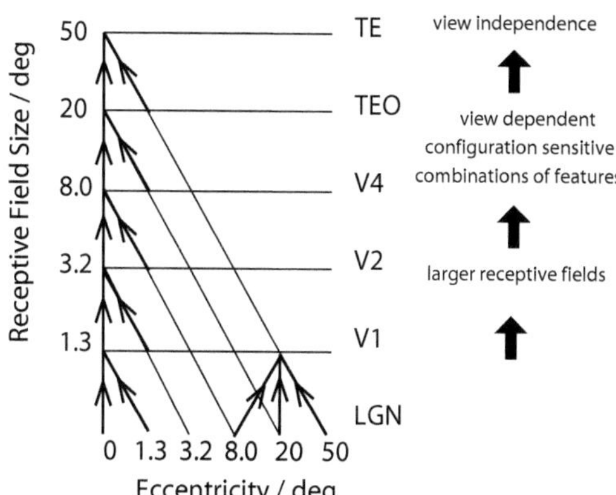

Fig. 4.7 Right. Schematic diagram showing convergence achieved by the forward projections in the visual system, and the types of representation that may be built by competitive networks operating at each stage of the system from the primary visual cortex (V1) to the inferior temporal visual cortex (area TE) (see text). LGN, lateral geniculate nucleus. Area TEO forms the posterior inferior temporal cortex. Left – as implemented in a biologically plausible working model of face and object identification, VisNet (Rolls, 2012). Convergence through the network is designed to provide fourth layer neurons in inferior temporal visual cortex area TE with information from across the entire input retina.

that is of reward vs punishment value, let alone of expected value including the type and amount of reward or punishment expected.) Nor do inferior temporal cortex neurons reflect reward value, in that the neuronal responses to the sight of food are not decreased by feeding to satiety (Rolls et al. 1977).

A great deal has now been discovered about how the visual pathways operate from the primary visual cortex to the inferior temporal cortex, to provide in the inferior temporal visual cortex representations of faces and object that provide the inputs in a very useful form for the emotion visual-to-reinforcer learning systems in the orbitofrontal cortex. As this visual processing provides a foundation for many of the emotion-related functions of the orbitofrontal cortex and amygdala, some of the discoveries are summarized next, with much fuller details, and indeed a complete biologically plausible theory of how this cortical visual system works, available elsewhere (Rolls 2012e, Rolls 2016c).

4.4.2.1 Pathways to the inferior temporal cortex (IT) in the primate visual system

A schematic diagram to indicate some of the pathways involved in object and face identification from the primary visual cortex, V1, through V2 and V4 to the posterior inferior temporal cortex (TEO) and the anterior inferior temporal cortex (TE) is shown in Fig. 4.7 (Rolls 2016c, Blumberg & Kreiman 2010, Orban 2011, Rolls 2011c, Rolls 2012e, Tsao & Livingstone 2008). Their approximate location on the brain of a macaque monkey is shown in Figs. 4.1 and 9.7. Similarly, in humans there are a number of separate visual representations of faces, other body parts, and objects (Spiridon, Fischl & Kanwisher 2006, Weiner & Grill-Spector 2013). An important point is that there is convergence from stage to stage over a four-layer network. This enables neurons in the inferior temporal visual cortex to reflect inputs from even large objects almost anywhere in the visual field, and at the same time enables the number of inputs to each neuron from the preceding stage of processing to be limited to about 10,000 synapses, as elucidated by Rolls (2016c).

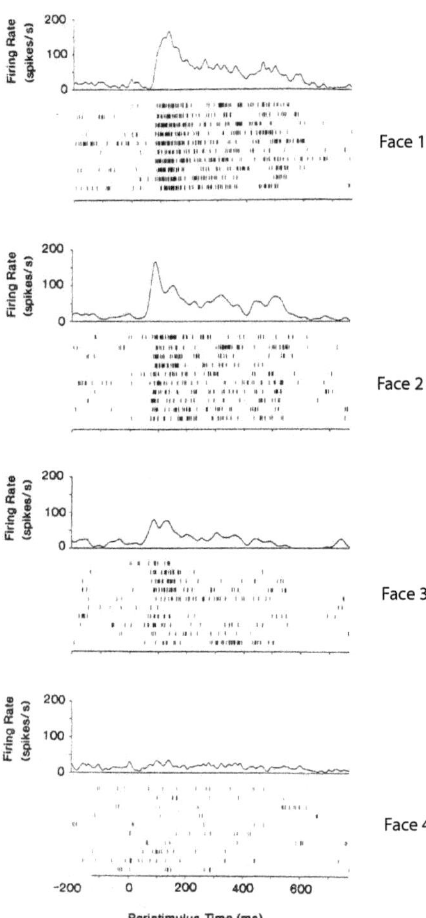

Fig. 4.8 Peristimulus time histograms and rastergrams showing the responses on different trials (originally in random order) of a face-selective neuron in the inferior temporal visual cortex to four different faces. (In the rastergrams each vertical line represents one spike from the neuron, and each row is a separate trial. Each block of the Figure is for a different face. A stimulus was presented at 0 ms for 500 ms on each trial.) (Reproduced from *Journal of Neurophysiology*, 70: 640–654, Information encoding and the responses of single neurons in the primate temporal visual cortex, M. J. Tovee, E. T. Rolls, A. Treves, and R. P. Bellis, doi.org/10.1152/jn.1993.70.2.640 © 1993, The American Physiological Society.)

4.4.2.2 Inferior temporal visual cortex neurons selective for face or object identity

We discovered neurons in the temporal lobe visual cortex that respond to face identity (Perrett, Rolls & Caan 1982, Rolls 2011c). These neurons respond to faces more than they respond to non-face stimuli. These neurons respond to combinations of features in the correct spatial arrangement, as shown, for example, with faces, for which it has been shown by masking out or presenting parts of the face (for example eyes, mouth, or hair) in isolation, or by jumbling the features in faces, that some cells in the cortex in IT/STS respond only if two or more features are present, and are in the correct spatial arrangement (Perrett, Rolls & Caan 1982, Rolls, Tovee, Purcell, Stewart & Azzopardi 1994b, Rolls 2011c).

The encoding scheme is **sparse distributed encoding**, which means that each neuron had a graded set of firing rates to a set of faces, with a few faces producing fast firing (Rolls &

Tovee 1995, Tovee, Rolls, Treves & Bellis 1993, Rolls, Treves, Tovee & Panzeri 1997c, Treves, Panzeri, Rolls, Booth & Wakeman 1999) (see example in Fig. 4.8). The sparseness facilitates **high capacity** in the stimulus-reinforcement association learning system in the orbitofrontal cortex implemented by pattern association (Rolls 2016c). The profiles of the responses of the neurons to a set of stimuli are different for each neuron. This means that the responses of different neurons are almost independent, and that the information available from a population of the neurons increases approximately linearly with the number of neurons (Rolls, Treves & Tovee 1997d). Moreover, much of the information available can be read by taking a weighted sum of the neuronal firing rates that reaches a neuron in for example the orbitofrontal cortex (Rolls et al. 1997d). This is termed dot product decoding, and is neuronally plausible. This beautiful and elegant coding scheme means that a neuron in for example the orbitofrontal cortex that receives the firing of inferior temporal visual cortex neurons can read quickly (in 20 ms) much information from the inferior temporal visual cortex about the identity of the face (Rolls & Treves 2011, Rolls 2016c). Moreover, because of this encoding scheme, and the dot product decoding, the receiving neurons can automatically **generalize** over small variations of the input, enabling correct identification even when the input produced by a particular face may be somewhat different on different occasions (Rolls & Treves 2011, Rolls 2016c). The same coding property provides for **graceful degradation**, i.e. relatively good performance even when the system is damaged by losing inputs to a neuron (Rolls 2016c). This whole body of evidence and theory about the encoding scheme used by neurons in the cortex, and how it is useful for processes such as emotion, is described in detail elsewhere (Rolls & Treves 2011, Rolls 2014b, Rolls 2016c).

These inferior temporal visual cortex face identity neurons are likely to be the major source of the inputs to the face identity selective neurons that we discovered in the orbitofrontal cortex (Rolls et al. 2006). We also discovered face-selective neurons in the amygdala (Leonard, Rolls, Wilson & Baylis 1985, Sanghera, Rolls & Roper-Hall 1979).

Similar neurons in other parts of the IT cortex encode the identity of objects using sparse distributed encoding (Rolls & Treves 2011, Rolls et al. 2003a), and these neurons also provide an important source of object information to the orbitofrontal cortex for visual stimulus to reinforcer association learning.

4.4.2.3 Inferior temporal visual cortex neurons have transform invariant representations

We discovered that IT neurons show many types of transform invariance, that is, the neuronal responses are relatively invariant (change little) if the face or object transforms in the world. This is crucial for what is supplied to the emotion learning system in the orbitofrontal cortex, for if on one occasion we learn an emotional association to for example a face, then we automatically can have the same emotional response if the face looks a little different on another occasion, perhaps because it is seen from a somewhat different view (Rolls 2014b, Rolls 2016c).

The types of invariance that we found include translation (i.e. position of the retina) (Tovee, Rolls & Azzopardi 1994, Rolls et al. 2003a), size (Rolls & Baylis 1986), contrast (Rolls & Baylis 1986), spatial frequency (underlying the ability to recognise a blurred face, or a line drawing of a face) (Rolls, Baylis & Leonard 1985, Rolls, Baylis & Hasselmo 1987), view (Hasselmo, Rolls, Baylis & Nalwa 1989b), and object-based motion (Hasselmo et al. 1989b).

There is also evidence that some neurons in the inferior temporal visual cortex have view-independent responses for objects, and these resulted from self-organizing learning occurring during natural experience of the objects without the need for training with rewards (Booth & Rolls 1998).

Brain design in primates including humans is that invariant object representations must be formed (by the inferior temporal cortex stage of processing) before any reward-related learning should occur (in the orbitofrontal cortex) in order that the correct generalization across transforms can be learned. Any alternative system by which associations are learned before invariant representations have been learned is far more fragile and likely to be disrupted by small variations in the stimulus from occasion to occasion (Rolls 2014b, Rolls 2016c).

We have developed a biologically plausible model of how these invariant representations are formed in the visual pathways leading to the inferior temporal visual cortex, based on a learning rule for synapses that takes into account inputs received over the time course of a second or two, during which objects may transform from one view or transform to another (Rolls 1992b, Wallis & Rolls 1997, Rolls 2012e, Rolls 2016c, Rolls & Webb 2014, Rolls & Mills 2018).

4.4.2.4 The importance of what is at the fovea

The receptive fields of IT neurons are large (70 degrees) if only one object is presented, but shrink to approximately 9 degrees in complex natural scenes (Rolls et al. 2003a). This is related to the greater emphasis given to objects at the fovea when there is competition from other objects in a scene. The advantage for emotion, and for the elicitation of action, is that IT passes on information primarily about what is close to the fovea in complex natural scenes, and this greatly simplifies the interface to emotion and action, because just the one or few objects near the fovea produce responses, so that we can respond to one or a few things, and not to every possible emotion-provoking object in a scene. Moreover, this greatly simplifies the interface to action, in that the goal for the action is where the fovea is pointing. Further, this greatly simplifies the interface to memory, in that we can remember what we have seen in different parts of a whole spatial scene (Rolls & Wirth 2018). The computational utility and basis for this are considered by Trappenberg, Rolls & Stringer (2002), Deco & Rolls (2004), Aggelopoulos & Rolls (2005) and Rolls & Deco (2006), and includes an advantage for what is at the fovea because of the large cortical magnification of the fovea, and shunting interactions between representations weighted by how far they are from the fovea.

4.4.2.5 Face expression neurons

We discovered neurons in the temporal lobe visual cortex in the superior temporal sulcus neurons that respond to face expression (Hasselmo, Rolls & Baylis 1989a). Some of these neurons respond only to moving heads, for example to heads that make social contact, or that break it. Some of these neurons are view-specific, which is important for example in knowing whether someone is looking at you. These IT face expression neurons are likely to be the major source of the inputs to the face expression selective neurons that we discovered in the orbitofrontal cortex (Rolls et al. 2006). The combination of the face identity and face expression information present in the orbitofrontal cortex is essential for providing an appropriate emotional response to a face expression being made by a particular individual (Hasselmo et al. 1989a, Rolls 2014b).

4.5 The orbitofrontal cortex and emotion

4.5.1 Historical background

The prefrontal cortex has for long been implicated in emotion, though it is only relatively recently that there has been a firm scientific foundation for understanding how it functions. Let us look first at some of the background.

4.5.1.1 Phineas Gage

One of the first indications that the prefrontal cortex is involved in emotion came from the remarkable case of Phineas Gage, who was working as a foreman for a railway development in Vermont in the USA (Harlow 1848). In 1848, he was tamping down explosives with a tamping iron when unexpectedly the tamping detonated the explosive. The tamping iron, a long bar like a crowbar approximately 3 ft 7 inches long, shot into the air and passed upwards through the front of Phineas Gage's brain (Damasio, Grabowski, Frank, Galaburda & Damasio 1994). Gage survived but from that time on became a changed person. Formerly he had held responsibility as a foreman, but after the operation he became less reliable, and did not appear to be so concerned about the consequences of his actions. Moreover, in his personal life, he was described as being a changed person ("No longer Gage", short-tempered, capricious and profane). However, these personality and emotional changes took place without other general changes in Phineas Gage's intellectual abilities and intelligence. Hannah and Antonio Damasio and colleagues have reconstructed the site of the brain damage from the fractures found in the skull, and have shown that there would have been considerable damage to the lower (or ventral) part of the frontal cortex, which is where the orbitofrontal cortex is located (Damasio et al. 1994, Damasio 1994)). (It is so-called because it is just above the orbit of the eye.) The case of Phineas Gage suggested that the prefrontal cortex is involved in some way in emotion and personality, and that these functions are dissociable in the brain from many other types of function.

4.5.1.2 Prefrontal leucotomy

Another historical line of evidence implicates the frontal lobes in emotion. During an investigation of the effects of frontal lobe lesions in non-human primates on a short-term spatial memory task, Jacobsen (1936) noted that after the operation one of his animals became calmer and showed less frustration when reward was not given. Hearing of this emotional change, Moniz, a Portuguese neurosurgeon, argued that anxiety, irrational fears, and emotional hyperexcitability in humans might be treated by damage to the frontal lobes. He operated on twenty patients and published an enthusiastic report of his findings (Moniz 1936) (see Fulton (1951)). This rapidly led to the widespread use of this surgical procedure, and more than 20,000 patients were subjected to prefrontal 'lobotomies' (in which a part of the frontal lobe was removed) or 'leucotomies' (in which some of the white matter connections of the frontal lobe were cut) of varying extent during the next 15 years. Although irrational anxiety or emotional outbursts were sometimes controlled, it was not clear that the surgery treated effectively the symptoms for which it was intended, side-effects were often apparent, and the effects were irreversible (Rylander 1948, Valenstein 1974). For these reasons these operations have been essentially discontinued. A lesson is that very careful and full assessment and follow-up of patients should be performed when a new neurosurgical (or any medical) procedure is being developed, before it is ever considered for widespread use. In relation to pain, patients who underwent a frontal lobotomy sometimes reported that after the operation they still had pain but that it no longer bothered them affectively (Freeman & Watts 1950, Melzack & Wall 1996).

4.5.2 Connections of the orbitofrontal cortex

The medial orbitofrontal cortex includes Area 13 caudally, Area 11 anteriorly, and Area 14 medially, and the lateral orbitofrontal cortex includes Area 12 (also known in

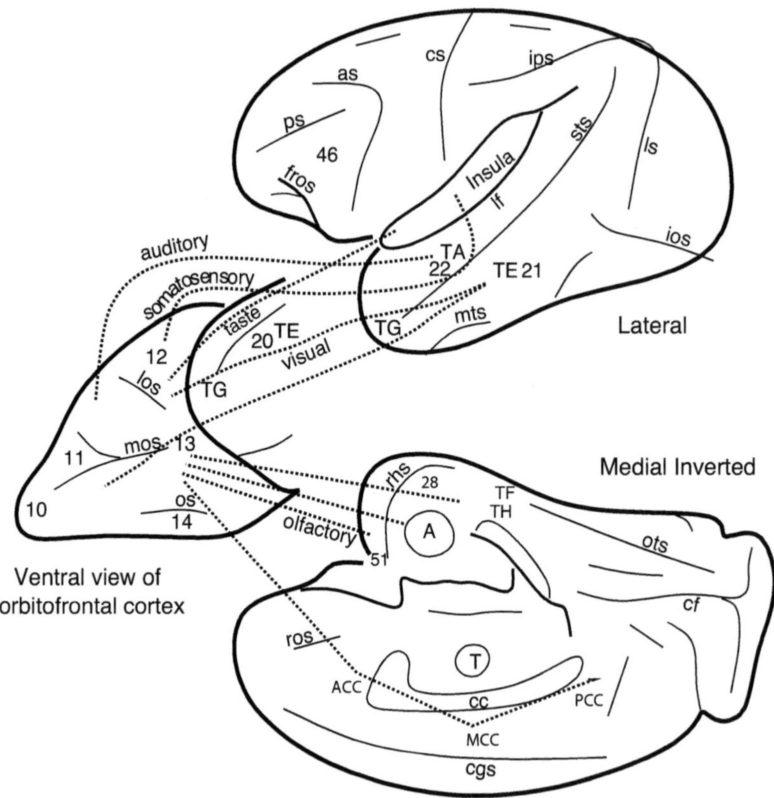

Fig. 4.9 Schematic diagram showing some of the gustatory, olfactory, and visual pathways to the orbitofrontal cortex, and some of the outputs of the orbitofrontal cortex. The secondary taste cortex and the secondary olfactory cortex are within the orbitofrontal cortex. V1, primary visual cortex. V4, visual cortical area V4. Abbreviations: as, arcuate sulcus; cc, corpus callosum; cf, calcarine fissure; cgs, cingulate sulcus; cs, central sulcus; ls, lunate sulcus; ios, inferior occipital sulcus; mos, medial orbital sulcus; os, orbital sulcus; ots, occipito-temporal sulcus; ps, principal sulcus; rhs, rhinal sulcus; sts, superior temporal sulcus; lf, lateral (or Sylvian) fissure (which has been opened to reveal the insula); A, amygdala; ACC, anterior cingulate cortex; INS, insula; MCC, mid-cingulate cortex; PCC, posterior cingulate/retrosplenial cortex; T, thalamus; TE (21), inferior temporal visual cortex; TA (22), superior temporal auditory association cortex; TF and TH, parahippocampal cortex; TG, temporal pole cortex; 12, 13, 11, orbitofrontal cortex; 28, entorhinal cortex; 51, olfactory (prepyriform and periamygdaloid) cortex.

humans as 12/47), as shown in Figs. 1.1 and 4.9. Some of the connections of the orbitofrontal cortex are shown schematically in Figs. 4.9, 4.1, and 4.2. The orbitofrontal cortex receives taste and probably visceral information from the anterior insular cortex; olfactory information from the primary olfactory (pyriform) cortex; somatosensory information from the mid-insula and other somatosensory areas; visual information from the inferior temporal visual cortex (and also the middle temporal gyrus in humans which has cortex which corresponds to some of that in the macaque superior temporal sulcus where there are face expression neurons); and auditory information from the superior temporal cortex. It is thus anatomically in an interesting position, because it receives information from the last processing stages for each sensory modality of 'what' is being represented in each sensory modality. (This is emphasized in Fig. 4.2.) Further, some of these sensory inputs provide information about what are represented as primary reinforcers in the orbitofrontal cortex (taste, pleasant touch, pain), and as secondary (learned) reinforcers (visual, auditory, and olfactory).

Important outputs of the orbitofrontal cortex are directed to the anterior cingulate cortex (for action-outcome learning), to the striatum (for stimulus-response habit learning); to the ventral anterior insula for autonomic output to influence heart rate etc (see Fig. 4.3), and to gateways to hippocampal memory systems in the entorhinal cortex and posterior cingulate cortex (Fig. 9.7).

Rolls, Yaxley & Sienkiewicz (1990) discovered a taste area in the primate orbitofrontal cortex by showing that neurons in it respond to taste placed into the mouth, and showed that this was the secondary taste cortex in that it receives a major projection from the primary taste cortex (Baylis, Rolls & Baylis 1994). More medially, there is an olfactory area (Rolls & Baylis 1994). Anatomically, there are direct connections from the primary olfactory cortex (pyriform cortex), to area 13a of the posterior orbitofrontal cortex, which in turn has onward projections to a middle part of the orbitofrontal cortex (area 11) (Price, Carmichael, Carnes, Clugnet & Kuroda 1991, Morecraft, Geula & Mesulam 1992, Barbas 1993, Carmichael, Clugnet & Price 1994) (see Fig. 4.9). Visual inputs reach the orbitofrontal cortex directly from the inferior temporal visual cortex, the cortex in the superior temporal sulcus, and the temporal pole, especially from areas TEav and the fundus and ventral bank of the superior temporal sulcus (Jones & Powell 1970, Barbas 1988, Barbas 1993, Barbas 1995, Petrides & Pandya 1988, Barbas & Pandya 1989, Seltzer & Pandya 1989, Morecraft et al. 1992, Carmichael & Price 1995b, Saleem, Kondo & Price 2008). There are corresponding auditory inputs (Barbas 1988, Barbas 1993), and somatosensory inputs from somatosensory cortical areas 1, 2 and SII in the frontal and pericentral operculum, and from the dysgranular insula area (Id) (Barbas 1988, Preuss & Goldman-Rakic 1989, Carmichael & Price 1995b, Saleem et al. 2008). The caudal orbitofrontal cortex has strong reciprocal connections with the amygdala (Price et al. 1991, Carmichael & Price 1995a, Barbas 2007).

Further details on the cytoarchitecture and connections of the orbitofrontal cortex including routes via the entorhinal and perirhinal cortex for reward information to reach the hippocampal memory system are available (Ongur & Price 2000, Ongur, Ferry & Price 2003, Price 2006, Barbas 2007, Saleem et al. 2008, Mackey & Petrides 2010, Barbas, Zikopoulos & Timbie 2011, Petrides, Tomaiuolo, Yeterian & Pandya 2012, Yeterian, Pandya, Tomaiuolo & Petrides 2012, Rolls 2014b, Saleem, Miller & Price 2014, Rolls 2017d, Rolls & Wirth 2018).

4.5.3 Neurophysiology and functional neuroimaging of the orbitofrontal cortex

The hypothesis that the orbitofrontal cortex is involved in representing reward value and rapidly updating these representations (Rolls 1999a, Rolls 2014b) has been investigated by making recordings from single neurons in the orbitofrontal cortex while macaques performed tasks known to be impaired by damage to the orbitofrontal cortex. It has been shown that some orbitofrontal cortex neurons respond to primary reinforcers such as taste and touch, and represent **outcome value**; that others respond to learned secondary reinforcers, such as the sight of a rewarded visual stimulus, and thus encode **expected value**; and that the rapid learning of associations between previously neutral visual stimuli and primary reinforcers to encode expected value is

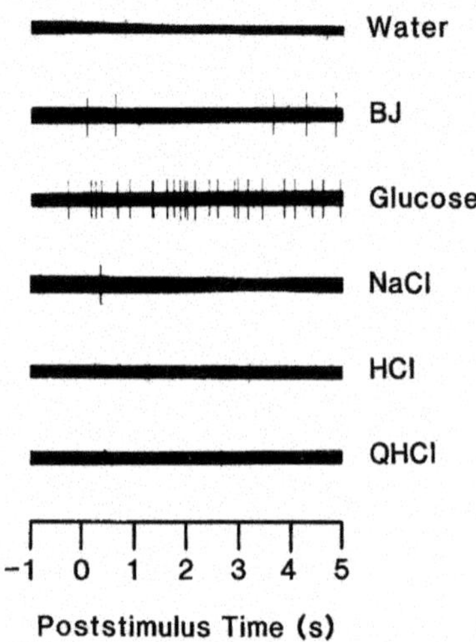

Fig. 4.10 Examples of the responses recorded from one orbitofrontal taste cortex neuron to the six taste stimuli, water, 20% blackcurrant juice (BJ), 1 M glucose, 1 M NaCl, 0.01 M HCl, and 0.001 M quinine HCl (QHCl). The stimuli were placed in the mouth at time 0. Each row is a single trial of a taste. The action potentials of the single neuron are the vertical spikes. (Reproduced from *Journal of Neurophysiology*, 64: 1055–1066, Gustatory responses of single neurons in the caudolateral orbitofrontal cortex of the macaque monkey, E. T. Rolls, S. Yaxley, Z. J. Sienkiewicz, © 1990, The American Physiological Society. doi.org/10.1152/jn.1990.64.4.1055)

reflected in the responses of orbitofrontal cortex neurons in primates. Because these findings are fundamental to understanding the function of the orbitofrontal cortex in emotion, these types of neuron, and extensions of these concepts using functional neuroimaging in humans, are highlighted next, with the fuller evidence described elsewhere (Rolls 2014b, Rolls 2017d).

4.5.3.1 Taste and oral texture: outcome value

One of the discoveries that has helped us to understand the functions of the orbitofrontal cortex in behaviour is that it contains a major cortical representation of taste (see also Chapter 5). Given that taste can act as a primary reinforcer, that is without learning as a reward or punisher, we now have the start for a fundamental understanding of the functions of the orbitofrontal cortex in stimulus–reinforcer association learning. We now know how one class of primary reinforcer reaches and is represented in the orbitofrontal cortex in terms of its value. A representation of primary reinforcers is essential for a system that is involved in learning associations between previously neutral stimuli and primary reinforcers, e.g. between the sight of an object, and its taste.

The most direct and precise evidence that taste is represented in the primate orbitofrontal cortex comes from recording the activity of single neurons in the macaque monkey orbitofrontal cortex (Kadohisa, Rolls & Verhagen 2005b, Rolls 2015c, Rolls 2016e, Rolls 2014b). It has been shown that different single neurons respond differently to the prototypical tastes sweet, salt, bitter, and sour (Rolls, Yaxley & Sienkiewicz 1990), to the 'taste' of water (Rolls, Yaxley & Sienkiewicz 1990), and to the taste of protein or umami (Rolls 2001, Rolls 2009a) as exemplified by monosodium glutamate (Baylis & Rolls 1991) and inosine monophosphate (Rolls, Critchley, Wakeman & Mason 1996b). An example of a single neuron that responds to the taste of glucose is shown in Fig. 4.10. Each neuron typically responds to more than one taste, but each taste can be clearly identified by considering the activity of a population of taste neurons (Rolls, Critchley, Verhagen & Kadohisa 2010a). This is called population encoding, and it has many very useful properties that are described by Rolls & Treves (2011) and Rolls (2016c). In addition, other neurons are tuned to respond best to astringency (which is a flavour characteristic of tea) as exemplified by tannic acid (Critchley & Rolls 1996a). The input in this case comes through the somatosensory (touch) rather than taste pathways, so astringency is a tactile contribution to flavour. The mouth feel of fat (which contributes to the pleasantness of many foods including chocolate and ice cream) also activates a different population of primate orbitofrontal cortex neurons (see Chapter 5) (Rolls et al. 1999a, Verhagen et al. 2003).

The orbitofrontal cortex has been shown anatomically to be the secondary taste cortex, in that it receives connections from the primary taste cortex just behind it in the insular/frontal opercular cortex (see Fig. 4.1) (Baylis, Rolls & Baylis 1994).

There is also evidence from functional neuroimaging that taste can activate the human orbitofrontal cortex. For example, Francis, Rolls, Bowtell, McGlone, O'Doherty, Browning, Clare & Smith (1999) showed that the taste of glucose can activate the human orbitofrontal cortex, and O'Doherty, Rolls, Francis, Bowtell & McGlone (2001b) showed that the taste of glucose and salt activate nearby but separate parts of the human orbitofrontal cortex. De Araujo, Kringelbach, Rolls & Hobden (2003a) showed that umami taste (the taste of protein) as exemplified by monosodium glutamate is represented in the human orbitofrontal cortex as well as in the primary taste cortex as shown by functional magnetic resonance imaging (fMRI). The taste effect of monosodium glutamate (present in e.g. tomato, green vegetables, fish, and human breast milk) was enhanced in an anterior part of the orbitofrontal cortex in particular by combining it with the nucleotide inosine monophosphate (present in e.g. meat and some fish including tuna), and this provides evidence that the activations found in the orbitofrontal cortex are closely related to subjectively reported taste effects (Rolls 2009a, Rolls & Grabenhorst 2008). Small and colleagues have also described activation of the orbitofrontal cortex by taste (Small, Zald, Jones-Gotman, Zatorre, Petrides & Evans 1999, Small, Bender, Veldhuizen, Rudenga, Nachtigal & Felsted 2007).

The nature of the representation of taste in the orbitofrontal cortex is that the reward value of the taste is represented. The evidence for this is that the responses of orbitofrontal cortex taste neurons are modulated by hunger in just the same way as is the reward value or palatability of a taste. In particular, it has been shown that orbitofrontal cortex taste neurons stop responding to the taste of a food with which the monkey is fed to satiety, and that this parallels the decline in the acceptability of the food (see Fig. 4.6) (Rolls et al. 1989b). In contrast, the representation of taste in the primary taste cortex (Scott, Yaxley, Sienkiewicz & Rolls 1986, Yaxley, Rolls & Sienkiewicz 1990) is not modulated by hunger (Rolls, Scott, Sienkiewicz & Yaxley 1988, Yaxley, Rolls & Sienkiewicz 1988). Thus in the primary taste cortex of primates (and at earlier stages of taste processing), the reward value of taste is not represented, and instead the identity of the taste is represented (Scott, Yan & Rolls 1995, Rolls & Scott 2003, Rolls 2015b).

In humans, there is also evidence that the reward value, and, what can be directly reported in humans, the subjective pleasantness, of food is represented in the orbitofrontal cortex. The evidence comes from an fMRI study in which humans rated the pleasantness of the flavour of chocolate milk and tomato juice, and then ate one of these foods to satiety. It was found that the pleasantness of the flavour of the food eaten to satiety decreased, and that this decrease in pleasantness was reflected in decreased activation in the orbitofrontal cortex (Kringelbach, O'Doherty, Rolls & Andrews 2003) (see Fig. 4.11). (This was measured

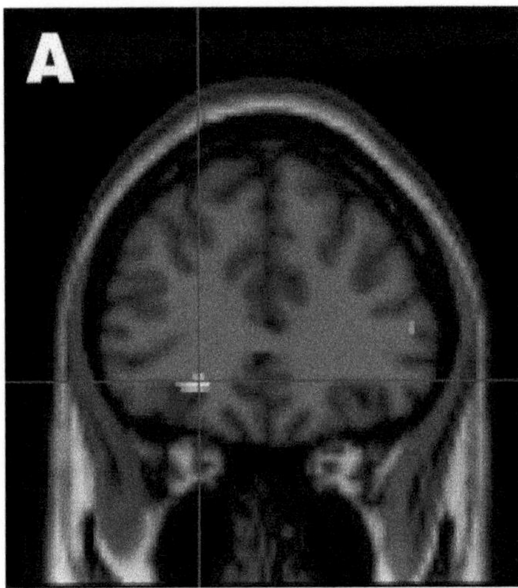

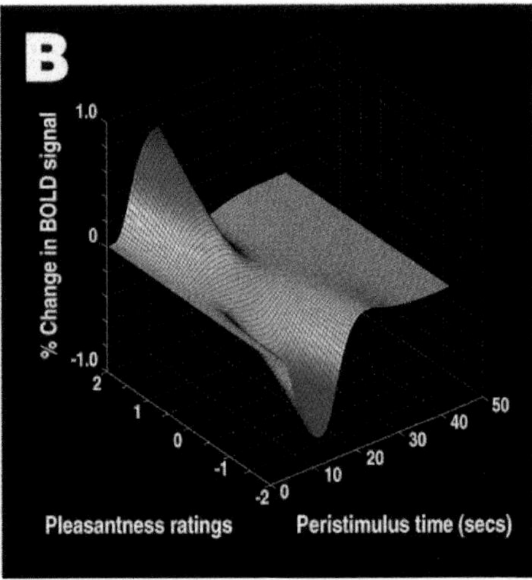

Fig. 4.11 Areas of the human orbitofrontal cortex with activations correlating with pleasantness ratings for food in the mouth. (A) Coronal section through the region of the orbitofrontal cortex from the random effects group analysis showing the peak in the left orbitofrontal cortex (Talairach co-ordinates X,Y,Z=[–22 34 –8], z-score=4.06), in which the BOLD signal in the voxels shown in yellow was significantly correlated with the subjects' subjective pleasantness ratings of the foods throughout an experiment in which the subjects were hungry and found the food pleasant, and were then fed to satiety with the food, after which the pleasantness of the food decreased to neutral or slightly unpleasant. The design was a sensory-specific satiety design, and the pleasantness of the food not eaten in the meal, and the BOLD activation in the orbitofrontal cortex, were not altered by eating the other food to satiety. The two foods were tomato juice and chocolate milk. (B) Plot of the magnitude of the fitted haemodynamic response from a representative single subject against the subjective pleasantness ratings (on a scale from –2 to +2) and peristimulus time in seconds. (This material was originally published in *Cerebral Cortex*, 13 (10) Activation of the Human Orbitofrontal Cortex to a Liquid Food Stimulus is Correlated with its Subjective Pleasantness, pp. 1064–1071 by M.L. Kringelbach, J. O'Doherty, E.T. Rolls, and C. Andrews and has been reproduced by permission of Oxford University Press http://cercor.oxfordjournals.org/content/13/10/1064.full.)

in a functional magnetic resonance imaging (fMRI) investigation in which the activation is measured by the blood oxygenation-level dependent (BOLD) signal, which reflects increased blood flow due to increased neuronal activity (Stephan, Weiskopf, Drysdale, Robinson & Friston 2007, Rolls, Grabenhorst & Franco 2009).) Further evidence that the pleasantness of flavour is represented here is that the flavour of the food not eaten to satiety showed very little decrease, and correspondingly the activation of the orbitofrontal cortex to this food not eaten in the meal showed little decrease. The phenomenon itself is called sensory-specific satiety, is an important property of reward systems, and is described in more detail in Chapter 5.

The experiment of Kringelbach, O'Doherty, Rolls & Andrews (2003) was with a whole food, but further evidence that the pleasantness of taste, or at least a stimulus very closely related to a taste, is represented in the human orbitofrontal cortex is that the orbitofrontal cortex is activated by water in the mouth when thirsty but not when satiated (De Araujo, Kringelbach, Rolls & McGlone 2003b). Thus, the neuroimaging findings with a whole food, and with water when thirsty, provide evidence that the activation to taste *per se* in the human orbitofrontal cortex is related to the subjective pleasantness or affective value of taste and flavour, that is, to *pleasure*. Further evidence on reward value for taste is that in fMRI investigations activations in the human orbitofrontal cortex are linearly related to the subjective pleasantness of the taste (Grabenhorst & Rolls 2008) (Fig. 4.21).

The orbitofrontal cortex also contains neurons that represent oral texture, including viscosity, fat texture, grittiness, capsaicin, and temperature, and some neurons combine this information with taste inputs, to provide a rich representation of **flavour**, as described in Section 5.3.1.2 (Rolls, Critchley, Browning, Hernadi & Lenard 1999a, Verhagen, Rolls & Kadohisa 2003, Rolls, Verhagen & Kadohisa 2003e, Kadohisa, Rolls & Verhagen 2004, Kadohisa, Rolls & Verhagen 2005b, Rolls 2011e). By responding to different combinations of these inputs (e.g. 5.4), and by showing selective effects of reward devaluation by feeding to satiety, these neurons provide evidence about the specific reward outcome value, not about general reward value converted to a common currency, and this is crucial for enabling different actions to be learned to obtain particular goals (outcomes), and for the mechanisms of sensory-specific satiety (Chapter 5).

4.5.3.2 An olfactory as well as a visual representation in the orbitofrontal cortex of expected value

We have seen in Section 4.4.1 that the expected value of visual stimuli is represented in the orbitofrontal cortex. In this section evidence that the expected value of olfactory stimuli is also represented in the orbitofrontal cortex is described. This is likely to be important in many affective states elicited by odours, including the pleasant smell of food (Chapter 5), but also the pleasant smell of perfumes, and even the recollection of pleasant memories from the past that were elicited in Marcel Proust by a madeleine and which triggered him to write *A la Recherche du Temps Perdu*. Some neurons may represent odours that may be primary (unlearned) reinforcers, such as the smell of flowers, which may be elaborated in some perfumes.

Some single neurons in the primate orbitofrontal cortex can respond to odours, and for 35% of the neurons, the odours to which a neuron responded were influenced by the taste (glucose or saline) with which the odour was associated (Critchley & Rolls 1996b). This convergence was built by olfactory to taste association, in that when the taste with which an odour was paired reversed, the olfactory responsiveness changed, and in some cases reversed in a similar way to that illustrated for visual-taste reversal in Fig. 4.5, though more slowly (Rolls, Critchley, Mason & Wakeman 1996a). Moreover, many of these olfactory neurons decreased their firing to zero as the reward value was decreased to zero by feeding to satiety, and indeed showed sensory-specific satiety (Critchley & Rolls 1996c) (e.g. Fig. 4.6). Consistent findings on olfactory sensory-specific satiety (Rolls & Rolls 1997) have been found in humans (O'Doherty et al. 2000, Gottfried et al. 2003). Thus many of these olfactory neurons illustrate the principles of learning to represent expected value by associative learning with a primary reinforcer (taste), and of value representation in the orbitofrontal cortex.

The orbitofrontal cortex is likely to be the first stage of processing in humans at which olfactory responses represent expected (reward) value and subjective pleasantness, as activations in primary olfactory cortical areas such as the pyriform cortex are related to the intensity but not the pleasantness of odours (Rolls, Grabenhorst, Margot, da Silva & Velazco 2008a). (In rodents the encoding may be different, in that an influence of reward-association learning on olfactory neuronal responses in the pyriform cortex (a primary olfactory cortical area) has been reported (Schoenbaum & Eichenbaum 1995)). In contrast to rodents, the fact that humans can still report accurately the intensity of an odour even when its reward value and pleasantness as influenced by feeding to satiety are decreased to zero (Rolls & Rolls 1997) provides evidence that modulation of processing to reflect reward value is not a general property of olfactory processing implemented at early stages in primates including humans, as described in Chapter 5 (Section 5.3.3).

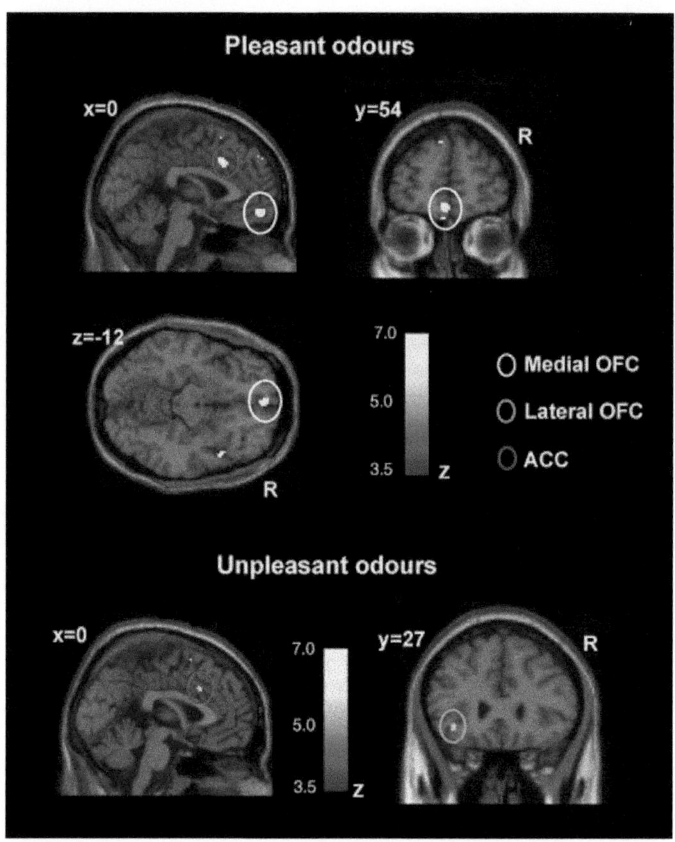

Fig. 4.12 The representation of pleasant and unpleasant odours in the human brain. Above : Group conjunction results for the 3 pleasant odours. Sagittal, horizontal and coronal views are shown at the levels indicated, all including the same activation in the medial orbitofrontal cortex, OFC [0 54 –12] z=5.23). Also shown is activation for the 3 pleasant odours in the anterior cingulate cortex, ACC [2 20 32] z=5.44). These activations were significant at $p<0.05$ fully corrected for multiple comparisons. Below : Group conjunction results for the 3 unpleasant odours. The sagittal view (left) shows an activated region of the anterior cingulate cortex [0 18 36] z=4.42, $p<0.05$, svc). The coronal view (right) shows an activated region of the lateral orbitofrontal cortex [–36 27 –8] z=4.23, $p<0.05$ svc). All the activations were thresholded at $p<0.00001$ to show the extent of the activations. (Reproduced from Edmund T. Rolls, Morten L. Kringelbach, and Ivan E. T. De Araujo, Different representations of pleasant and unpleasant odours in the human brain, *European Journal of Neuroscience*, 18 (3) pp. 695–703, doi.org/10.1046/j.1460-9568.2003.02779.x Copyright © 2003, John Wiley and Sons.)

In humans, pleasant odours are represented in the medial orbitofrontal cortex in that 3 pleasant odours (linalyl acetate [floral, sweet], geranyl acetate [floral], and alpha-ionone [woody, slightly food-related]) had overlapping activations in the medial orbitofrontal cortex. Three unpleasant odours (hexanoic acid, octanol, and isovaleric acid) activated the lateral orbitofrontal cortex (Rolls, Kringelbach & De Araujo 2003c) (see Fig. 4.12). Moreover, activation of the medial orbitofrontal cortex was correlated with the subjective pleasantness ratings of the odours, and activation of the lateral orbitofrontal cortex with the subjective unpleasantness ratings of the odours (Rolls, Kringelbach & De Araujo 2003c). Other studies have also shown activation of the human orbitofrontal cortex by odour (Zatorre, Jones-Gotman, Evans & Meyer 1992, Zatorre, Jones-Gotman & Rouby 2000, Royet, Zald, Versace, Costes, Lavenne, Koenig, Gervais, Routtenberg, Gardner & Huang 2000, Anderson, Christoff,

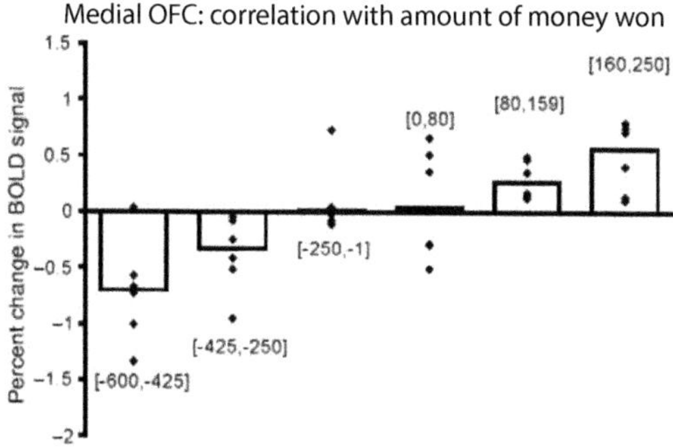

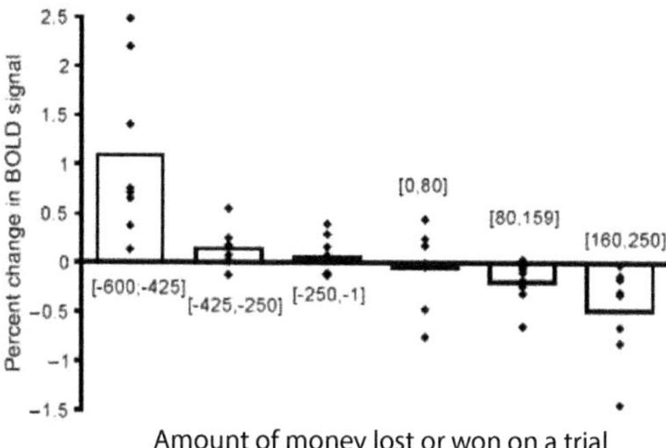

Fig. 4.13 Correlation of brain activations in the medial orbitofrontal cortex with the amount of money won (above), and in the lateral orbitofrontal cortex with the amount of money lost (below). The activations were measured in humans in a visual discrimination reversal task with probabilistic monetary reward and loss. The mean percent change in the BOLD signal from baseline across subjects for 6 different category ranges of monetary loss (negative values) or gain (positive values) shown along the abscissa. The signal was averaged across a category range within each subject and then the average signal change from each category was averaged across subjects. This is plotted for voxels in the medial OFC that significantly correlated with reward (monetary gain) and for voxels in the lateral OFC that significantly correlated with punishment (monetary loss). (Modified from *Nature Neuroscience*, 4 (1), J. O'Doherty, M. L. Kringelbach, E. T. Rolls, J. Hornak, and C. Andrews, Abstract reward and punishment representations in the human orbitofrontal cortex, pp. 95–102, Figure 4b, doi: 10.1038/82959 © 2001, Springer Nature.)

Stappen, Panitz, Ghahremani, Glover, Gabrieli & Sobel 2003, Grabenhorst, Rolls, Margot, da Silva & Velazco 2007, Rolls, Grabenhorst, Margot, da Silva & Velazco 2008a).

4.5.3.3 Representations of many types of reward and punisher in the orbitofrontal cortex, including monetary reward

When we extended our investigations of reward systems in the brain to human neuroimaging, one of the first studies we performed was on monetary reward and loss. We discovered that monetary reward is represented in the human medial orbitofrontal cortex, and monetary loss in the lateral orbitofrontal cortex. In addition, we show that many different rewards are represented in the medial orbitofrontal cortex, where activations are linearly correlated with subjective pleasantness; and that many different punishers and non-reward are represented in the lateral orbitofrontal cortex, where activations are correlated with the subjective unpleasantness of stimuli. Single neuron studies described in more detail in Chapter 5 show that different neurons represent different types of reward, so that there is no common currency, but there is a common scale of reward value, which facilitates decision-making. The area of monetary reward and loss, and the factors that affect the value of a good, has now developed into the field of neuroeconomics (Glimcher & Fehr 2013, Rolls 2014b).

In humans, it has been possible to extend the types of visual conditioned reinforcers represented in the orbitofrontal cortex to quite abstract reinforcers such as monetary reward. In an fMRI study, O'Doherty, Kringelbach, Rolls, Hornak & Andrews (2001a) used a visual discrimination task in which one stimulus was associated with monetary reward, and a different visual stimulus with monetary loss (punishment). The actual amounts of money won on reward trials and lost on punishment trials were probabilistic. This part of the design, and the fact that unexpected visual discrimination reversals occurred so that there were trials on which money was lost, enabled us to show that the magnitude of the activation of the medial orbitofrontal cortex (measured by the BOLD signal) was correlated with the amount of money won on each trial, and the magnitude of the activation of the lateral orbitofrontal cortex was correlated with the amount of money lost on each trial, as shown in Fig. 4.13.

Consistent with the finding of outcome value and expected value neurons in the same parts of the primate orbitofrontal cortex, the monetary outcome value and the expected monetary value produced activations on the same scale and in the same part of the medial orbitofrontal cortex in humans, when the probability of obtaining the reward was varied to signal different expected values (Rolls, McCabe & Redoute 2008e). The effects on expected value and on decision-making of the probability of obtaining a reward, the delay before the reward will become available, the trade-offs made between rewards of different value, etc, have developed into the field of neuroeconomics (Glimcher & Fehr 2013, Rolls 2014b).

Many different types of reward are represented in the medial orbitofrontal cortex, and many types of punisher and non-reward in the lateral orbitofrontal cortex (Kringelbach & Rolls 2004, Rolls & Grabenhorst 2008, Grabenhorst & Rolls 2011, Rolls 2014b). These include pleasant, painful and neutral somatosensory stimulation (Rolls et al. 2003d, McCabe et al. 2008, Rolls et al. 2008b); pleasant vs unpleasant odours (Rolls et al. 2003c, Grabenhorst et al. 2007, Rolls et al. 2008a); pleasant flavours (Kringelbach, O'Doherty, Rolls & Andrews 2003, McCabe & Rolls 2007, Rolls & McCabe 2007, Grabenhorst, Rolls & Bilderbeck 2008a, Grabenhorst & Rolls 2008); face attractiveness (O'Doherty et al. 2003); non-reward, on trials on which an expected reward was not obtained; monetary reward vs loss as described above (O'Doherty, Kringelbach, Rolls, Hornak & Andrews 2001a, Rolls, McCabe & Redoute 2008e); not obtaining an expected social reward in a visual discrimination reversal task (Kringelbach & Rolls 2003) (Fig. 4.18); and conditioned stimuli associated with drug self-administration in addicts (Childress, Mozley, McElgin, Fitzgerald, Reivich & O'Brien 1999), and also the administration of amphetamine to drug-naive human subjects (Voellm, De Araujo, Cowen, Rolls, Kringelbach, Smith, Jezzard, Heal & Matthews 2004).

Very interestingly, at sites where positive value, produced by a reward, is represented, there is often an almost linear relation with the subjective emotional state measured by the subjective pleasantness or unpleasantness rating provided on each trial. Fig. 4.14 shows the peaks of the correlations found in many different investigations related to these subjective states of pleasantness (yellow) and of unpleasantness (white) for both the orbitofrontal and the cingulate and ventromedial prefrontal cortices (see also Section 4.7) (Grabenhorst & Rolls 2011). The activations related to pleasantness tend to be found in the medial orbitofrontal cortex and pregenual anterior cingulate cortex; and the activations related to unpleasantness

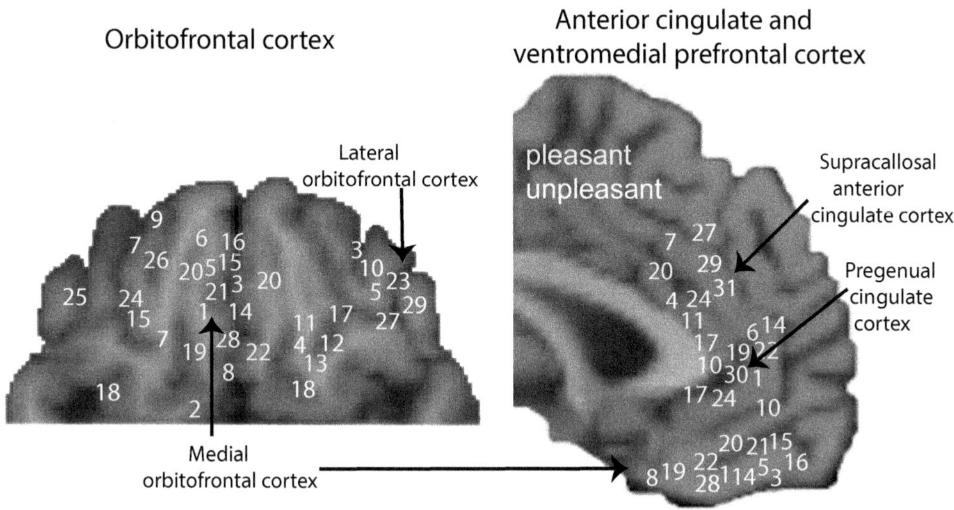

Fig. 4.14 Maps of subjective pleasure in the human orbitofrontal cortex (ventral view) and anterior cingulate and ventromedial prefrontal cortex (sagittal view). Yellow: sites where activations correlate with subjective pleasantness. White: sites where activations correlate with subjective unpleasantness. The numbers refer to effects found in specific studies. Taste: 1, 2; odor: 3-10; flavor: 11-16; oral texture: 17, 18; chocolate: 19; water: 20; wine: 21; oral temperature: 22, 23; somatosensory temperature: 24, 25; the sight of touch: 26, 27; facial attractiveness: 28, 29; erotic pictures: 30; laser-induced pain: 31. (Reprinted from *Trends in Cognitive Sciences*, 15 (2), Fabian Grabenhorst and Edmund T. Rolls, Value, pleasure and choice in the ventral prefrontal cortex, pp. 56–67, doi.org/10.1016/j.tics.2010.12.004. Copyright © 2011 Elsevier Ltd. All rights reserved.)

or non-reward in the lateral orbitofrontal cortex and supracallosal cingulate cortex.

The neuronal recording studies in macaques show clearly that there is an exquisite representation of the detailed properties of these different stimuli, with different neurons by virtue of their different tuning to each of these properties and to combinations of these properties providing information about all the individual properties of each particular stimulus. For example, as a population, different orbitofrontal cortex neurons in macaques have different responses to the following properties of oral stimuli, with some neurons encoding each property independently, and others responding to different combinations of them: taste, fat texture, viscosity, astringency, grittiness, capsaicin content, odour, and sight (see above and Chapter 5).

So why are so many of these different types of specific reward represented in the same medial part of the orbitofrontal cortex? I suggest that part of the functional utility of this is that there can be comparison of the magnitudes of what may be quite different types of reward, implemented by the local lateral inhibition mediated via the inhibitory interneurons. This may also help in setting up different rewards to be on the same scale (Rolls 2014b).

4.5.3.4 A representation of faces in the orbitofrontal cortex

Another type of information represented in the orbitofrontal cortex is information about faces. Some of the orbitofrontal cortex face-selective neurons first described by Thorpe, Rolls & Maddison (1983), then by Rolls et al. (2006), respond to face identity, with different responses to different faces as is evident in Fig. 4.15, and others

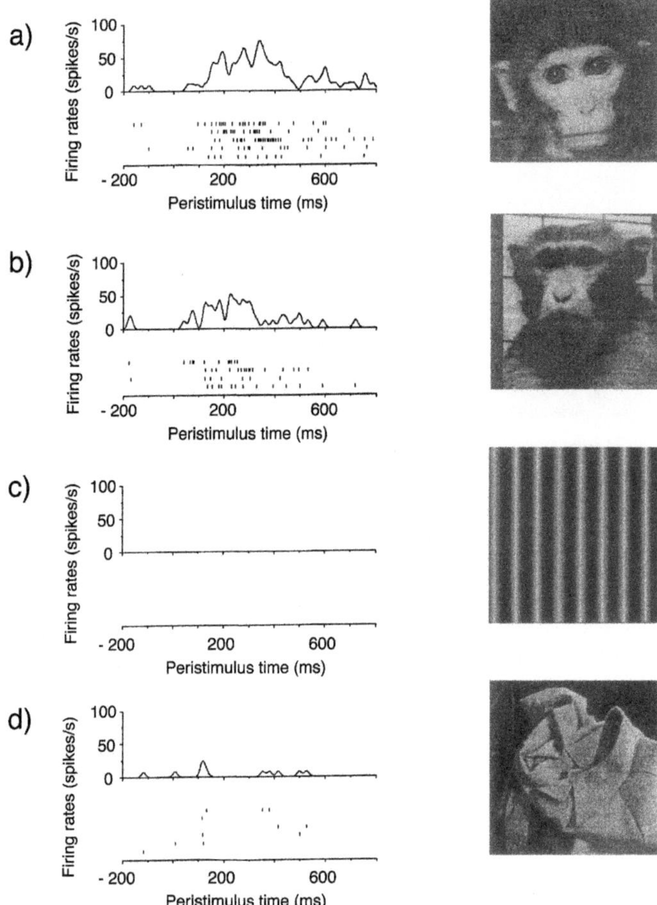

Fig. 4.15 Orbitofrontal cortex face-selective neuron as found in macaques. Peristimulus rastergrams and time histograms are shown. Each trial is a row in the rastergram. Several trials for each stimulus are shown. The ordinate is in spikes/s. The neuron responded best to face (a), also responded, though less to face (b), had different responses to other faces (not shown), and did not respond to non-face stimuli (e.g. (c) and (d)). The stimulus appeared at time 0 on a video monitor. (Reproduced from *Experimental Brain Research*, 170: 743–787. Edmund T. Rolls, Hugo D. Critchley, Andrew S. Browning, and Kazuo Inoue. Face-selective and auditory neurons in the primate orbitofrontal cortex. doi.org/10.1007/s00221-005-0191-y. Springer Verlag 2006.)

respond to face expression. Some also respond only to moving heads, for example when a face moves to break social contact Rolls et al. (2006). The significance of the neurons is likely to be related to the fact that faces convey information that is important in emotion and social behaviour, by encoding information about which individual is present, and what their face expression is, both of which are needed to have the correct emotion or social response (Rolls et al. 2006, Rolls 2011c). Other neurons in the primate orbitofrontal cortex are tuned to vocalization, which is also important in social communication (Rolls et al. 2006).

Consistent with these findings in macaques, and as described above, in humans, activation of the lateral orbitofrontal cortex occurs when a rewarding smile expression is expected, but an angry face expression is obtained, in a visual discrimination reversal task (Kringelbach & Rolls 2003). This is an example of the operation of a social reinforcer, and, consistent with these results, Farrow, Zheng, Wilkinson, Spence, Deakin, Tarrier, Griffiths & Woodruff (2001) have found that activation of the orbitofrontal cortex is found when humans are making social judgements. In addition, activation of the medial orbitofrontal cortex is correlated with face attractiveness (O'Doherty et al. 2003). Further, as described in Section 4.5.4, we have shown that humans with orbitofrontal damage are impaired at decoding the emotional expression of faces and vocalizations.

Auditory stimuli may have similar representations in the human orbitofrontal cortex related to their affective value. For example, Blood et al. (1999) found a correlation between subjective ratings of dissonance and consonance of musical chords and the activations produced in the orbitofrontal cortex (see also Blood & Zatorre (2001) and Frey, Kostopoulos & Petrides (2000)). The transition of harmony towards a pleasant resolution also activates the orbitofrontal cortex (Fujisawa & Cook 2011).

4.5.3.5 Non-reward, error, neurons in the orbitofrontal cortex

Some neurons in the orbitofrontal cortex respond when an expected reward is not obtained. They may fire for several seconds when an error is made resulting in no reward. Many of these neurons respond if a reward such as a food stops approaching, or is moved away. These error neurons are related to correcting the expected value of a stimulus, and not to correcting actions, for actions are not represented in the orbitofrontal cortex. In humans, activations occur in the lateral orbitofrontal cortex if an expected reward such as a smiling face is not obtained, indicating that the face is no longer rewarding, and that choices should change to another stimulus or face. These neurons are likely to be important in the emotions including sadness and the altered choices that are produced by non-reward, for both are impaired by damage to the orbitofrontal cortex. The theory is developed in Chapter 9 that oversensitivity of this non-reward system may contribute to depression.

Some neurons (3.5%) in the orbitofrontal cortex detect different types of non-reward, i.e. negative reward prediction error, when the reward outcome value is less than the expected value (Thorpe, Rolls & Maddison 1983). For example, some neurons responded in extinction, immediately after a lick had been made to a visual stimulus that had previously been associated with fruit juice reward, but no juice reward was obtained. Other neurons responded in a reversal task, immediately after the monkey had responded to the previously rewarded visual stimulus, but had obtained the punisher of salt taste rather than fruit juice reward (see example in Fig. 4.16). Other neurons respond to the removal of a formerly approaching taste reward. Some of these neurons respond for several seconds after non-reward, as illustrated in Fig. 4.16.

The finding that different non-reward neurons respond to different types of non-reward potentially enables context-specific extinction or reversal to occur. Thus the error neurons can be specific to different tasks, and this could provide a mechanism for reversal in one task to be implemented, while at the same time not reversing behaviour in another task (Rolls & Grabenhorst 2008). Also, it provides evidence that these neurons did not respond simply as a function of arousal, or just in relation to a general frustrative non-reward/error signal.

The existence of neurons in the macaque orbitofrontal cortex that respond to non-reward (Thorpe, Rolls & Maddison 1983) (originally described by Thorpe, Maddison & Rolls (1979) and Rolls (1981a)) is confirmed by recordings that revealed 10 such non-reward neurons (of 140 recorded, or approximately 7%) found in delayed match to sample and delayed response

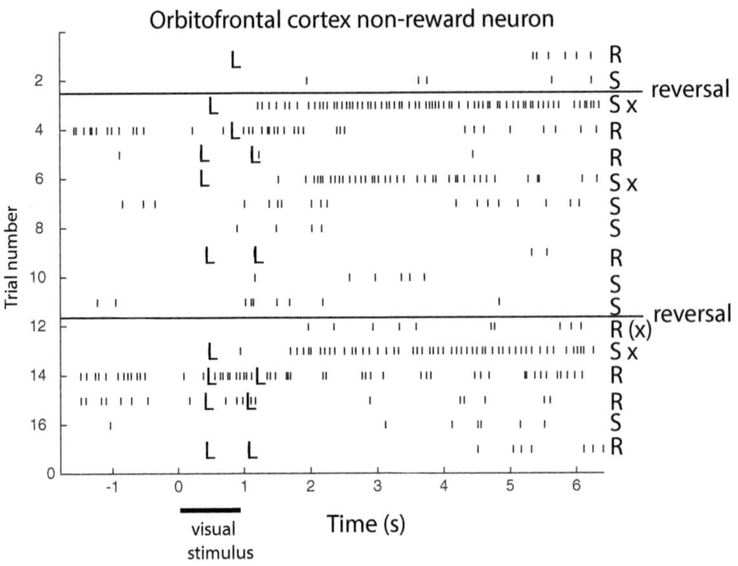

Fig. 4.16 Error neuron: Responses of an orbitofrontal cortex neuron that responded only when the monkey licked to a visual stimulus during reversal, expecting to obtain fruit juice reward, but actually obtained the taste of aversive saline because it was the first trial of reversal (trials 3, 6, and 13, where each trial is a separate row). Each vertical line represents an action potential; each L indicates a lick response in the Go–NoGo visual discrimination task. The visual stimulus was shown at time 0 for 1 s. The neuron did not respond on most reward (R) or saline (S) trials, but did respond on the trials marked Sx, which were the first or second trials after a reversal of the visual discrimination on which the monkey licked to obtain reward, but actually obtained saline because the task had been reversed. The two times at which the reward contingencies were reversed are indicated. After responding to non-reward, when the expected reward was not obtained, the neuron fired for many seconds, and was sometimes still firing at the start of the next trial. It is notable that after an expected reward was not obtained due to a reversal contingency being applied, on the very next trial the macaque selected the previously non-rewarded stimulus. This shows that rapid reversal can be performed by a non-associative process, and must be rule-based. (Data from *Experimental Brain Research*, 49: 93–115, The orbitofrontal cortex: Neuronal activity in the behaving monkey, S. J. Thorpe, E. T. Rolls, and S. Maddison 1983.)

tasks by Joaquin Fuster and colleagues (Rosenkilde, Bauer & Fuster 1981).

The presence of these orbitofrontal cortex non-reward or negative reward prediction error neurons is fully consistent with the hypothesis that they are part of the mechanism by which the orbitofrontal cortex enables very rapid reversal of behaviour by stimulus–reinforcer association relearning when the association of stimuli with reinforcers is altered or reversed (Rolls 1990a, Rolls 2014b, Rolls 2017d). This information appears to be necessary for primates to rapidly alter behavioural responses when reinforcement contingencies are changed, as shown by the effects of damage to the orbitofrontal cortex.

To the extent that the firing of some dopamine neurons may reflect error signals (Waelti, Dickinson & Schultz 2001) (see Section 6.2.5), one might ask where the error information comes from, given that the dopamine neurons themselves may not receive information about expected rewards (e.g. a visual stimulus associated with the sight of food), reward outcomes (e.g. taste), and would not be able to compute an error from these signals. On the other hand, the orbitofrontal cortex does have all three types of neuron and the required neuroanatomically

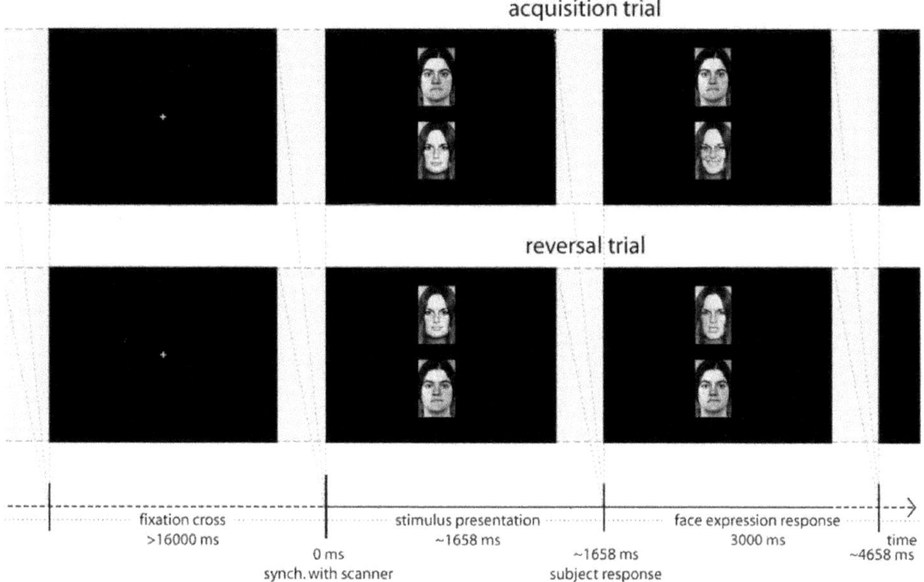

Fig. 4.17 Social reversal task: The trial starts synchronized with the scanner and two people with neutral face expressions are presented to the subject. The subject has to select one of the people by pressing the corresponding button, and the person will then either smile or show an angry face expression for 3000 ms depending on the current mood of the person. The task for the subject is to keep track of the mood of each person and choose the 'happy' person as much as possible (upper row). Over time (after between 4 and 8 correct trials) this will change so that the 'happy' person becomes 'angry' and vice versa, and the subject has to learn to adapt her choices accordingly (bottom row). Randomly intermixed trials with either two men, or two women, were used to control for possible gender and identification effects, and a fixation cross was presented between trials for at least 16000 ms. (Reprinted from *Neuroimage* 20 (2), Morten L. Kringelbach and Edmund T. Rolls, Neural correlates of rapid reversal learning in a simple model of human social interaction, pp. 1371–83. Copyright © 2003 Elsevier Inc. All rights reserved.)

defined inputs, and this is an important site in the brain for computing reward error signals. Pathways via brain regions such as the ventral striatum and habenula by which the reward-related and error information computed in the orbitofrontal cortex could reach and influence brainstem dopamine and serotonin neurons are described in Section 9.7.1 (Rolls 2017b) (Fig. 9.14 on page 9.14).

We have also been able to obtain evidence that non-reward used as a signal to reverse behavioural choice is represented in the human orbitofrontal cortex. Kringelbach & Rolls (2003) used the faces of two different people, and if one face was selected then that face smiled, and if the other was selected, the face showed an angry expression. After good performance was acquired, there were repeated reversals of the visual discrimination task (see Fig. 4.17). Kringelbach & Rolls (2003) found that activation of a lateral part of the orbitofrontal cortex in the fMRI study was produced on the error trials, that is when the human chose a face, and did not obtain the expected reward (see Fig. 4.18). Control tasks showed that the response was related to the error, and the mismatch between what was expected and what was obtained, in that just showing an angry face expression did not selectively activate this part

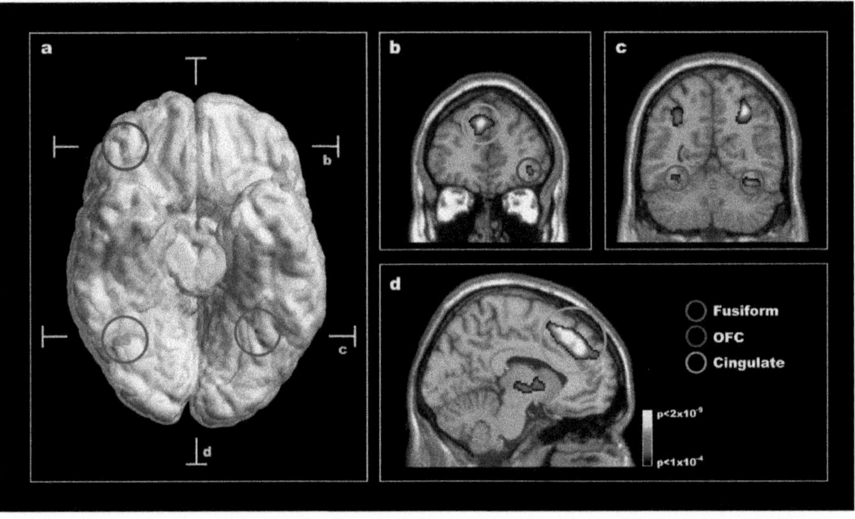

Fig. 4.18 Evidence that the human lateral orbitofrontal cortex is activated by non-reward. Activation of the lateral orbitofrontal cortex in a visual discrimination reversal task on reversal trials, when a face was selected but the expected reward was not obtained, indicating that the subject should select the other face in future to obtain the reward. a) A ventral view of the human brain with indication of the location of the two coronal slices (b,c) and the transverse slice (d). The activations with the red circle in the lateral orbitofrontal cortex (OFC, peaks at [42 42 -8] and [-46 30 -8]) show the activation on reversal trials compared to the non-reversal trials. For comparison, the activations with the blue circle show the fusiform face area produced just by face expressions, not by reversal, which are also indicated in the coronal slice in (c). b) A coronal slice showing the activation in the right orbitofrontal cortex on reversal trials. Activation is also shown in the supracallosal anterior cingulate region (Cingulate, green circle) that is also known to be activated by many punishing, unpleasant, stimuli (see Grabenhorst and Rolls (2011)). (From Neuroimage 20 (2), Morten L. Kringelbach and Edmund T. Rolls, Neural correlates of rapid reversal learning in a simple model of human social interaction, pp. 1371–83, Copyright, 2003, with permission from Elsevier.)

of the lateral orbitofrontal cortex. An interesting aspect of this study that makes it relevant to human social behaviour is that the conditioned stimuli were faces of particular individuals, and the unconditioned stimuli were face expressions. Moreover, the study reveals that the human orbitofrontal cortex is very sensitive to social feedback when it must be used to change behaviour (Kringelbach & Rolls 2003, Kringelbach & Rolls 2004).

Consistent with this human neuroimaging evidence and with the macaque neurophysiology (Thorpe, Rolls & Maddison 1983, Rolls 2014b), the macaque lateral orbitofrontal cortex has now been shown to be activated by non-reward during a reward reversal task as shown by fMRI (Chau, Sallet, Papageorgiou, Noonan, Bell, Walton & Rushworth 2015) (Fig. 9.2c).

4.5.3.6 Cognitive influences on the orbitofrontal cortex

How does cognition including language interact with emotion? Is it only when emotions enter high-level linguistic systems? Here we show that cognitive influences, originating from as high in processing as linguistic representations, can reach down into the first part of the brain in which emotion, affective, hedonic or reward value is made explicit in the representation, the orbitofrontal cortex, to modulate the responses there

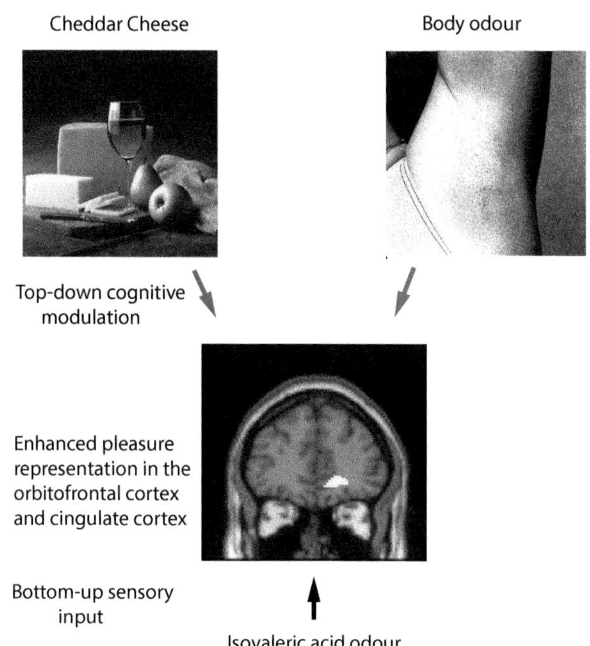

Fig. 4.19 Cognition even at the level of words can have a top-down influence to enhance and bias affective representations in the orbitofrontal cortex and anterior cingulate cortex produced by bottom-up inputs. In this experiment, the test odour (isovaleric acid, which smells a bit like brie: it might be pleasant, or not, depending on the context) was paired in different trials with a label of either 'Cheddar cheese' or 'Body odour'. (No pictures were shown in the experiment.) (After de Araujo, Rolls et al 2005.)

to affective inputs. These affective inputs include taste, olfactory, flavour, somatosensory, and visual stimuli. The investigations thus show that linguistic representations can influence how emotional states are represented and thus experienced. It is in this very direct way that cognition can have a powerful effect on emotional states, emotional behaviour, and emotional experience, because the emotional representations in the first cortical area in which affective value is represented, the orbitofrontal cortex, are altered.

These findings emphasize the importance of cognitive influences on emotion, and show how, in situations that might range from enjoying food, to listening to music, to a romantic evening, the cognitive top-down influences can play an important role in influencing affective representations in the brain. Indeed, these findings lend support to the hypothesis that an interesting role for cognitive systems in emotion is to help set up the optimal conditions in terms of the reinforcers available and contextual surroundings for reinforcers to produce affective states, as treated further in the hypothesis of multiple routes to emotional responses described in Chapter 10.

An example of such cognitive influences on the reward/aversive states that are elicited by stimuli was revealed in a study of olfaction described by De Araujo, Rolls, Velazco, Margot & Cayeux (2005). In this investigation, a standard test odour, isovaleric acid, was used as the test olfactory stimulus delivered during functional

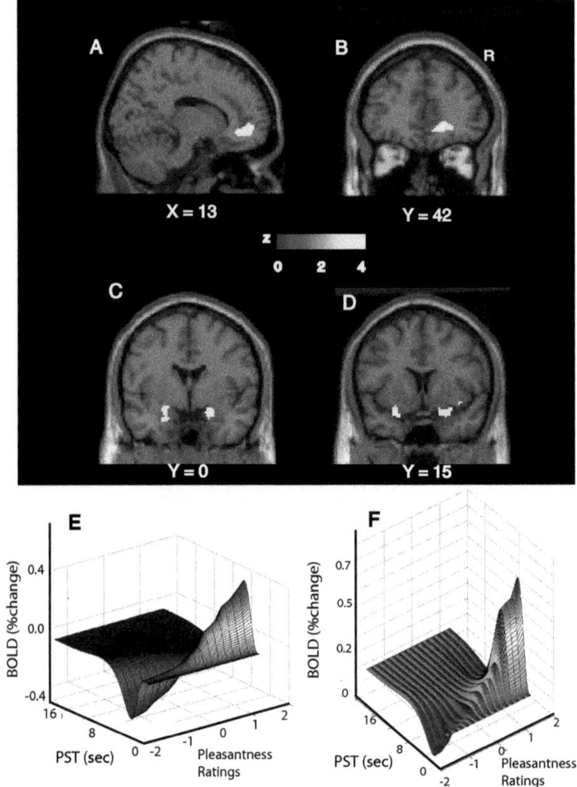

Fig. 4.20 Effects of cognition on emotion. The brain regions where the activation (measured by the BOLD signal) was correlated with pleasantness ratings given to the test odour, and where the activation were increased by the word label 'Cheddar Cheese' which enhanced the pleasantness rating, are shown. (A) Activations in the rostral anterior cingulate cortex, in the region adjoining the medial OFC, shown in a sagittal slice. (B) The same activation shown coronally. (C) Bilateral activations in the amygdala. (D) These activations extended anteriorly to the primary olfactory cortex. (E) Plots to show how if the word label was Cheddar Cheese and the pleasantness rating of the isovaleric acid was increased, the BOLD signal was increased; and how if the label was 'Body odour' and the pleasantness was decreased, there was a small BOLD signal. This is for the regions shown in A and B. PST - Post-stimulus time (s) after the odour was delivered. (F) The same as for E, but for the amygdala region shown in C. (Reprinted from *Neuron*, 46 (4), Ivan E. de Araujo, Edmund T. Rolls, Maria Inés Velazco, Christian Margot, and Isabelle Cayeux, Cognitive Modulation of Olfactory Processing, pp. 671–679. Copyright © 2005 Elsevier Inc. All rights reserved.)

neuroimaging with fMRI (De Araujo et al. 2005) (Fig. 4.19). This odour is somewhat ambiguous, and might be interpreted as the odour emitted by a cheese (rather like brie), or might be interpreted as a rather pungent and unpleasant body odour. A word was shown during the 8 s odour delivery. On some trials, the test odour was accompanied by the visually presented word 'Cheddar cheese'. On other trials, the test odour was accompanied by the visually presented word 'Body odour'. A word label was used rather than a picture label to make the modulating input reflect high-order cognition at the level of language. It was found that the word label 'Cheddar Cheese' increased the subjective pleasantness rating of the isovaleric acid, and the word label 'Body odour' decreased the pleasantness rating of the isovaleric acid.

Very interestingly, we discovered that the word label modulated the activation to the odour in brain regions where the pleasantness of odours is represented such as the orbitofrontal cortex (secondary olfactory cortex), anterior cingulate cortex, and amygdala. For example, in the medial orbitofrontal cortex the word label 'Cheddar cheese' caused a larger activation to be produced to the test odour than when the word label 'Body odour' was being presented.

The implication is that cognition at the word level, the language level, reaches down into the orbitofrontal cortex to influence affective / emotional states related to subjective pleasantness in this first stage of emotion-related processing.

This study has been extended to taste and flavour, for which the representations related to subjective pleasantness in the orbitofrontal / anterior cingulate cortex were modulated by word-level descriptors (Grabenhorst, Rolls & Bilderbeck 2008a).

Similar cognitive modulation of affective touch is also found. We applied hand cream by slow gentle rubbing to the forearm, and found that the activations in the anterior cingulate/orbitofrontal cortex were enhanced in pleasantness-related areas by the word label 'Rich moisturizing cream', and decreased by the word label 'Basic cream' (McCabe, Rolls, Bilderbeck & McGlone 2008).

Another example of what could be a similar phenomenon is that colour can have a strong influence on olfactory judgements. This was demonstrated when a white wine was artificially coloured red with an odourless dye, and it was found that participants (undergraduates at the Faculty of Oenology of the University of Bordeaux) described the wine using the descriptors normally used for red wine (Morrot, Brochet & Dubourdieu 2001).

The mechanisms by which cognitive states have top-down effects on emotion are probably similar to the biased competition (Desimone & Duncan 1995, Deco & Rolls 2005b, Rolls 2016c) and biased activation (Rolls 2013a, Grabenhorst & Rolls 2010, Rolls 2016c) mechanisms of selective attention described in Section 4.5.3.7.

4.5.3.7 Attentional modulation of affective vs sensory processing

Attentional instructions at a very high, linguistic, level, e.g. 'pay attention to and rate pleasantness' can increase responses in brain regions that represent the pleasantness of stimuli, such as the orbitofrontal cortex. The instruction 'pay attention to and rate intensity' can increase responses in brain regions that represent the perceptual intensity and identity of stimuli in structures in Tier 1 of Fig. 4.2, such as the primary taste and olfactory cortex.

The implication is that even the brain systems that preferentially process stimuli can be biased between affective / emotional streams and sensory / perceptual streams. This has important applications for emphasizing or de-emphasizing emotional states, for the development and testing of stimuli (including for example new foods, perfumes, etc), and for marketing products.

This modulation of affective processing has been shown for olfactory stimuli (Rolls, Grabenhorst, Margot, da Silva & Velazco 2008a). When subjects were instructed to remember and rate the pleasantness of a jasmine odour, activations in an fMRI investigation were greater in the medial orbitofrontal and pregenual cingulate cortex than when subjects were instructed to remember and rate the intensity of the odour. When the subjects were instructed to remember and rate the intensity, activations were greater in the pyriform primary olfactory cortex and inferior frontal gyrus.

This modulation of affective processing has also been shown for taste processing. When

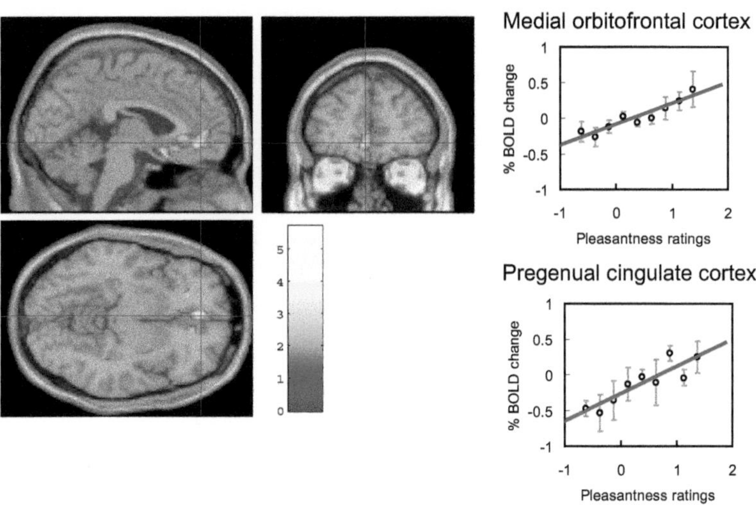

Fig. 4.21 Top-down attention and emotion. Effect of paying attention to the pleasantness of a taste. Left: A significant difference related to the taste period was found in the medial orbitofrontal cortex at [-6 14 -20] z=3.81 p<0.003 (towards the back of the area of activation shown) and in the pregenual cingulate cortex at [-4 46 -8] z=2.90 p<0.04 (at the cursor). Right upper: The correlation between the subjective pleasantness ratings and the activation (% BOLD change) in the orbitofrontal cortex (r=0.94, df=8, p<<0.001). Right lower: The correlation between the pleasantness ratings and the activation (% BOLD change) in the pregenual cingulate cortex r=0.89, df=8, p=0.001). The taste stimulus, monosodium glutamate, was identical on all trials. (Reproduced from Fabian Grabenhorst and Edmund T. Rolls, Selective attention to affective value alters how the brain processes taste stimuli, *European Journal of Neuroscience*, 27 (3) pp. 723–729. doi.org/10.1111/j.1460-9568.2008.06033.x. Copyright © 2008, John Wiley and Sons.)

participants were instructed to remember and rate the pleasantness of a savoury taste stimulus, 0.1 M monosodium glutamate, activations were greater in the medial orbitofrontal and pregenual cingulate cortex than when subjects were instructed to remember and rate the intensity of the taste (Grabenhorst & Rolls 2008) (Fig. 4.21). When the subjects were instructed to remember and rate the intensity, activations were greater in the insular taste cortex and a mid-insular cortex region (Fig. 4.22). Thus, depending on the context in which tastes are presented and whether affect is relevant, the brain responds to a taste differently.

A possible source for the top-down attentional modulation is the lateral prefrontal cortex, a region implicated in attentional control (Corbetta & Shulman 2002, Meehan, Bressler, Tang, Astafiev, Sylvester, Shulman & Corbetta 2017, Rolls 2016c), which has a greater correlation with the orbitofrontal and pregenual cingulate cortex when attention is to pleasantness compared with when attention is to intensity (Grabenhorst & Rolls 2010, Ge, Feng, Grabenhorst & Rolls 2012).

These interaction effects reflect the underlying mechanism, that a weak top-down effect can have a large, non-linear, effect on bottom-up inputs when the bottom-up inputs are weak or ambiguous, as shown by an integrate-and-fire neuronal model of the mechanisms of selective attention (Deco & Rolls 2005b), which describes a mechanism for top-down attention (Desimone & Duncan 1995, Rolls 2013a, Rolls 2016c).

One way in which top-down attention may operate is by biased competition (Fig. 4.23b.) For example in visual selective attention (Desimone & Duncan 1995), within an area, e.g. a cortical region, some neurons receive a weak top-down input that increases their response to the bottom-up stimuli (Desimone & Duncan 1995), potentially supralinearly if the bottom-up stimuli are weak (Deco & Rolls 2005b, Rolls 2016c). The enhanced firing of the biased

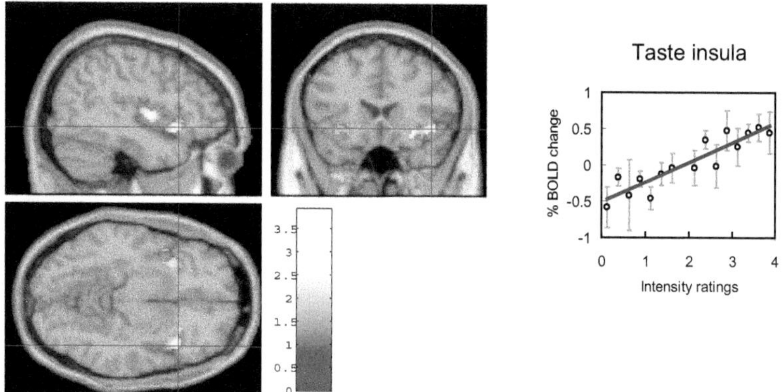

Fig. 4.22 Top-down attention and emotion. Left: Effect of paying attention to the intensity of a taste. Top: A significant difference related to the taste period was found in the taste insula at [42 18 -14] z=2.42 p<0.05 (indicated by the cursor) and in the mid insula at [40 -2 4] z=3.03 p<0.025. Right: The correlation between the intensity ratings and the activation (% BOLD change) in the taste insula (r=0.91, df=14, p<<0.001). The taste stimulus, monosodium glutamate, was identical on all trials. (Reproduced from Fabian Grabenhorst and Edmund T. Rolls, Selective attention to affective value alters how the brain processes taste stimuli, *European Journal of Neuroscience*, 27 (3) pp. 723–729. doi.org/10.1111/j.1460-9568.2008.06033.x. Copyright © 2008, John Wiley and Sons.)

neurons then, via the local inhibitory neurons, inhibits the other neurons in the local area from responding to the bottom-up stimuli. This is a local mechanism, in that the inhibition in the neocortex is primarily local, being implemented by cortical inhibitory neurons that typically have inputs and outputs over no more than a few mm (Douglas, Markram & Martin 2004, Rolls 2016c).

This type of locally implemented 'biased competition' situation may not apply in the case of top-down attention on emotional vs perceptual processing, where we have facilitation of processing in a whole cortical area (e.g. orbitofrontal cortex, or pregenual cingulate cortex) or even cortical processing stream (e.g. the linked orbitofrontal and pregenual cingulate cortex). So the attentional effect might more accurately be described in this case as biased activation, without local competition being part of the effect. I have therefore proposed a *biased activation theory and model of attention*, illustrated in Fig. 4.23a (Rolls 2013a, Grabenhorst & Rolls 2010, Rolls 2016c). In this case, the short-term memory systems implemented by an attractor network in for example the prefrontal cortex that holds in short-term memory the property to which attention should be paid provides top-down inputs which bias the activations in whole processing streams. Biased activation as a mechanism for top-down selective attention may be widespread in the brain, and may be engaged when there is segregated processing of different attributes of stimuli. It may apply not only for affective, value-based vs sensory processing, but also to the dorsal vs ventral visual system in vision, and to the 'what' vs 'where' systems for visual processing (Rolls & Deco 2002, Rolls 2016c, Rolls 2013a). The sources cited above including Deco & Rolls (2005b) provide biologically plausible computational models of how this biased competition works. Understanding at this level of the operation of the brain has many implications for not only understanding how our brains work, but also for treating some disorders of brain function (Rolls 2016c).

These findings show that, when attention is paid to affective value, the brain systems engaged to represent stimuli are in part different from those engaged when attention is directed to the physical properties of a stimulus such as its intensity. This has many implications

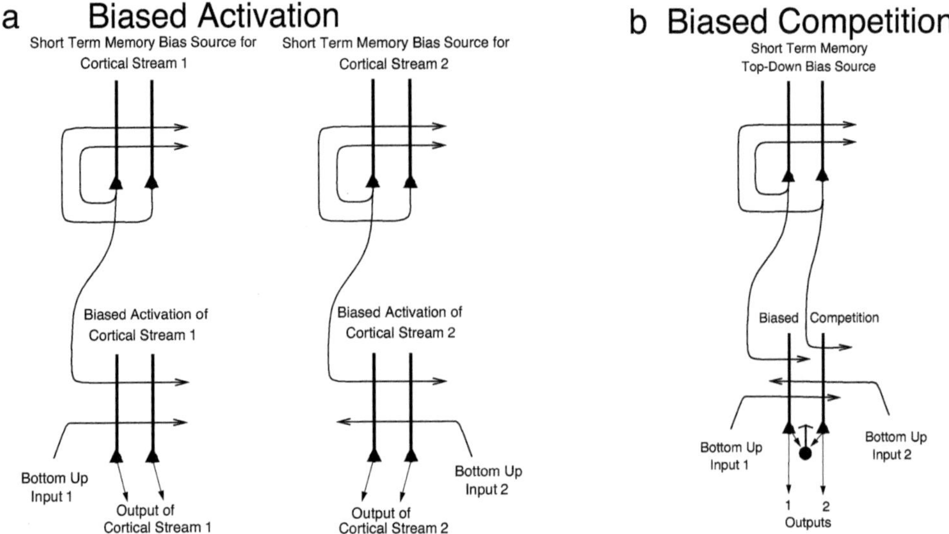

Fig. 4.23 Mechanisms for top-down attention. (a) Biased activation. The short-term memory systems that provide the source of the top-down activations may be separate (as shown), or could be a single network with different attractor states for the different selective attention conditions. The top-down short-term memory systems hold what is being paid attention to active by continuing firing in an attractor state, and bias separately either cortical processing system 1, or cortical processing system 2. This weak top-down bias interacts with the bottom up input to the cortical stream and produces an increase of activity that can be supralinear (Deco and Rolls 2005c). Thus the selective activation of separate cortical processing streams can occur. In the example, stream 1 might process the affective value of a stimulus, and stream 2 might process the intensity and physical properties of the stimulus. The outputs of these separate processing streams then must enter a competition system, which could be for example a cortical attractor decision-making network that makes choices between the two streams, with the choice biased by the activations in the separate streams (see text). (b) Biased competition. There is usually a single attractor network that can enter different attractor states to provide the source of the top-down bias (as shown). If it is a single network, there can be competition within the short-term memory attractor states, implemented through the local GABA inhibitory neurons. The top-down continuing firing of one of the attractor states then biases in a top-down process some of the neurons in a cortical area to respond more to one than the other of the bottom-up inputs, with competition implemented through the GABA inhibitory neurons (symbolized by a filled circle) which make feedback inhibitory connections onto the pyramidal cells (symbolized by a triangle) in the cortical area. The thick vertical lines above the pyramidal cells are the dendrites. The axons are shown with thin lines and the excitatory connections by arrow heads. (After Rolls 2013a.)

for understanding the effects of many stimuli and recalled memories too, and has many implications for sensory testing. These insights have implications for a number of areas related to neuroeconomics and decision-making, including the design of studies in which attentional instructions may influence which brain systems become engaged, as well as situations in which affective processing may be usefully modulated (for example in the control of the effects of the reward value of food and its role in obesity (Chapter 5), and in addiction (Chapter 6)) (Rolls 2014b, Rolls 2012c).

Another implication is that paying attention to pleasantness, and also cognitive top-down modulation, may be used to enhance pleasant emotional and aesthetic experiences.

4.5.4 The human orbitofrontal cortex

4.5.4.1 Overview

In Section 4.5.3 we considered evidence from neurophysiology and neuroimaging on the functions of the orbitofrontal cortex in emotion and motivation. In this section we consider complementary evidence from the effects of damage to the human orbitofrontal cortex, which highlights the importance of the orbitofrontal cortex in human emotion, and which helps to reveal some of the underlying processes.

Patients with orbitofrontal cortex damage are rated as having problems in behaviours such as emotion recognition in others (e.g. their sad, angry, or disgusted mood); in interpersonal relationships (such as not caring what others think, and not being close to the family); emotional empathy (e.g. when others are happy, are not happy for them); interpersonal relationships (e.g. do not care what others think, and are not close to their family); public behaviour (are uncooperative); antisocial behaviour (are critical of and impatient with others); impulsivity (do things without thinking); and sociability (are not sociable, and have difficulty making or maintaining close relationships). In relation to these problems, carers may describe the personality as having changed after the orbitofrontal cortex damage. The patients may report subjective changes in sadness, anger, fear and happiness. The patients may be relatively unconcerned about their condition, and more generally in the consequences of their actions. The patients may complain about the flavour of food. All of these changes could reflect less behavioural sensitivity to different types of punishment and reward.

In tests to analyse the bases for the changes in these patients, it has been found that the patients fail on a visual discrimination reversal task, in that they keep choosing the previously reward stimulus even when it is no longer being rewarded. This insensitivity to non-reward may contribute to the social and behavioural problems just described in these patients, in that they are failing to respond correctly to non-rewarding or punishing stimuli that would normally check and change behaviour. Indeed, the patients who fail in the visual discrimination reversal task have most of the problems just described. Gambling tasks may also require sensitivity to not receiving rewards, and are also impaired in these patients.

Many of these patients also have deficits in identifying correctly the emotional expression on a face, or the emotional expression in a voice. These failures to decode socially relevant stimuli are also likely to contribute to the social and related problems in patients with orbitofrontal cortex damage or dysfunction.

All these problems are consistent with the theory that the orbitofrontal cortex is important in representing reward and punisher value, and in updating the expected value based on errors between what is expected and what is obtained.

4.5.4.2 Orbitofrontal cortex damage impairs reward reversal learning in humans

Humans with frontal lobe damage can show impairments in a number of tasks in which an alteration of behavioural strategy is required in response to a change in environmental reinforcement contingencies (Goodglass & Kaplan 1979, Jouandet & Gazzaniga 1979, Kolb & Whishaw 2015, Zald & Rauch 2006). Frontal patients may be able to verbalize the correct rules yet may be unable to correct their behavioural sets or strategies based on the rewards being received.

Some of the personality changes that can follow frontal lobe damage may be related to a similar type of dysfunction. For example, the euphoria, irresponsibility, lack of affect, and lack of concern for the present or future that can follow frontal lobe damage (see Zald & Rauch (2006) and Section 4.5.1 on page 66) may also be related to a dysfunction in altering behaviour appropriately in response to a change in reinforcement contingencies. A failure to correct stimulus–reinforcer associations when they become inappropriate might be reflected in effects such as impulsive behaviour, and a failure to respond appropriately to corrective feedback received from the environment.

To examine these hypotheses, we measured the performance of patients with damage to the orbitofrontal cortex in a visual discrimination reversal task, in which patients could learn to obtain points by touching one stimulus when it appeared on a video monitor, but had to withhold a response when a different visual stimulus appeared, otherwise a point was lost. After the participants had acquired the visual discrimination, the reinforcement contingencies unexpectedly reversed. The patients with ventral frontal / orbitofrontal cortex lesions made more errors in the reversal task (or in a similar extinction task in which no reward as delivered), and completed fewer reversals, than control patients with damage elsewhere in the frontal lobes or in other brain regions (Rolls, Hornak, Wade & McGrath 1994a). A reversal deficit in a similar task in patients with ventromedial frontal cortex damage was also reported by Fellows & Farah (2003).

An important aspect of the findings of Rolls et al. (1994a) was that the reversal learning impairment correlated highly with the socially inappropriate or disinhibited behaviour of the patients, and also with their subjective evaluation of the changes in their emotional state since the brain damage. The behaviours that were correlated with the impairment in reversal learning included disinhibited or socially inappropriate behaviour; misinterpretation of other people's moods; impulsiveness; unconcern about or underestimation of the seriousness of their condition; and lack of initiative. It is of interest that the patients could often verbalize the correct response, yet committed the incorrect action. This is consistent with the hypothesis that the orbitofrontal cortex is normally involved in executing behaviour when the behaviour is performed by evaluating the reinforcement associations of environmental stimuli.

To seek positive confirmation that effects on stimulus–reinforcer association learning and reversal were related to orbitofrontal cortex damage rather than to any other associated pathology, a new reversal-learning task was used with a group of patients with discrete, surgically produced, lesions of the orbitofrontal cortex, performed for example to remove tumours. In the new visual discrimination task, two stimuli were always present on the video monitor and the patient obtained 'monetary' reward by touching the correct stimulus, and lost 'money' by touching the incorrect stimulus. This design controls for an effect of the lesion in simply increasing the probability that any response will be made. The task also used probabilistic amounts of reward and punishment on each trial, to make it harder to use a verbal strategy with an explicit rule. The task also had the advantage that it was the same as that used in our human functional neuroimaging study that had showed activation of the orbitofrontal cortex by monetary gain or loss (O'Doherty et al. 2001a). It was found that a group of patients with bilateral orbitofrontal cortex lesions were severely impaired at the reversal task, in that they accumulated less money (Hornak, O'Doherty, Bramham, Rolls, Morris, Bullock & Polkey 2004). These patients often failed to switch their choice of stimulus after a large loss; and often did switch their choice even though they had just received a reward, and this has been quantified in more recent studies (Berlin, Rolls & Kischka 2004, Berlin, Rolls & Iversen 2005).

The importance of the failure to rapidly learn about the value of stimuli from negative feedback has been confirmed as a critical difficulty for patients with orbitofrontal cortex lesions (Fellows 2007, Wheeler & Fellows 2008, Fellows 2011), and has been contrasted with the effects of lesions to the anterior cingulate cortex which impair the use of feedback to learn about actions (Fellows 2011, Camille, Tsuchida & Fellows 2011) (see Section 4.7). In addition, Bechara and colleagues also have findings that are consistent with those described above in patients with frontal lobe damage when they perform a gambling task (Bechara, Damasio, Damasio & Anderson 1994, Bechara, Tranel, Damasio & Damasio 1996, Bechara, Damasio, Tranel & Damasio 1997, Damasio 1994, Bechara, Damasio, Tranel & Damasio 2005, Glascher, Adolphs, Damasio, Bechara, Rudrauf, Calamia, Paul & Tranel 2012). In the gambling task, impairments could often be related to a failure to not learn to avoid choices on which losses were being made.

It is important that the patients with bilateral orbitofrontal cortex damage who were impaired at the visual discrimination reversal task (Hornak et al. 2004) had high scores on parts of a Social Behaviour Questionnaire in which the patients were rated on behaviours such as emotion recognition in others (e.g. their sad, angry, or disgusted mood); in interpersonal relationships (such as not caring what others think, and not being close to the family); emotional empathy (e.g. when others are happy, is not happy for them); interpersonal relationships (e.g. does not care what others think, and is not close to his family); public behaviour (is uncooperative); antisocial behaviour (is critical of and impatient with others); impulsivity (does things without thinking); and sociability (is not sociable, and has difficulty making or maintaining close relationships) (Hornak, Bramham, Rolls, Morris, O'Doherty, Bullock & Polkey 2003), all of which could reflect less behavioural sensitivity to different types of punishment and reward. Further, in a Subjective Emotional Change Questionnaire in which the patients reported on any changes in the intensity and/or frequency of their own experience of emotions, the bilateral orbitofrontal cortex lesion patients with deficits in the visual discrimination reversal task reported a number of changes, including changes in sadness, anger, fear and happiness (Hornak et al. 2003).

These results on the effects of brain damage to the orbitofrontal cortex, complemented by the neuroimaging results described above in Section 4.5.3, provide evidence that at least part of the function of the orbitofrontal cortex in emotion, social behaviour, and decision-making is related to representing reinforcers, detecting changes in the reinforcers being received, using these changes to rapidly reset stimulus–reinforcer associations, and rapidly changing behaviour as a result.

The more general impact on the behaviour of these patients is that their irresponsibility tended to affect their everyday lives. For example, if such patients had received their brain damage in a road traffic accident, and compensation had been awarded, the patients often tended to spend their money without appropriate concern for the future, sometimes, for example, buying a very expensive car. Such patients often find it difficult to invest in relationships too, and are sometimes described by their family as having changed personalities, in that they care less about a wide range of social and emotional factors than before the brain damage. The suggestion that follows from this is that the orbitofrontal cortex may normally be involved in much social behaviour, and the ability to respond rapidly and appropriately to social reinforcers is, of course, an important aspect of primate social behaviour.

4.5.4.3 Orbitofrontal cortex damage impairs face and voice expression identification

To investigate the possible significance of face-related inputs to the orbitofrontal cortex visual neurons described above, we also tested the responses of these patients to faces. We included tests of face (and also voice) expression decoding, because these are ways in which the reinforcing quality of individuals is often indicated. Impairments in the identification of facial and vocal emotional expression were demonstrated in a group of patients with ventral frontal lobe damage who had socially inappropriate behaviour (Hornak, Rolls & Wade 1996, Rolls 1999c). The expression identification impairments could occur independently of perceptual impairments in facial recognition, voice discrimination, or environmental sound recognition. The face and voice expression problems did not necessarily occur together in the same patients, providing an indication of separate processing. Poor performance on both expression tests was correlated with the degree of alteration of emotional experience reported by the patients. There was also a strong positive correlation between the degree of altered emotional experience and the severity of the behavioural problems (e.g. disinhibition) found in these patients. Later findings confirm that face emotion recognition is impaired following ventromedial, but not dorsal or lateral, prefrontal cortex damage (Heberlein, Padon, Gillihan, Farah & Fellows 2008).

These findings have been extended, and it has been found that patients with face expression decoding problems do not necessarily have impairments at visual discrimination reversal, and vice versa (Hornak, Bramham, Rolls, Morris, O'Doherty, Bullock & Polkey 2003, Hornak, O'Doherty, Bramham, Rolls, Morris, Bullock & Polkey 2004). This is consistent with some topography in the orbitofrontal cortex (see Section 4.5.1.2 and Rolls & Baylis (1994)).

To obtain clear evidence that the changes in face and voice expression identification, emotional behaviour, and subjective emotional state were related to orbitofrontal cortex damage itself, and not to damage to surrounding areas which is present in many closed head injury patients, we performed these assessments in patients with circumscribed lesions made surgically in the course of treatment (Hornak, Bramham, Rolls, Morris, O'Doherty, Bullock & Polkey 2003). We found that some patients with bilateral lesions of the orbitofrontal cortex had deficits in voice and face expression identification, and the group had impairments in social behaviour, and significant changes in their subjective emotional state (Hornak et al. 2003). The same group of patients had deficits on the probabilistic monetary reward task (Hornak et al. 2004). Some patients with unilateral damage restricted to the orbitofrontal cortex also had deficits in voice expression identification. In all cases in which voice expression identification was impaired, there were no deficits in control tests of the discrimination of unfamiliar voices and the recognition of environmental sounds.

These results (Hornak et al. 2003) thus confirm that damage restricted to the orbitofrontal cortex can produce impairments in face and voice expression identification, which may be primary reinforcers.

It is possible to relate psychiatric types of symptom to orbitofrontal cortex function is frontotemporal dementia, which is a progressive neurodegenerative disorder attacking the frontal lobes and producing major and pervasive behavioural changes in personality and social conduct resembling those produced by orbitofrontal cortex lesions (Rahman, Sahakian, Hodges, Rogers & Robbins 1999, Rascovsky, Hodges & al. 2011). Patients appear either socially disinhibited with facetiousness and inappropriate jocularity, or apathetic and withdrawn. Many patients show mental rigidity and inability to appreciate irony or other subtle aspects of language. They tend to engage in ritualistic and stereotypical behaviour, and their planning skills are invariably impaired. The dementia is accompanied by gradual withdrawal from all social interactions. Memory is usually intact but patients have difficulties with working memory and concentration. Interestingly, given the anatomy and physiology of the orbitofrontal cortex, frontotemporal dementia causes profound changes in eating habits, with escalating desire for sweet food coupled with reduced satiety, which is often followed by enormous weight gain (Piguet 2011).

4.5.5 A neurophysiological and computational basis for stimulus–reinforcer association learning and reversal in the orbitofrontal cortex

We now consider how stimulus–reinforcer association learning and its reversal may be implemented in the orbitofrontal cortex. The suggested process for the initial association is

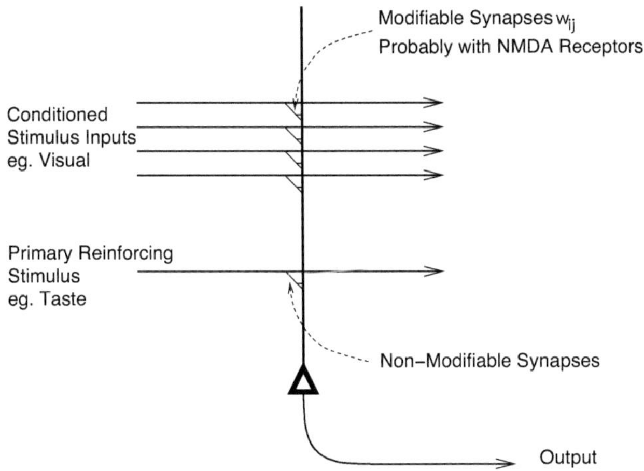

Fig. 4.24 Pattern association between a primary reinforcer, such as the taste of food, which activates neurons through non-modifiable synapses, and a potential secondary reinforcer, such as the sight of food, which has modifiable synapses on to the same neurons. The modifiable synapses increase in strength when there is concurrent activity between the firing of the presynaptic neuron conveying the conditioned stimulus inputs and the firing of the post-synaptic neuron activated by the primary reinforcing stimulus. This pattern association mechanism learns the association between the input and the output, and leads the neuron to respond to expected value. Such a mechanism appears to be implemented in the orbitofrontal cortex and amygdala.

illustrated in Fig. 4.24. If the visual input (e.g. the sight of food) is present at the same time (or just before) the primary reinforcer (e.g. taste) is activating the postsynaptic neuron, then the set of synapses that are driven by the conditioned stimulus become strengthened by the associative process of long-term synaptic potentiation (LTP). The LTP occurs only if the post-synaptic neuron is strongly activated, because the NMDA receptors activated by the presynaptic release of the transmitter glutamate only become unblocked to allow Ca^{2+} entry when the postsynaptic neuron is sufficiently depolarized (Rolls 2016c). This pattern association network can learn many associations between conditioned stimuli and primary reinforcers, in fact in the order of the number of synapses per neuron, which is in the order of 5,000–10,000 (Rolls 2016c, Rolls & Treves 1990). This type of learning also has many other desirable properties, including generalization to similar conditioned stimuli, and graceful degradation (fault tolerance) if the system sustains some damage (Rolls 2016c)).

Next, we need a mechanism to account for reversal learning set, the process by which during repeated reversal learning, performance gradually improves until reversal can occur in one trial. Even more, the mechanism has to account for the fact that after reversal learning set has been acquired, when the contingency is reversed, the individual (human or non-human primate) makes a response to the current S+ expecting to get reward, but instead obtains the punisher. On the very first subsequent trial on which the pre-reversal S– is shown, the individual will perform a response to it expecting now to get reward, *even though the post-reversal S+ has not since the reversal been associated with reward to produce LTP for the post-reversal S+*. (This is in fact illustrated in Fig. 4.16 on page 80.) To implement this very rapid stimulus–reinforcer association reversal, a rule-based process, requires the current rule to be held in mind, in short-term memory. This, and non-reward neurons that maintain their firing for many seconds as illustrated in Fig. 4.16, may be developments provided for by the evolution of granular orbitofrontal cortex areas in primates (see Section 1.3).

It is this rule-based, one-trial, visual reversal learning that is the type of emotion-related learning to which the primate including human orbitofrontal cortex makes an important contribution. Claims that the orbitofrontal cortex is not involved in reversal learning (Stalnaker, Cooch & Schoenbaum 2015) have not adequately dealt with this point, and it is not clear that this type of learning occurs in rodents. Moreover, when assessing the effects of lesions of the orbitofrontal cortex on this type of learning in primates, it appears to be important that the lateral orbitofrontal cortex is included in the lesion (which it not always is (Murray & Izquierdo 2007, Rudebeck & Murray 2014)), because that is where a focus appears to be of the non-reward reversal-related effects in primates including humans in tasks that often involve probabilistic situations (Kringelbach & Rolls 2003, O'Doherty et al. 2001a, Chau et al. 2015). Indeed, earlier research in which the lesions included the lateral orbitofrontal cortex did demonstrate reversal learning and extinction deficits (Iversen & Mishkin 1970, Butter 1969). In addition, more recent research is showing that lateral orbitofrontal cortex lesions (sometimes termed ventrolateral prefrontal cortex, VLPFC, or inferior prefrontal convexity cortex) does impair choices based on probabilities of reward (Rudebeck, Saunders, Lundgren & Murray 2017), which benefits from sensitivity to non-reward and the ability to remember previous rewards and non-rewards received for a choice. This is in line with the importance of the cortex for holding items in short-term memory in attractor networks (Rolls 2016c), which is what I propose contributes to the rule based non-reward-related functionality of the lateral orbitofrontal cortex, with these short-term memories also useful for probabilistic reward-related learning.

A model for how the very rapid, one-trial, reversal could be implemented has been developed (Deco & Rolls 2005a). The model uses a short-term memory autoassociation attractor network with associatively modifiable synaptic connections to hold the neurons representing the current rule active. When non-reward neurons fire, they quench this attractor by the competition implemented by inhibitory neurons, and the non-adapted set of neurons representing the opposite rule then can emerge as the winning new attractor. The rule attractor then biases other neurons of the type found in the orbitofrontal cortex to implement the reversal (Deco & Rolls 2005a).

This model also provides a computational account of why the orbitofrontal cortex may play a more important role in rapid reversal learning than the amygdala. The account is based on the fact that a feature of cortical architecture is a highly developed set of local (within 1–2 mm) recurrent collateral excitatory associatively modifiable connections between pyramidal cells (Rolls 2016c). These provide the basis for short-term memory attractor networks, and thus the basis for the rule attractor model which is at the heart of my suggestion for how rapid reversal learning is implemented (Deco & Rolls 2005a). In contrast, the amygdala is thought to have a much less well developed set of recurrent collateral excitatory connections, and thus may not be able to implement rapid reversal learning in the way described using competition biased by a rule module. Instead, the amygdala would need to rely on synaptic relearning, and this would be likely to be a slower process, and would certainly not lead to correct choice of the new to be rewarded but not yet rewarded stimulus the first time it is presented after a punishment trial when the reversal contingency changes.

The generation of the firing of the non-reward neurons has also been modelled. In the model one set of neurons in an attractor responds to high expected value, and another set of neurons responds when the reward is less than expected. If the reward outcome is high as expected, this maintains the firing in the high expected reward value neurons. If the reward outcome is low, this does not support the high expected reward value neurons, and due to adaptation their firing rates decrease, and release from inhibition the non-reward neurons into activity. This model accounts for extinction as well as reversal (Rolls & Deco 2016).

4.6 The amygdala and emotion

4.6.1 Overview of the functions of the amygdala in emotion

The amygdala is an evolutionarily old subcortical structure with parts of it present in amphibia and reptiles. This is in contrast with the orbitofrontal cortex, which develops greatly in primates including humans as shown in Fig. 1.1.

The connections of the amygdala are similar to those of the orbitofrontal cortex, as shown in Figs. 4.1 and 4.2, and the amygdala connections do involve many with the orbitofrontal cortex.

The amygdala does have neurons that respond to primary reinforcers such as the taste, flavour, and smell of food; touch; and aversive stimuli. The amygdala also has neurons that learn associations between visual and auditory stimuli, and primary reinforcers. However, this learning does not support rule-based one-trial reversal learning, so the amygdala is less good at this rapid emotion-related learning than the orbitofrontal cortex. The primate amygdala also contains a population of neurons specialized to respond to faces, and damage to the human amygdala can alter the ability to discriminate between different facial expressions, though this may be related to how faces are fixated.

Classically conditioned responses such as autonomic, freezing, and startle responses to auditory stimuli can depend on outputs from the amygdala to structures such as the hypothalamus and ventral striatum. Bilateral damage to the amygdala can produce a deficit in learning to associate visual and other stimuli with a primary (i.e. unlearned) reward or punisher. For example, monkeys with damage to the amygdala when shown foods and non-foods pick up both and place them in their mouths. When such visual or auditory discrimination learning is tested more formally, it is found that primates including humans with amygdala damage have difficulty in associating the sight or sound of a stimulus with whether it produces a reward, or is noxious and should be avoided. Sensory-specific satiety (the reduced choice of a food devalued by feeding to satiety) is impaired by damage to the amygdala (as is also the case for the orbitofrontal cortex).

In humans and other primates the amygdala does not appear to play such an important role in emotional and social behaviour as the orbitofrontal cortex, with the changes to emotion much more subtle after amygdala damage. Further, the deficits described after amygdala damage involve fear conditioning (with classical conditioning of for example autonomic responses and effects on startle especially studied), and somewhat subtle aspects of face expression processing. In evolution, the balance may have moved to the orbitofrontal cortex, which has evolved much more recently, and may allow more powerful computations, such as those involved in rapid reversal learning and rapid correction of behaviour, to be implemented, as described in Section 4.5.

Indeed, LeDoux, who has performed research on the amygdala, is, with colleagues, now suggesting that the amygdala may have little to do with subjective feelings of emotion (LeDoux, Brown, Pine & Hofmann 2018). In contrast, the orbitofrontal cortex may be much more closely related to emotional feelings, in that activations in it are linearly related to subjective affective ratings of pleasantness, and damage to the orbitofrontal cortex impairs subjective emotional feelings, as described in Section 4.5. In Chapter 10 it is suggested that the orbitofrontal cortex is en route to the brain processes that implement conscious feelings.

A much fuller analysis of the functions of the amygdala in emotion in primates including humans is provided by (Rolls 2014b), with further human studies described in Whalen & Phelps (2009). The rodent literature and how it has focussed on conditioned responses and not on emotional feelings is described more fully elsewhere (LeDoux 2012, LeDoux & Pine 2016).

4.6.2 The amygdala and the associative processes involved in emotion-related learning

The amygdala is implicated in some learning processes involved in emotion including some classically conditioned effects, but not in other learning processes involved in emotion. To clarify this, I briefly summarize some of these learning processes, with a much fuller analysis provided elsewhere (Cardinal et al. 2002, Rolls 2014b).

When a conditioned stimulus (CS) (such as a tone) is paired with a primary reinforcer or unconditioned stimulus (US) (such as a painful stimulus), then there are opportunities for a number of types of association to be formed.

Some of these involve 'classical conditioning' or 'Pavlovian conditioning', in which no action is performed that affects the contingency between the conditioned stimulus and the unconditioned stimulus. Typically an unconditioned response (UR), for example an alteration of heart rate, is produced by the US, and will come to be elicited by the CS as a conditioned response (CR). These responses are typically autonomic (such as the heart beating faster), or endocrine (for example the release of adrenaline (epinephrine in American usage) by the adrenal gland).

In addition, the organism may learn to perform an instrumental response with the skeletal muscles in order to alter the probability that the primary reinforcer will be obtained. In our example, the experimenter might alter the contingencies so that when the tone sounded, if the organism performed an action such as pressing a lever, then the painful stimulus could be avoided. This is confirmed to be instrumental learning if the response learned is arbitrary, for example performing the opposite response, such as raising the lever to avoid the painful stimulus.

In the instrumental learning situation there are still opportunities for many classically conditioned responses including emotional states such as fear to occur. For example, in Pavlovian–instrumental transfer, if a stimulus that predicts the arrival of sucrose as a result of Pavlovian conditioning is provided during an instrumental task such as working to obtain sucrose, the responding (e.g. lever pressing) can be enhanced. Further, approach to a food may be under Pavlovian rather than instrumental control. Finally, we must beware of the facts that after overtraining, habits may be formed in which stimuli may become inflexibly linked to responses, with the reward value of the goal no longer directly influencing behaviour, as shown by the fact that the response may continue for at least one trial after the goal has been devalued by for example feeding to satiety. This had led to some confusion in the literature (Berridge & Robinson 1998, Berridge, Robinson & Aldridge 2009), for when the goal controls the behaviour wanting is driven by liking, and what happens during habits is not an exception, as habits are stimulus-response associations and have little to do with wanting or liking a goal (Rolls 2014b, Rolls 2013d).

4.6.3 Connections of the amygdala

The amygdala is a subcortical region in the anterior part of the temporal lobe. It receives massive projections in the primate from the overlying temporal lobe cortex (Van Hoesen 1981, Amaral, Price, Pitkanen & Carmichael 1992, Ghashghaei & Barbas 2002, Freese & Amaral 2009) (see Fig. 4.25). Via these inputs, the amygdala receives inputs about objects

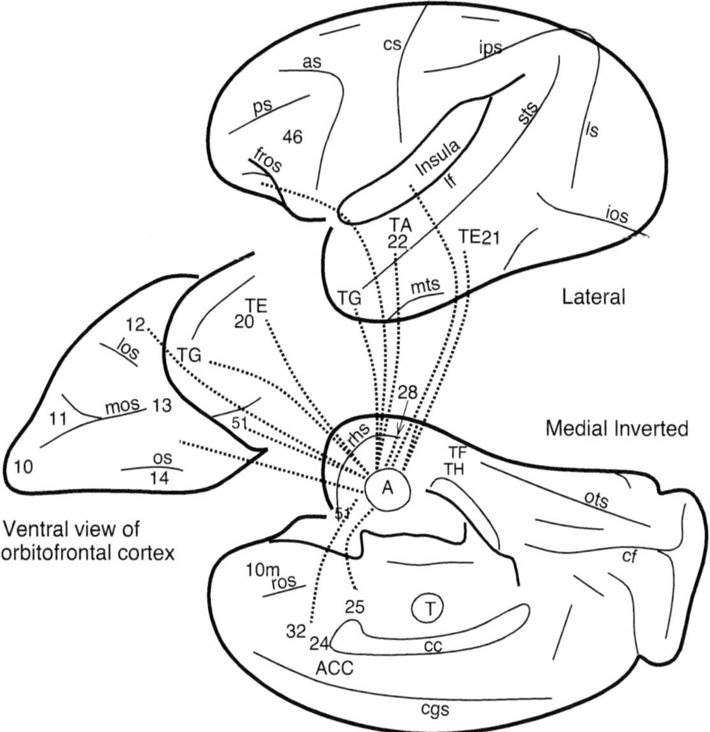

Fig. 4.25 Connections of the amygdala shown on lateral, ventral, and medial inverted views of the monkey brain. Abbreviations: as, arcuate sulcus; cc, corpus callosum; cf, calcarine fissure; cgs, cingulate sulcus; cs, central sulcus; ls, lunate sulcus; ios, inferior occipital sulcus; mos, medial orbital sulcus; os, orbital sulcus; ots, occipito-temporal sulcus; ps, principal sulcus; rhs, rhinal sulcus; sts, superior temporal sulcus; lf, lateral (or Sylvian) fissure (which has been opened to reveal the insula); A, amygdala; ACC, anterior cingulate cortex; INS, insula; T, thalamus; TE (21), inferior temporal visual cortex; TA (22), superior temporal auditory association cortex; TF and TH, parahippocampal cortex; TG, temporal pole cortex; 12, 13, 11, orbitofrontal cortex; 24, 32, parts of the anterior cingulate cortex; 25, subgenual cingulate cortex; 28, entorhinal cortex; 51, olfactory (prepyriform and periamygdaloid) cortex. The cortical connections shown provide afferents to the amygdala, but are reciprocated. (Reproduced from G. W. Van Hoesen, The differential distribution, diversity and sprouting of cortical projections to the amygdala in the rhesus monkey, in Y. Ben-Ari (ed.), *The Amygdaloid Complex*, pp. 77–90 © 1981 Elsevier, with permission.)

and faces that could become secondary reinforcers, as a result of pattern association in the amygdala with primary reinforcers. The amygdala also receives inputs that are potentially about primary reinforcers, e.g. taste inputs (from the insula, and from the secondary taste cortex in the orbitofrontal cortex), and somatosensory inputs, potentially about the rewarding or painful aspects of touch (from the somatosensory cortex via the insula). The amygdala receives strong projections from the posterior orbitofrontal cortex (see Fig. 4.25, areas 12 and 13) where there are value representations, and from the anterior cingulate cortex (Carmichael & Price 1995a, Ghashghaei & Barbas 2002, Freese & Amaral 2009).

Although there are some inputs from early on in some sensory pathways, for example auditory inputs from the medial geniculate nucleus (LeDoux 1992, Pessoa & Adolphs 2010), this route is unlikely to be involved in most emotions, for which cortical analysis of the stimulus is likely to be required. Emotions are usually elicited to environmental stimuli analysed to the object level (including other organisms), and not to retinal arrays of spots or the frequency (tone) of a sound as represented in the cochlea.

Some of the outputs of the amygdala relevant to different types of response in rodents are shown in Fig. 4.26, and in addition there are backprojections to the neocortical areas that project to the amygdala.

4.6.4 Effects of amygdala lesions

4.6.4.1 Amygdala lesions in primates

Bilateral removal of the amygdala in monkeys produces striking behavioural changes which include tameness, a lack of emotional responsiveness, excessive examination of objects, often with the mouth, and eating of previously rejected items such as meat (Weiskrantz 1956). These behavioural changes comprise much of the Kluver–Bucy syndrome which is produced in monkeys by bilateral anterior temporal lobectomy (Kluver & Bucy 1939). In analyses of the bases of these behavioural changes, it has been observed that there are deficits in some types of learning. For example, Larry Weiskrantz (1956) found that bilateral ablation of the amygdala in the monkey produced a deficit on learning an active avoidance task. The monkeys failed to learn to make a response when a light signalled that shock would follow unless the response was made. He was perhaps the first to suggest that these monkeys had difficulty with forming associations between stimuli and reinforcers, when he suggested that "the effect of amygdalectomy is to make it difficult for reinforcing stimuli, whether positive or negative, to become established or to be recognized as such" (Weiskrantz 1956). In this avoidance task, associations between a stimulus and punishers were impaired.

It has been confirmed with the more selective type of neurotoxic amygdala lesion that non-foods as well as foods are picked up and eaten, and also that emotional responses to snakes and human intruders are impaired (Murray & Izquierdo 2007), but there are relatively minor changes in social behaviour (Amaral 2003, Bliss-Moreau, Moadab, Bauman & Amaral 2013), and this is consistent with the trend for the orbitofrontal cortex to become relatively more important in emotion and social behaviour in primates including humans. The amygdala is implicated by lesion studies in learning associations between visual stimuli and rewards, and devaluation by feeding to satiety is impaired too (Murray & Izquierdo 2007).

A difference between the effects of selective amygdala lesions and orbitofrontal cortex lesions in monkeys is that selective amygdala lesions have no effect on object reversal learning, whereas orbitofrontal cortex lesions do impair object reversal learning (Murray & Izquierdo 2007) (see further Section 4.4.1). Further, and consistently, orbitofrontal but not selective amygdala lesions impair instrumental extinction (i.e. they showed a large number of choices of the previously rewarded object when it was no longer rewarded) (Murray & Izquierdo 2007). This is consistent with the evidence described in Section 4.5 that the orbitofrontal cortex is important in rapid, one-trial, learning and reversal between visual stimuli and primary reinforcers using both associative and rule-based mechanisms, and its representations of outcome value, expected value, and negative reward prediction error (Thorpe, Rolls & Maddison 1983, Rolls 2014b, Rolls & Grabenhorst 2008). These contributions of the orbitofrontal cortex are facilitated by its neocortical architecture, which can operate using attractors that are important in many functions including short-term memory, attention, rule-based operation with switching, long-term memory, and decision-making which may help it to compute and utilize non-reward to reset value representations in the orbitofrontal cortex (Rolls 2014b).

4.6.4.2 Amygdala lesions in rats

In rats, there is also evidence that the amygdala is involved in behaviour to stimuli learned as being associated with reward as well as with punishers. We may summarize these investigations in the rat as follows. The central nuclei of the amygdala encode or express Pavlovian S–R (stimulus–response, CS–UR) associations (including conditioned suppression, conditioned orienting, conditioned autonomic and endocrine responses, and Pavlovian–instrumental transfer); and modulate perhaps by arousal the associability of representations stored elsewhere in the brain (Gallagher & Holland 1994, Gallagher & Holland 1992, Holland & Gallagher 1999). In contrast, the basolateral amygdala (BLA) encodes or retrieves the affective value of the predicted US, and can use this to influence action–outcome learning via pathways to brain regions such as the nucleus accumbens and prefrontal cortex including the orbitofrontal cortex (Cardinal et al. 2002). We shall see below that the nucleus accumbens is not involved in action–outcome learning itself, but does allow the affective states retrieved by the BLA to conditioned stimuli to influence instrumental behaviour by for example Pavlovian–instrumental transfer, and facilitating locomotor approach to food which appears to be in rats a Pavlovian process (Cardinal et al. 2002, Cardinal & Everitt 2004, Everitt & Robbins 2013, Rolls 2014b). This leaves parts of the prefrontal and cingulate cortices as strong candidates for action–outcome learning.

In a different model of fear-conditioning in the rat, Davis and colleagues (Davis 2006), have used the fear-potentiated startle test, in which the amplitude of the acoustic startle reflex is increased when elicited in the presence of a stimulus previously paired with shock. Lesions of either the central nucleus or the lateral and basolateral nuclei of the amygdala block the expression of fear-potentiated startle. These latter amygdala nuclei may be the site of plasticity for fear conditioning, because local infusion of the NMDA (N-methyl-d-aspartate) receptor antagonist AP5 (which blocks long-term potentiation, an index of synaptic plasticity) blocks the acquisition but not the maintenance of fear-potentiated startle (Davis 2006). These investigations have now been extended to primates, in which similar effects are found, with ibotenic acid-induced lesions of the amygdala preventing the acquisition of fear-potentiated startle, though, remarkably, not the expression of fear-potentiated startle when fear conditioning was carried out prior to the lesion (Davis, Antoniadis, Amaral & Winslow 2008).

Reconsolidation refers to a process in which after a memory has been stored, it may be weakened or lost if recall is performed during the presence of a protein synthesis inhibitor (Debiec, LeDoux & Nader 2002, Debiec, Doyere, Nader & LeDoux 2006). The implication that has been drawn is that whenever a memory is recalled, some reconsolidation process requiring protein synthesis may be needed. The computational utility of reconsolidation is considered by Rolls (2016c). Here, it is of interest that this applies to fear association mechanisms in the amygdala (Doyere, Debiec, Monfils, Schafe & LeDoux 2007), and drug-associated memories in the amygdala (Milton, Lee, Butler, Gardner & Everitt 2008). The findings have interesting implications for the treatment of fear-associated memories. For example, in humans old fear memories can be updated with non-fearful information provided during the reconsolidation window. As a consequence, fear responses are no longer expressed, an effect that can last at least a year and is selective only to reactivated memories without affecting other memories (Schiller, Monfils, Raio, Johnson, LeDoux & Phelps 2010), although success has so far been limited (Kroes, Schiller, LeDoux & Phelps 2016). Procedures that influence the extinction of fear memory may also be useful in the treatment of fear states (Davis 2011).

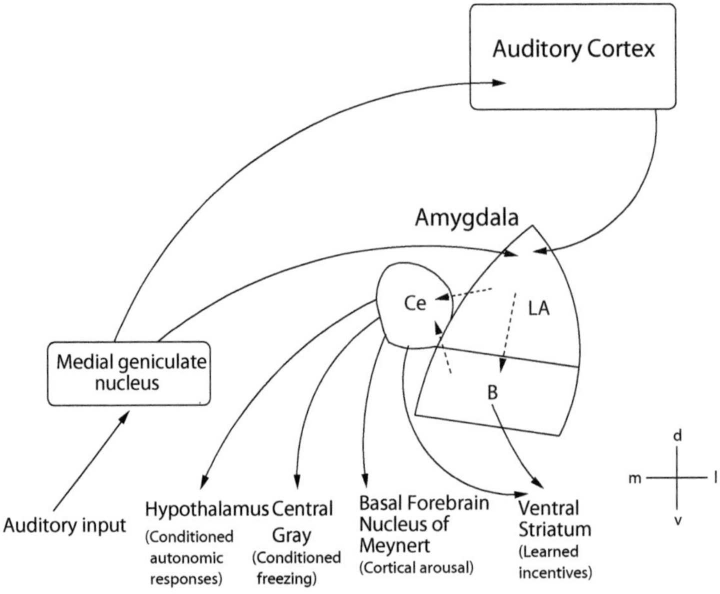

Fig. 4.26 The pathways for fear-conditioning to pure-tone auditory stimuli associated with footshock in the rat. The lateral amygdala (LA) receives auditory information directly from the medial part of the medial geniculate nucleus (the auditory thalamic nucleus), and from the auditory cortex. Intra-amygdala projections (directly and via the basal and basal accessory nuclei, B) end in the central nucleus (Ce) of the amygdala. Different output pathways from the central nucleus and the basal nucleus mediate different conditioned fear-related effects. d, dorsal; v, ventral; m, medial; l, lateral. (Reproduced from G. J. Quirk, J. L. Armony, J. C. Repa, X. F. Li, and J. E. LeDoux, Emotional memory: a search for sites of plasticity, *Cold Spring Harbor Symposia on Quantitative Biology*, 61, pp. 247–257, figure 1b © 1996, Cold Spring Harbor Laboratory Press.)

4.6.5 Neuronal activity in the primate amygdala to reinforcing stimuli

There is clear evidence that some neurons in the primate amygdala respond to stimuli that are potentially primary reinforcers. For example, Sanghera, Rolls & Roper-Hall (1979) found some amygdala neurons with taste responses. In an extensive study of 1416 macaque amygdala neurons, Kadohisa, Rolls & Verhagen (2005a) showed that a very rich and detailed representation of the stimulus (such as food) that is in the mouth is provided by neurons that respond to oral stimuli. An example of a macaque single amygdala orally-responsive neuron is shown in Fig. 4.27. The neuron had different responses to different tastes, different temperatures of what was in the mouth, and different viscosities, but had no response to the texture of fatty oils. Other amygdala neurons were selective for even one modality, responding for example only to the oral texture of fat (Kadohisa, Rolls & Verhagen 2005a). 3.1% of the recorded amygdala neurons responded to oral stimuli. Of the orally responsive neurons, some (39%) represent the viscosity of oral stimuli, tested using carboxymethyl-cellulose in the range 1–10,000 centiPoise. Other neurons (5%) responded to fat in the mouth by encoding its texture (shown by the responses of these neurons to a range of fats, and also to non-fat oils such as silicone oil ($Si(CH_3)_2O)_n$) and mineral oil (pure hydrocarbon), but no or small responses to the cellulose viscosity series or to the fatty acids linoleic acid and lauric acid). Some neurons (7%) responded to gritty texture (produced by microspheres suspended in carboxymethyl cellulose). Some neurons (41%) responded to the temperature of the liquid in the mouth. Some amygdala neurons responded to capsaicin, and some to fatty acids (but not to fats in the mouth). Some amygdala neurons respond to taste, texture and temperature unimodally,

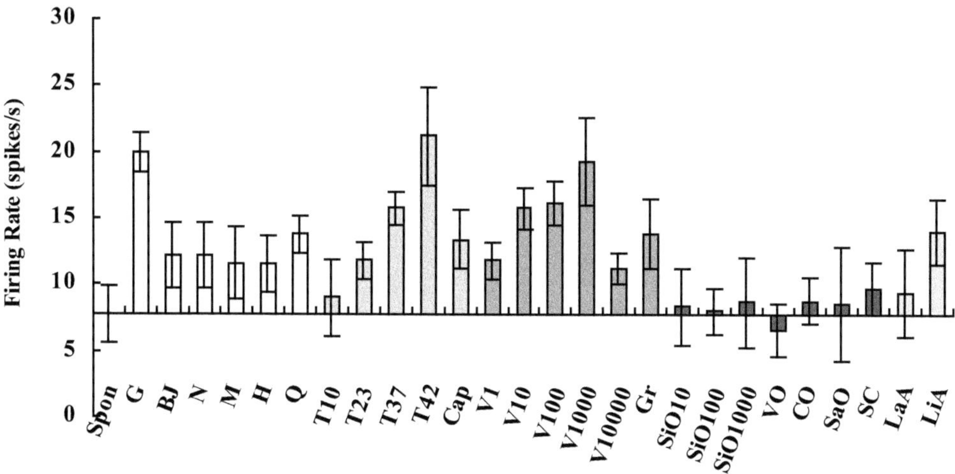

Fig. 4.27 The responses of an amygdala neuron (bo217) with differential responses to taste, temperature and viscosity. The neuron did not respond to fat texture. The mean (± the standard error of the mean, sem) firing rate responses to each stimulus calculated in a 1 s period over 4–6 trials are shown. The spontaneous (Spon) firing rate is shown. G, N, M, H and Q are the taste stimuli. T10–T42 are the temperature stimuli. V1 - V10,000 are the CMC viscosity series with the viscosity in cP. The fat texture stimuli were SiO10, SiO100, SiO1000 (silicone oil with the viscosity indicated), vegetable oil (VO), coconut oil (CO) and safflower oil (SaO). BJ is fruit juice; Cap is 10 μM capsaicin; LaA is 0.1 mM lauric acid; LiA is 0.1 mM linoleic acid; Gr is the gritty stimulus. (Reprinted from *Neuroscience*, 132 (1), M. Kadohisa, J. V. Verhagen, and E. T. Rolls, The primate amygdala: Neuronal representations of the viscosity, fat texture, temperature, grittiness and taste of foods, pp. 33–48. doi.org/10.1016/j.neuroscience.2004.12.005 Copyright © 2005 IBRO. Published by Elsevier Ltd. All rights reserved.)

but others combine these inputs. An interesting difference is that in terms of best responses to different tastes, 57% of the orbitofrontal cortex taste neurons had their best responses to glucose, whereas 21% of the amygdala neurons had their best response to glucose (Kadohisa, Rolls & Verhagen 2005b). (More amygdala neurons had their best responses to sour (HCl) (18%) and monosodium glutamate (14%) (Kadohisa, Rolls & Verhagen 2005b).)

These results show that a very detailed representation of substances in the mouth, which are likely to be primary reinforcers, is present in the primate amygdala (Kadohisa, Rolls & Verhagen 2005a). Less is known about whether it is though the reinforcer value of the stimuli that is represented. It has been shown that satiety produces a rather modest (on average 58%) reduction in the responses of amygdala neurons to taste (Yan & Scott 1996, Rolls & Scott 2003), in comparison to the essentially complete reduction of responsiveness found in orbitofrontal cortex taste neurons (Rolls, Sienkiewicz & Yaxley 1989b). Further, the representation in the amygdala of these oral stimuli does not appear to be on any simple hedonic basis, in that no direction in the multidimensional taste space in Fig. 7 of Kadohisa, Rolls & Verhagen (2005a) reflected the measured preference of the monkeys for the stimuli, nor were the response profiles of the neurons to the set of stimuli closely related to the preferences of the macaques for the stimuli (Kadohisa, Rolls & Verhagen 2005a). The failure to find very strong effects of satiety on the responsiveness of amygdala taste neurons (Yan & Scott 1996, Rolls & Scott 2003) mirrors the earlier finding of Sanghera, Rolls & Roper-Hall (1979) of inconsistent effects of feeding to satiety on the responses of amygdala visual neurons responding to the sight of food.

Recordings from single neurons in the amygdala of the monkey have shown that some neurons do respond to visual stimuli, consistent with the inputs from the temporal lobe visual cortex (Sanghera, Rolls & Roper-Hall 1979). Other neurons responded to auditory, gustatory, olfactory, or somatosensory stimuli, or in relation to movements. In tests of whether the neurons responded on the basis of the association of stimuli with reinforcers, it was found that approximately 20% of the neurons with visual responses had responses that occurred primarily to stimuli associated with reinforcers, for example to food and to a range of stimuli which the monkey had learned signified food in a visual discrimination task for food reward (Sanghera, Rolls & Roper-Hall 1979, Rolls 1981c, Wilson & Rolls 1993, Wilson & Rolls 2005, Rolls 2000c). Many of these neurons responded more to the positive discriminative stimulus (S+) than to the negative visual discriminative stimulus (S–) in the Go/NoGo visual discrimination task (Rolls 2000c, Wilson & Rolls 2005). However, none of these neurons (in contrast with some neurons in the orbitofrontal cortex) responded exclusively to rewarded stimuli, in that all responded at least partly to one or more neutral, novel, or aversive stimuli.

The degree to which the visual responses of these amygdala neurons are associated with reinforcers has been assessed in learning tasks. When the association between a visual stimulus and an instrumental reinforcer was altered by reversal (so that the visual stimulus formerly associated with juice reward became associated with aversive saline and vice versa), it was found that 10 of 11 neurons did not reverse their responses (and for the other neuron the evidence was not clear) (Sanghera, Rolls & Roper-Hall 1979, Rolls 1992a, Rolls 2000c).

Although more investigations would be useful, the evidence now available indicates that primate amygdala neurons do not alter their activity flexibly and rapidly (in one or even a few trials) in visual discrimination reversal learning (Rolls 1992a, Rolls 2000c, Rolls 2014b). What has been found in contrast is that neurons in the orbitofrontal cortex do show very rapid, often one-trial, reversal of their responses in visual discrimination reversal, and it therefore seems likely that the orbitofrontal cortex is especially involved when repeated relearning and re-assessment of stimulus–reinforcer associations are required, as described above, rather than initial learning, in which the amygdala may be involved. (It is noted that some other studies do not address the issue convincingly of rapid reversal, for they were not studying one-trial reversal with instrumental learning, but instead slow classical conditioning (Paton, Belova, Morrison & Salzman 2006, Morrison, Saez, Lau & Salzman 2011). However, more recent studies in that series are in fact consistent with the discoveries we have made that the orbitofrontal cortex updates reward value representations more rapidly and flexibly than the amygdala, in that neural responses to reward-predictive cues updated more rapidly in the orbitofrontal cortex than amygdala, and activity in the orbitofrontal cortex but not the amygdala was modulated by recent reward history (Saez, Saez, Paton, Lau & Salzman 2017).

Evidence that primate amygdala neurons encode reward value is that while monkeys chose between saving liquid reward with interest and spending the accumulated reward, some of the neurons reflected the accumulating value (Grabenhorst, Hernadi & Schultz 2012) and reflect whether a macaque will perform economic saving (Zangemeister, Grabenhorst & Schultz 2016). Overall, there is thus evidence that some amygdala neurons reflect reward value, yet do not reverse their value-related responses rapidly (in the one trial shown by orbitofrontal cortex neurons), and the evidence from the effects of selective amygdala lesions (Murray & Izquierdo 2007) is consistent with this.

4.6.6 Responses of primate amygdala neurons to novel stimuli that are reinforcing

Wilson & Rolls (2005) (see Rolls (2000c)) discovered that some amygdala neurons with reward-related responses also responded to relatively novel visual stimuli. When the monkeys are given such relatively novel stimuli outside the task, they will reach out for and explore the objects, and in this respect the novel stimuli are reinforcing. Repeated presentation of the stimuli results in habituation of the neuronal response and of behavioural approach, if the stimuli are not associated with a primary reinforcer. It is thus suggested that the amygdala neurons described operate as filters that provide an output if a stimulus is associated with a positive reinforcer, or is positively reinforcing because of relative unfamiliarity, and that provide no output if a stimulus is familiar and has not been associated with a positive primary reinforcer or is associated with a punisher. The functions of this output may be to influence the interest shown in a stimulus, whether it is approached or avoided, whether an affective response occurs to it, and whether a representation of the stimulus is made or maintained (see Rolls (2014b)).

It is an important adaptation to the environment to explore relatively novel objects or situations, for in this way advantage due to gene inheritance can become expressed and selected for. This function appears to be implemented in the amygdala in this way. Lesions of the amygdala impair the operation of this mechanism, in that objects are approached and explored indiscriminately, relatively independently of whether they are associated with reinforcers (including punishers), or are novel or familiar.

4.6.7 Neuronal responses in the amygdala to faces

Another interesting group of neurons in the amygdala responds primarily to faces (Rolls 1981c, Leonard, Rolls, Wilson & Baylis 1985). Each of these neurons responds to some but not all of a set of faces, and thus across an ensemble could convey information about the identity of the face (see Fig. 4.28). These neurons are found especially in the basal accessory nucleus of the amygdala (Leonard, Rolls, Wilson & Baylis 1985), a part of the amygdala that develops markedly in primates (Amaral et al. 1992). Similar neurons have been further analysed (Gothard, Battaglia, Erickson, Spitler & Amaral 2007, Gothard, Mosher, Zimmerman, Putnam, Morrow & Fuglevand 2018), and, as with face-selective neurons in the orbitofrontal cortex (Rolls, Critchley, Browning & Inoue 2006), some neurons respond to face identity, some to face expression, and some to combinations of identity and expression. In addition, some neurons in the primate amygdala respond during social interactions, some may respond preferentially to eyes (as do some neurons in the temporal lobe visual cortex (Perrett, Rolls & Caan 1982)), and their output may influence face expression (Brothers & Ring 1993, Gothard et al. 2018). Face-selective neurons have also been found now in the human amygdala (Rutishauser, Tudusciuc, Neumann, Mamelak, Heller, Ross, Philpott, Sutherling & Adolphs 2011, Rutishauser, Mamelak & Adolphs 2015).

4.6.8 Evidence from humans

In relation to neurons in the macaque amygdala with responses selective for faces and social interactions (Leonard, Rolls, Wilson & Baylis 1985, Gothard, Mosher, Zimmerman, Putnam, Morrow & Fuglevand 2018), a patient (DR) has been described who has bilateral damage to or disconnection of the amygdala, and has an impairment of face-expression matching and identification, but not of matching face identity or in discrimination (Young, Aggleton, Hellawell, Johnson, Broks & Hanley 1995, Young, Hellawell, Van de Wal & Johnson 1996). This patient is also impaired at detecting whether someone is gazing at the patient, another important social signal (Perrett, Smith, Potter, Mistlin, Head, Milner & Jeeves 1985). The same patient is also impaired at the auditory recognition of fear and anger (Scott, Young, Calder, Hellawell, Aggleton & Johnson 1997).

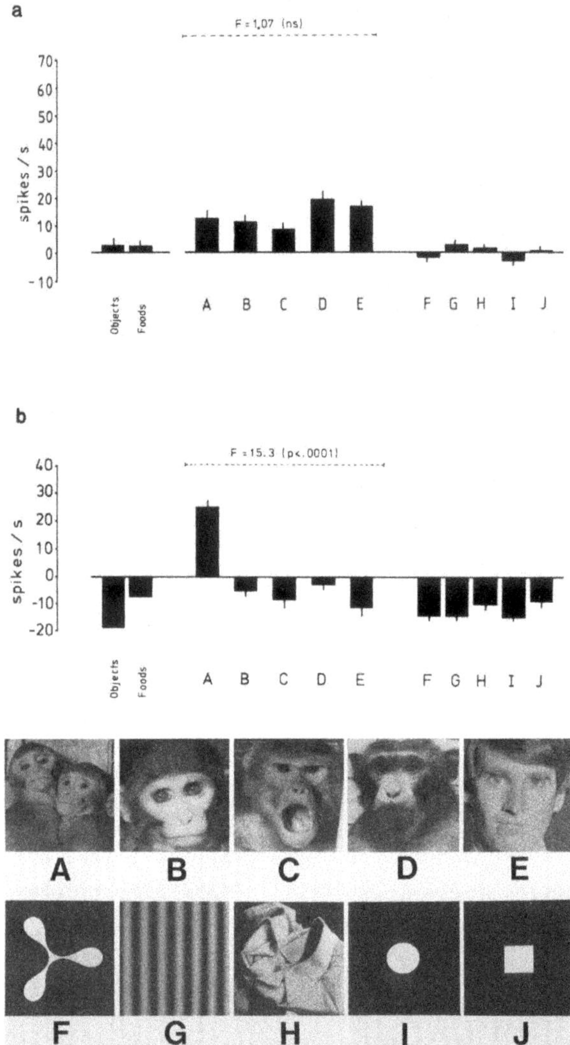

Fig. 4.28 The responses of two neurons (a,b) in the amygdala to a variety of monkey and human face stimuli (A–E), and to non-face stimuli (F–J, objects, and foods). Each bar represents the mean response above baseline with the standard error calculated over 4 to 10 presentations. The F ratio for an analysis of variance calculated over the face sets indicates that the neurons shown range from very selective between faces (neuron b, Y0809) to relatively non-selective (neuron A, Z0264). Some stimuli produced inhibition below the spontaneous firing rate. (Reprinted from *Behavioural Brain Research*, 15 (2), C. M. Leonard, E. T. Rolls, F. A. W. Wilson, and G. C. Baylis, Neurons in the amygdala of the monkey with responses selective for faces, pp. 159–76. doi.org/10.1016/0166-4328(85)90062-2. Copyright © 1985 Published by Elsevier B.V.)

Adolphs, Tranel, Damasio & Damasio (1994) also found face expression but not face identity impairments in a patient (SM) with bilateral damage to the amygdala, and extended this to other patients (Adolphs, Tranel & Baron-Cohen 2002). The bilateral amygdala patient SM was especially impaired at recognizing the face expression of fear, and also rated expressions of fear, anger, and surprise as less intense than control subjects. It has been shown that SM's impairment stems from an inability to make normal use of information from the eye region of faces when judging emotions, which in turn is related to a lack of spontaneous fixations on the eyes during free viewing of faces (Adolphs, Gosselin, Buchanan, Tranel, Schyns & Damasio 2005), though this is mainly evident just for the first fixation (Kennedy & Adolphs 2011). Although SM fails to look normally at the eye region in all facial expressions, her selective impairment in recognizing fear is explained by the fact that the eyes are the most important feature for identifying this emotion. Indeed, SM's recognition of fearful faces became entirely normal when she was instructed explicitly to look at the eyes. This finding provides a mechanism to explain the amygdala's role in fear recognition, and points to new approaches for the possible rehabilitation of patients with defective emotion perception.

The changes in emotion in patients with amygdala lesions are much less marked than those in patients with orbitofrontal cortex damage, and special tests, analogous in some cases to those developed in rodent studies, are necessary to reveal deficits (Phelps & LeDoux 2005). For example, patients with amygdala lesions are impaired at learning conditioned skin conductance responses when a blue square is associated with a shock, and are also impaired in acquiring the same autonomic response to fear by verbally instructed learning or by observational learning (Phelps 2004, Phelps, O'Connor, Gatenby, Gore, Grillon & Davis 2001, Phelps 2006, Whalen & Phelps 2009). The human amygdala has been described as being important mainly for some fear responses to some stimuli, such as whether an individual backs off in a social encounter (Adolphs 2003, Adolphs et al. 2005, Phelps 2004, Schiller et al. 2010, Feinstein, Adolphs, Damasio & Tranel 2011). Interestingly, the amygdala was involved during aversive conditioning with primary reinforcers (electric shock) and less so with a secondary reinforcer (money), as suggested by both an fMRI analysis and a follow-up case study with a patient with bilateral amygdala damage (Delgado, Jou & Phelps 2011).

A very interesting clarification is provided by the finding that personality interacts with whether particular stimuli activate the human amygdala. For example, happy face expressions are more likely to activate the human amygdala in extraverts than in introverts (Canli et al. 2002). In addition, positively affective pictures interact with extraversion to produce activation of the amygdala (Canli et al. 2001). This supports the conceptually important point described in section 2.5 that part of the basis of personality may be differential sensitivity to different rewards and punishers, and omission and termination of rewards and punishers. It has additionally been found that negative pictures interact with neuroticism in producing differential activation of the human amygdala (Canli et al. 2001). Further, FFFS and BIS-related personality traits related to an anxiety-related 'Behavioural Inhibition System', and to a fear-related 'Fight, Flight, Freeze System', are positively correlated to activity in the amygdala in response to negative stimuli (Kennis, Rademaker & Geuze 2013).

4.7 The cingulate cortex and emotion

4.7.1 Introduction and overview of the anterior cingulate cortex

The orbitofrontal cortex is involved in representing the value of stimuli. It is in a sense an output region for all the sensory systems, including taste, olfaction, visual, auditory, and somatosensory, that represent 'what' a stimulus is, and uses that information to build what are frequently multimodal representations but in value space rather than 'what' or stimulus identity space. Orbitofrontal cortex neurons focus on value representations for stimuli, and know little about actions.

The anterior cingulate cortex receives inputs from the orbitofrontal cortex about the value of stimuli, that is about goals including the value of outcomes (the reward received) and the expected value. The anterior cingulate cortex in combination with the midcingulate motor area, which contains representations of actions, interfaces

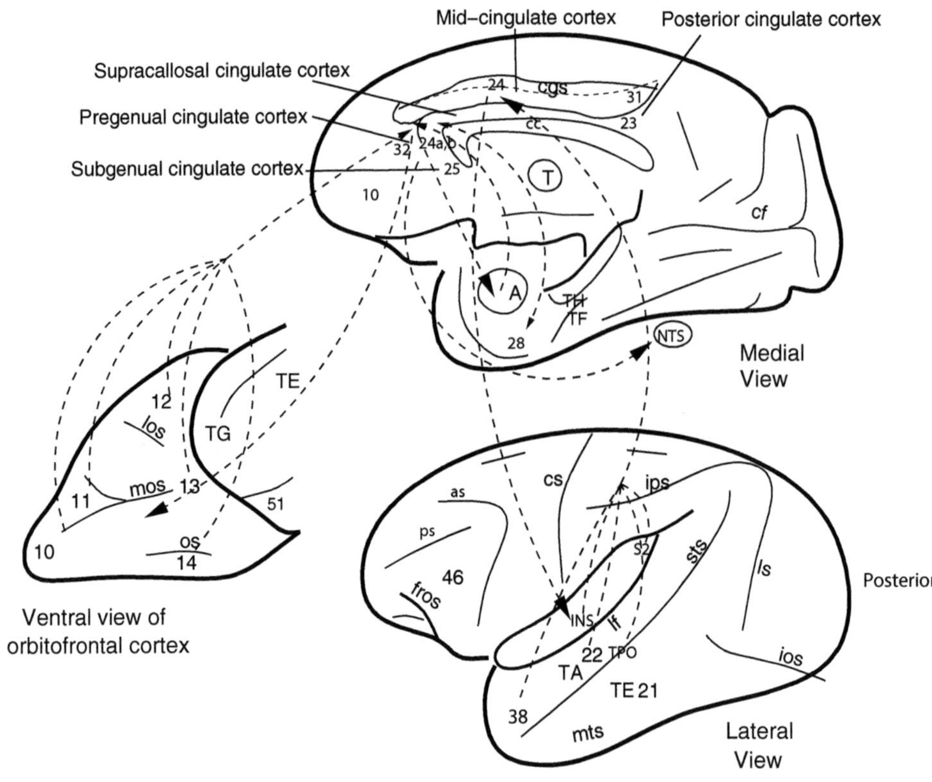

Fig. 4.29 Connections of the anterior cingulate and midcingulate cortical areas (shown on views of the primate brain). The anterior cingulate cortex includes the supracallosal/dorsal anterior, pregenual, and subgenual parts. The cingulate sulcus (cgs) has been opened to reveal the cortex in the sulcus, with the dashed line indicating the depths (fundus) of the sulcus. The cingulate cortex is in the lower bank of this sulcus, and in the cingulate gyrus which hooks above the corpus callosum and around the corpus callosum at the front and the back. The anterior cingulate cortex extends from cingulate areas 32, 24a and 24b to subgenual cingulate area 25. (The cortex is called subgenual because it is below the genu (knee) formed by the anterior end of the corpus callosum, cc.) The perigenual cingulate cortex tends to have connections with the amygdala and orbitofrontal cortex, whereas area 24c tends to have connections with the somatosensory insula (INS), the auditory association cortex (22, TA), and with the temporal pole cortex (38). The midcingulate areas include area 24d, which is part of the cingulate motor area. Abbreviations: as, arcuate sulcus; cc, corpus callosum; cf, calcarine fissure; cgs, cingulate sulcus; cs, central sulcus; ls, lunate sulcus; ios, inferior occipital sulcus; mos, medial orbital sulcus; os, orbital sulcus; ps, principal sulcus; sts, superior temporal sulcus; lf, lateral (or Sylvian) fissure (which has been opened to reveal the insula); A, amygdala; INS, insula; NTS, autonomic areas in the medulla, including the nucleus of the solitary tract and the dorsal motor nucleus of the vagus; TE (21), inferior temporal visual cortex; TA (22), superior temporal auditory association cortex; TF and TH, parahippocampal cortex; TPO, multimodal cortical area in the superior temporal sulcus; 28, entorhinal cortex; 38, TG, temporal pole cortex; 12, 13, 11, orbitofrontal cortex; 51, olfactory (prepyriform and periamygdaloid) cortex.

actions to outcomes (rewards or punishers received) using action–outcome learning, and also takes into account the cost of actions to obtain the goal when selecting actions. The anterior and midcingulate cortical areas are thus relevant to emotion, for they implement the instrumental goal-directed actions that the instrumental reinforcers involved in emotion produce. In the context of its representations of value, damage to the anterior cingulate areas does influence emotion.

The anterior cingulate cortex operates as a system that is aiming to obtain goals, and is taking into account the outcomes received after actions, in that it is sensitive to devaluation of the goal, and will not select an action if the goal has been devalued. This is in contrast to the basal ganglia, which implement a stimulus–motor response mapping which becomes automated as a habit after much learning, and is not sensitive to devaluation of the goal, as described in Chapter 6 and Section 4.6.2.

The posterior cingulate cortex has different functions, for it is not activated in the same way as the anterior cingulate cortex by rewards and punishers, and is involved in spatio-topographical and related memory functions with its connections to parietal structures such as the precuneus and with the hippocampus that are involved in these functions (Vogt 2009, Cavanna & Trimble 2006, Rolls 2015d, Rolls 2018, Rolls & Wirth 2018). However, the posterior cingulate cortex does have connectivity with the lateral orbitofrontal cortex which is increased in depression, and this may contribute to the increased negative rumination in depression (Cheng, Rolls, Qiu, Xie, Wei, Huang, Yang, Tsai, Li, Meng, Lin, Xie & Feng 2018b) (see Section 9.4.4).

In more detail, the pregenual and the adjoining dorsal anterior cingulate areas can be conceptualized as a relay that allows information about rewards and outcomes to be linked, via longitudinal connections running in the cingulum fibre bundle, to information about actions represented in the mid-cingulate cortex. Bringing together information about specific rewards with information about actions, and the costs associated with actions, is important for associating actions with the value of their outcomes and for selecting the correct action that will lead to a desired reward (Walton, Bannerman, Alterescu & Rushworth 2003, Rushworth, Buckley, Behrens, Walton & Bannerman 2007, Rolls 2009b, Rushworth, Noonan, Boorman, Walton & Behrens 2011, Grabenhorst & Rolls 2011, Rolls 2014b, Kolling, Wittmann, Behrens, Boorman, Mars & Rushworth 2016). Indeed, consistent with its strong connections to motor areas (Morecraft & Tanji 2009), lesions of the anterior cingulate cortex impair reward-guided action selection (Kennerley, Walton, Behrens, Buckley & Rushworth 2006, Rudebeck, Behrens, Kennerley, Baxter, Buckley, Walton & Rushworth 2008), neuroimaging studies have shown that the anterior cingulate cortex is active when outcome information guides choices (Walton, Devlin & Rushworth 2004), and single neurons in the anterior cingulate cortex encode information about both actions and outcomes including reward prediction errors for actions (Matsumoto, Matsumoto, Abe & Tanaka 2007, Luk & Wallis 2009, Kolling et al. 2016). For example, Luk & Wallis (2009) found that in a task where information about three potential outcomes (three types of juice) had to be associated on a trial-by-trial basis with two different responses (two lever movements), many neurons in the anterior cingulate cortex encoded information about both specific outcomes and specific actions.

4.7.2 Anterior cingulate cortex anatomy and connections

The anterior cingulate areas occupy approximately the anterior one third of the cingulate cortex (see Fig. 4.29) and are involved in emotion. They may be distinguished from a mid-cingulate area (i.e. further back than the anterior cingulate region and occupying approximately the middle third of the cingulate cortex) which has been termed the cingulate motor area (Vogt, Derbyshire & Jones 1996, Vogt 2009) and may be involved in action selection (Rushworth, Walton, Kennerley & Bannerman 2004, Rushworth et al. 2011). The anterior cingulate cortex includes area 32 the pregenual (or perigenual, meaning around the genu of the corpus callosum) cingulate cortex, area 25 the subgenual cingulate cortex, and part of area 24 (Figs. 4.29 and 4.9) (Price 2006, Ongur, Ferry & Price 2003, Ongur & Price 2000).

As shown in Fig. 4.29, the anterior cingulate cortex receives strong inputs from the orbitofrontal cortex (Carmichael & Price 1995a, Morecraft & Tanji 2009, Vogt 2009). A very interesting finding in relation to what follows is that the medial orbitofrontal cortex has strong functional connectivity with the pregenual cingulate cortex, in both of which rewards are represented; and that the lateral orbitofrontal cortex has strong functional connectivity with the supracallosal, more dorsal, anterior cingulate cortex area, both of which are activated by unpleasant aversive stimuli (Rolls, Cheng, Qiu, Zhou, Zhang, Lyu, Ruan, Wei, Huang, Yang, Tsai, Cheng, Meng, Lin, Xie & Feng 2018b).

The outputs of the anterior cingulate cortex reach further back in the cingulate cortex towards the midcingulate cortex, which includes the cingulate motor area (Vogt et al. 1996, Morecraft & Tanji 2009, Vogt 2009). The anterior cingulate cortex also projects forwards to medial prefrontal cortex area 10 (Price 2006, Ongur & Price 2000). Another route for output is via the projections to the striatum / basal ganglia system. The anterior cingulate cortex, including the subgenual cingulate cortex area 25, has outputs that can influence autonomic/visceral function via the hypothalamus, midbrain periaqueductal gray, and insula, as does the orbitofrontal cortex (Rempel-Clower & Barbas 1998, Price 2006, Ongur & Price 2000, Critchley & Harrison 2013).

4.7.3 Anterior cingulate cortex functional neuroimaging and neuronal activity

In early functional neuroimaging investigations, Vogt et al. (1996) showed that pain produced an increase in regional cerebral blood flow (rCBF, measured with positron emission tomography, PET) in an area of perigenual cingulate cortex which included parts of areas 25, 32, 24a, 24b and/or 24c. Vogt et al. suggested that activation of the anterior part of the cingulate area is related to the affective aspect of pain. Lane, Fink, Chau & Dolan (1997a) found increased regional blood flow in a PET study in a far anterior part of the cingulate cortex where it adjoins prefrontal cortex when humans paid attention to the affective aspects of pictures they were being shown which contained pleasant images (e.g. flowers) and unpleasant pictures (e.g. a mangled face and a snake).

Functional magnetic resonance neuroimaging (fMRI) studies are now showing that there are rather separate representations of positively affective, pleasant, stimuli in the pregenual cingulate cortex (yellow in Fig. 4.14); and of negative, unpleasant, stimuli just posterior to this above the corpus callosum in the anterior cingulate cortex (white in Fig. 4.14) (Rolls 2009b, Grabenhorst & Rolls 2011). The area activated by pain is typically 10–30 mm behind and above the most anterior (i.e. pregenual) part of the anterior cingulate cortex (see e.g. Rolls, O'Doherty, Kringelbach, Francis, Bowtell & McGlone (2003d), Fig. 4.4, and Vogt & Sikes (2000)). Pleasant touch was found to activate the most anterior part of the anterior cingulate cortex, just in front of the (genu or knee of the) corpus callosum (i.e. pregenual cingulate cortex) (Rolls, O'Doherty, Kringelbach, Francis, Bowtell & McGlone 2003d, McCabe, Rolls, Bilderbeck & McGlone 2008) (Fig. 4.4). Pleasant temperature applied to the hand also produces a linear activation related to the degree of subjective pleasantness in the pregenual cingulate cortex (Grabenhorst, Rolls & Parris 2008b). Oral somatosensory stimuli such as viscosity and the pleasantness of fat texture also activate this pregenual part of the anterior cingulate cortex (De Araujo & Rolls 2004, Grabenhorst, Rolls, Parris & D'Souza 2010b). More than just somatosensory stimuli are represented, however, in that (pleasant) sweet taste also activates the pregenual anterior cingulate cortex (De Araujo & Rolls 2004, De Araujo, Kringelbach, Rolls & Hobden 2003a) where attention to pleasantness (Grabenhorst & Rolls 2008) and cognition (Grabenhorst, Rolls & Bilderbeck 2008a) also enhances activations, as do pleasant odours (Rolls, Kringelbach & De Araujo 2003c) (Fig. 4.12, and cognitive inputs that influence the pleasantness of odours (De Araujo et al. 2005) (Fig. 4.20, and also top-down inputs that produce selective attention to odour pleasantness (Rolls, Grabenhorst, Margot, da Silva & Velazco 2008a). Unpleasant odours activate further back in the anterior cingulate cortex (Rolls, Kringelbach & De Araujo 2003c) (Fig. 4.12). Activations in the pregenual cingulate cortex are also produced by the taste of water when it is rewarding because of thirst (De Araujo, Kringelbach, Rolls & McGlone 2003b), by the flavour of food (Kringelbach, O'Doherty, Rolls & Andrews 2003), and by monetary reward (O'Doherty, Kringelbach, Rolls, Hornak & Andrews 2001a) (Fig. 4.13). Moreover, the outcome value and the expected value of monetary reward activate the pregenual cingulate cortex (Rolls, McCabe & Redoute 2008e). The locations of some of these activations are shown in Fig. 4.14.

In these studies, the anterior cingulate activations were linearly related to the subjective pleasantness or unpleasantness of the stimuli, providing evidence that the anterior cingulate cortex provides a representation of value on a continuous scale. Moreover, evidence was found that there is a common scale of value in the pregenual cingulate cortex, with the affective pleasantness of taste stimuli and of thermal stimuli applied to the hand producing identically scaled BOLD activations (Grabenhorst, D'Souza, Parris, Rolls & Passingham 2010a). The implication is that the anterior cingulate cortex contains a value representation used in decision-making, but that the decision itself may be made elsewhere. Decisions about actions that reflect the outcomes represented in the anterior cingulate cortex may be made further posterior towards the mid-cingulate cortex. Decisions about the value of stimuli may be made in the medial prefrontal cortex area 10 (or ventromedial prefrontal cortex, VMPFC), which receives inputs from the orbitofrontal cortex and also from the anterior cingulate cortex.

Value representations in the pregenual cingulate cortex are confirmed by recording studies in monkeys (Rolls 2008b, Rolls 2009b, Kolling et al. 2016). For example, Gabbott, Verhagen, Kadohisa and Rolls found neurons in the pregenual cingulate cortex that respond to taste and it was demonstrated that the representation is of reward value, for devaluation by feeding to satiety selectively decreased neuronal responses to the food with which the animal was satiated (Rolls 2008b).

Some single neuron studies indicating encoding of actions and outcomes have often involved rather dorsal recordings above the pregenual cingulate cortex in the dorsal anterior cingulate cortex (dorsal bank of the cingulate sulcus) (Matsumoto et al. 2007, Luk & Wallis 2009, Kolling et al. 2016). In a similar area, action–outcome associations appear to be represented, in that in tasks in which there were different relations between actions and rewards, it was found that even before a response was made, while the monkey was looking at a visual cue, the activity of anterior cingulate cortex neurons depended on the expectation of reward or non-reward (25%), the intention to move or not (25%), or a combination of movement intention and reward expectation (11%) (Matsumoto, Suzuki & Tanaka 2003). Luk & Wallis (2013) described recordings in the same dorsal anterior cingulate cortex area that reflected the outcomes when monkeys made a choice of a left or right lever response to obtain a reward outcome, and also described a weak dissociation for more stimulus-outcome neurons in the orbitofrontal cortex, that is when monkeys had to choose the reward outcome based on which visual stimulus was shown. In the same dorsal anterior cingulate area neurons were more likely to take into account the costs of the actions required to obtain rewards, as well as the probability of obtaining the reward, than were neurons in the orbitofrontal cortex (Kennerley & Wallis 2009, Kennerley, Behrens & Wallis 2011, Kolling et al. 2016). In the dorsal anterior cingulate cortex, neurons may reflect evidence about the several most recent rewards, and use this to help guide choices (Kolling et al. 2016). More ventrally in the anterior cingulate cortex, neurons are more likely to reflect reward outcome rather than primarily actions (Cai & Padoa-Schioppa 2012).

Foraging studies also implicate the anterior cingulate cortex in representing value, and in taking into account costs. Hayden, Pearson & Platt (2011) taught monkeys a simple computerized foraging task in which they could chose to continue foraging in the same patch for diminishing returns, or seek an alternative patch at the expense of paying a cost of a travel delay before foraging could resume. Single neurons in the anterior cingulate cortex that fire to reward receipt did so at an increasing rate as monkeys moved towards leaving a known patch to search for a new one. Patch moving was initiated when the anterior cingulate cortex activity reached a threshold. The threshold firing rate that had to be reached was proportional to the search costs that were to be incurred by switching away from the current foraging patch.

In a neuroimaging study that provides evidence that the anterior cingulate cortex is active when outcome information guides choices made by the individual (Walton et al. 2004), the activations were relatively far back in the anterior cingulate cortex (y=22) towards the midcingulate cortex. This is consistent with the hypothesis that the reward value information in the pregenual cingulate cortex and the negative value representations just behind and dorsal to this in the anterior cingulate cortex are projected posteriorly towards the midcingulate area for interfacing to action.

4.7.4 Anterior cingulate cortex lesion effects

Lesion studies in monkeys (Rudebeck et al. 2008) and humans (Camille, Tsuchida & Fellows 2011), have demonstrated a dissociation in the role of the anterior cingulate cortex in action–outcome associations to guide behaviour; and of the orbitofrontal cortex in stimulus–outcome associations to update expected value (Rushworth, Kolling, Sallet & Mars 2012). Lesions of the anterior cingulate cortex in rats impair he ability to take into account the costs of actions, and this is supported by a neuroimaging study in humans (Croxson, Walton, O'Reilly, Behrens & Rushworth 2009).

An investigation more closely related to the understanding of emotion showed that patients with selective surgical lesions of the antero-ventral part of the anterior cingulate cortex (ACC) and/or medial BA9 were in some cases impaired on voice and face expression identification, had some change in social behaviour, such as inappropriateness, and had significant changes in their subjective emotional state (Hornak, Bramham, Rolls, Morris, O'Doherty, Bullock & Polkey 2003).

There is also neuroimaging evidence that complements the effects of lesions (Hornak et al. 2003) in suggesting a role for certain medial regions in the subjective experience of emotion. In neuroimaging studies with normal human subjects bilateral activations in Medial BA9 were found as subjects viewed emotion-laden stimuli, and in both Medial BA9 as well as in ventral ACC during self-generated emotional experience (i.e., in the absence of a stimulus) as subjects recalled emotions of sadness or happiness (Lane, Reiman, Ahern, Schwartz & Davidson 1997b, Lane, Reiman, Bradley, Lang, Ahern, Davidson & Schwartz 1997c, Lane, Reiman, Axelrod, Yun, Holmes & Schwartz 1998, Phillips, Drevets, Rauch & Lane 2003). On the basis of a review of imaging studies which consistently emphasize the importance of anterior and ventral regions of the anterior cingulate cortex for emotion, Bush, Luu & Posner (2000) argue that the anterior cingulate cortex can be divided into a ventral 'affective' division (which includes the subcallosal region and the part anterior to the corpus callosum), and a dorsal 'cognitive' division, a view strengthened by the demonstration of reciprocally inhibitory interactions between these two regions.

The subgenual part (area 25) of the anterior cingulate cortex is, via its outputs to the hypothalamus and brainstem autonomic regions, involved in the autonomic component of emotion (Koski & Paus 2000, Barbas & Pandya 1989, Ongur & Price 2000, Gabbott, Warner, Jays & Bacon 2003, Vogt 2009). The anterior cingulate cortex is also activated in relation to autonomic events, and Nagai, Critchley, Featherstone, Trimble & Dolan (2004) have shown that there is a correlation with skin conductance, a measure of autonomic activity related to sympathetic activation, in the anterior cingulate cortex and related areas. The dorsal anterior and mid-cingulate cortical areas may be especially related to blood pressure, pupil size, heart rate, and electrodermal activity, whereas the subgenual cingulate cortex, with ventromedial prefrontal cortex, appears antisympathetic (and parasympathetic) (Critchley & Harrison 2013).

A current working hypothesis is that the affective part of the anterior cingulate cortex receives inputs about expected rewards and punishers, and about the rewards and punishers received, from the orbitofrontal cortex and amygdala. There is some segregation of the areas that receive these inputs. The anterior cingulate cortex may compare these signals, take into account the cost of actions, and utilize the value representations in action–outcome learning.

4.7.5 Mid-cingulate cortex, the cingulate motor area, and action–outcome learning

The anterior or perigenual cingulate area[3] may be distinguished from a mid-cingulate area (i.e. further back than the perigenual cingulate region and occupying approximately the middle third of the cingulate cortex), which has been termed the cingulate motor area (Vogt et al. 1996, Vogt, Berger & Derbyshire 2003, Vogt 2009). (Both may be included in what anatomically is sometimes designated as the anterior cingulate cortex (Vogt 2009).) This area is also activated by pain but, because this area is also activated in response selection tasks such as divided attention and Stroop tasks (which involve cues that cause conflict such as the word red written in green when the task is to make a response to the green colour), it is suggested that activation of this mid-cingulate area by painful stimuli was related to the response selection processes initiated by painful stimuli (Vogt et al. 1996, Derbyshire, Vogt & Jones 1998). Both the perigenual and the mid-cingulate areas may be activated in functional neuroimaging studies not only by physical pain, but also by social pain, for example being excluded from a social group (Eisenberger & Lieberman 2004).

The mid-cingulate area may be divided into an anterior or rostral cingulate motor area (24c′) concerned with skeletomotor control which may be required in avoidance and fear tasks, and a posterior or caudal cingulate motor area (24d) which may be more involved in skeletomotor orientation (Vogt et al. 2003).

In human imaging studies it has been found that the anterior/mid-cingulate cortex is activated when there is a change in response set or when there is conflict between possible responses, but it is not activated when only stimulus selection is at issue (van Veen, Cohen, Botvinick, Stenger & Carter 2001, Rushworth, Hadland, Paus & Sipila 2002).

Some anterior/mid-cingulate neurons respond when errors are made (Niki & Watanabe 1979, Kolling et al. 2016), or when rewards are reduced (Shima & Tanji 1998) (and activations are found in corresponding imaging studies, (Bush, Vogt, Holmes, Dales, Greve, Jenike & Rosen 2002)). In humans, an event-related potential (ERP), called the error related negativity (ERN), may originate in the area 24c′ (Ullsperger & von Cramon 2001), and many studies provide evidence that errors made in many tasks activate the anterior/mid-cingulate cortex,

[3] Perigenual cingulate cortex refers to anterior cingulate cortex around the genu of the corpus callosum.

whereas tasks with response conflict activate the superior frontal gyrus (Rushworth et al. 2004, Kolling et al. 2016).

Correspondingly, in rodents a part of the medial prefrontal / anterior cingulate cortex termed the prelimbic cortex is involved in learning relations between behavioural responses and reinforcers, that is between actions and outcomes (Balleine & Dickinson 1998, Cardinal et al. 2002, Killcross & Coutureau 2003). Balleine & Dickinson (1998) showed that the sensitivity of instrumental behaviour to whether a particular action was followed by a reward was impaired by prelimbic cortex lesions. When making decisions about actions, it is important to take into account the costs as well as the benefits. There is some evidence implicating the rodent anterior cingulate cortex (prelimbic cortex) in this, in that rats with prelimbic cortex lesions were impaired in a task that required decisions about an action with a large reward but a high barrier to climb, vs an action with a lower reward but no barrier (Walton, Bannerman & Rushworth 2002, Walton et al. 2003).

4.8 Insula

There is some evidence that the face expression of disgust involves special processing by the insula. Not only is there some evidence that the insula can be differentially activated by the face expression of disgust (Phillips 2004, Phillips, Williams, Heining, Herba, Russell, Andrew, Bullmore, Brammer, Williams, Morgan, Young & Gray 2004), but also patient NK with an insular lesion is impaired on disgust face and voice expression identification, and on self-experience of disgust (Calder, Keane, Manes, Antoun & Young 2000). However, to place this into perspective, we have described a patient with a right amygdala lesion with an impairment of the recognition of disgust face expressions (Gallo, Gamiz, Perez-Garcia, Del Moral & Rolls 2014).

In a neuroeconomics study with monetary reward, it was found that expected value was negatively correlated with activations in the anterior insula [–38 24 16] in a region that has been implicated in disgust, and interestingly, the activations here were also correlated with the uncertainty of the magnitude of the reward that would be obtained (Rolls, McCabe & Redoute 2008e). Effectively there was more insula activation in situations that might be described as aversive. In a bargaining game which is a probe for fairness, the ultimatum game (Montague, King-Casas & Cohen 2006), insula activation was produced by unfair offers (Sanfey, Rilling, Aronson, Nystrom & Cohen 2003). [In the one-round ultimatum game, a pair of players is given an endowment, say $100. The first player proposes a split of the money to the second player, who can respond by either accepting the proposal (take it) or rejecting it (leave it). If the proposal is rejected, neither player receives any money. A rational agent model predicts that proposers should offer as little as possible, and responders should accept whatever they are offered because something is better than nothing. However, responders routinely reject offers less than about 20% of the endowment, and, correspondingly, proposers routinely offer significant amounts. Thus humans routinely act with a sense of 'fairness' in the ultimatum game. While this is not in their short-term interest, it is a strategy or heuristic that may have evolved to promote reciprocation and in the long run mutual benefit for reciprocators.]

Craig has suggested that not only are the human insular cortices involved in processing body feelings (such as pain, pleasure, and temperature) and feelings of emotions (Craig, Chen, Bandy & Reiman 2000, Damasio, Grabowski, Bechara, Damasio, Ponto, Parvizi & Hichwa 2000), but further, that the insular cortices are the necessary and sufficient platform for feeling states in humans and are, in effect, the sole source of their experience (Craig 2009, Craig 2011).

Damasio has suggested in his somatic marker hypothesis of emotion (Damasio 1996) that the insula and related somatosensory cortical areas play a crucial role in emotion and decision-making, by receiving feedback from the periphery that results in an emotion-related decision being made. However, feelings and sentience persist after bilateral damage of the insula (Damasio, Damasio & Tranel 2013).

Menon & Uddin (2010) have suggested that the insula is part of a 'salience' network. They postulate that the insula is sensitive to salient events, and that its core function is to mark such events for additional processing and initiate appropriate control signals.

These observations and thoughts (Berntson, Norman, Bechara, Bruss, Tranel & Cacioppo 2011) lead one to ask whether the insula is a crucial computational centre for emotion, decision-making, and even saliency. The following parsimonious points may be made.

First, the anterior part of the insula contains the primary taste cortex (Fig. 4.2), where neurons fire to tastes independently of hunger, where activations are linearly related to the intensity but not the pleasantness of the taste, and where some neurons respond also to oral viscosity, to oral temperature, and to fat texture in the mouth, but do not respond to visual or olfactory stimuli in discrimination tasks in which a taste or flavour is the reward (Sections 5.3.1.1 and 4.5.3.1, and Chapter 5). Thus the primary taste cortex contains a representation of what the taste is, and not of its outcome value, expected value, or emotional / affective properties (Rolls 2016b). In an even more anterior part of the insula (agranular cortex), there is a region that responds to both taste and odour stimuli (De Araujo, Rolls, Kringelbach, McGlone & Phillips 2003c, McCabe & Rolls 2007).

Second, there is a visceral / autonomic part of the anterior insula that is probably just ventral to the taste insula. This receives visceral inputs from the thalamus (ventral posteromedial nucleus (Carmichael & Price 1995b)), and projects to the orbitofrontal cortex. (The visceral insular cortex neurons are probably the ventral group of insular cortex cells found by Baylis, Rolls & Baylis (1994)). Some of the connections of this insular cortical region, including its connections with the anterior cingulate cortex, are shown in Fig. 4.30, which indicates that this part of the anteroventral insula may be thought of as the primary visceral cortex, with important functions on the efferent side in regulating autonomic output via the vagus and sympathetic nerves. This part of the insula has activations that are related to visceral / autonomic function, for example to heart and stomach responses during disgust-associated nausea (Harrison, Gray, Gianaros & Critchley 2010, Critchley & Harrison 2013, Nagai et al. 2004, Hassanpour, Simmons, Feinstein, Luo, Lapidus, Bodurka, Paulus & Khalsa 2018). Further, Krolak-Salmon, Henaff, Isnard, Tallon-Baudry, Guenot, Vighetto, Bertrand & Mauguiere (2003) found that electrical stimulation in the antero-ventral insula produced feelings related to disgust, including viscero-autonomic feelings. Moreover, it is of course to be expected, and is the case, that the autonomic output and the corresponding visceral insular activity will be different for different emotional states, e.g. when eating a food vs when reacting to the disgusting bitter taste of quinine or to pain or the sight of aversive or unpleasant stimuli (Harrison et al. 2010, Critchley & Harrison 2013).

Based on evidence of this type, I make the parsimonious hypothesis that the role of the anterior insula in emotion, disgust including face expressions of disgust, and salience, is that it receives inputs from cortical areas such as the anterior cingulate cortex and orbitofrontal cortex that are involved in the fundamental computations for emotion, and, as the 'head ganglion' of the autonomic nervous system, the anteroventral insula is involved in producing autonomic responses, via pathways of the type illustrated in Fig. 4.30.

Third, the mid- and posterior insula has somatosensory representations of the body (Mufson & Mesulam 1982). A property that may be special about these somatosensory cortical representations is that activations are produced by touch to the body but, in con-

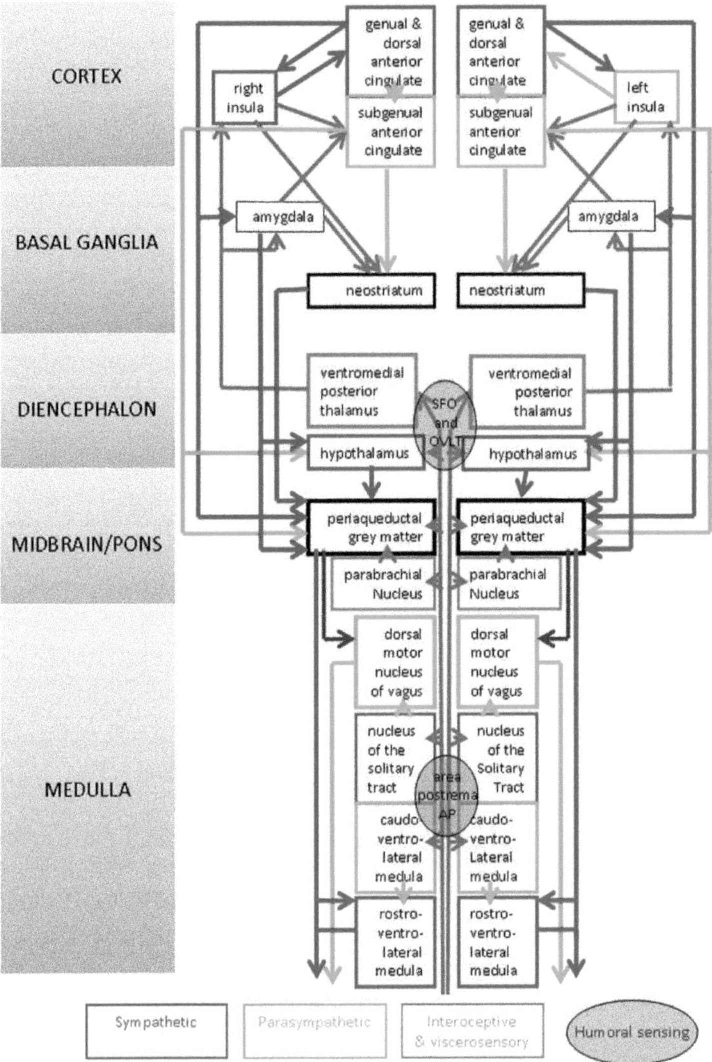

Fig. 4.30 Afferent and efferent neural pathways mediating autonomic system function. Brain regions are linked according to their association with visceral afferent sympathetic and parasympathetic function. SFO: Subfornical organ. OVLT: organum vasculosum of the lamina terminalis. (Reprinted from *Neuron*, 77 (4), Hugo D. Critchley and Neil A. Harrison, Visceral Influences on Brain and Behavior, pp. 624–638. Figure 3, doi.org/10.1016/j.neuron.2013.02.008.)

trast to many other somatosensory cortical areas, not by the sight of touch (McCabe, Rolls, Bilderbeck & McGlone 2008). It was therefore suggested that insular cortex activation thus allows an individual to know that it is touch to the person's body, and not that someone else's body is about to be touched (McCabe, Rolls, Bilderbeck & McGlone 2008). The insular somatosensory cortex may thus provide evidence about what is happening to one's own body (Rolls 2010c). The same might be said of the insular primary taste cortex, which when activated leaves no doubt that one is tasting, and not seeing someone else tasting. So, in a sense, feelings associated with activations of the insular cortex (and they are: the subjective intensity of taste is linearly related to the activation of the primary taste cortex) do inform one about the state of one's own body, and this relates to Craig's suggestions (2009, 2011)

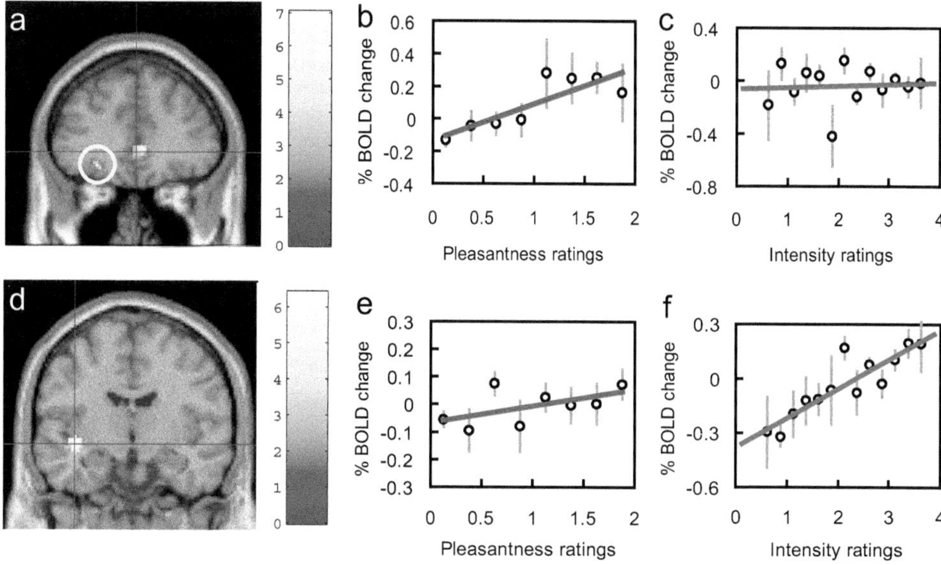

Fig. 4.31 Representation of the pleasantness but not intensity of thermal stimuli in the orbitofrontal cortex (top), and of the intensity but not the pleasantness in the mid ventral (somatosensory) insular cortex (bottom). a. SPM analysis showing a correlation in the mid orbitofrontal cortex (blue circle) at [-26 38 -10] between the BOLD signal and the pleasantness ratings of four thermal stimuli. Correlations are also shown in the pregenual cingulate cortex. For this mid orbitofrontal cortex region, (b) shows the positive correlation between the subjective pleasantness ratings and the BOLD signal ($r=0.84$, $df=7$, $p<0.01$), and (c) shows that there is no correlation between the subjective intensity ratings and the BOLD signal ($r=0.07$, $df=12$, $p=0.8$). d. SPM analysis showing a correlation with intensity in the posterior ventral insula with peak at [-40 -10 -8] between the BOLD signal and the intensity ratings for the four thermal stimuli. For this ventral insula cortex region, (e) shows no correlation between the subjective pleasantness ratings and the BOLD signal ($r=0.56$, $df=7$, $p=0.15$), and (f) shows a positive correlation between the subjective intensity ratings and the BOLD signal ($r=0.89$, $df=12$, $p<0.001$). (Reprinted from *Neuroimage* 41, Edmund T. Rolls, Fabian Grabenhorst and Benjamin A. Parris, Warm pleasant feelings in the brain, pp. 1504–1513, doi.org/10.1016/j.neuroimage.2008.03.005.)

about interoceptive feelings. However, this does not mean that the insular cortex is necessary for body feelings, and indeed that seems to be ruled out by the finding that a patient with extensive bilateral damage to the insular cortex reported normal body / emotional feelings (Damasio et al. 2013).

Finally, the insular somatosensory representations do not appear to be affective, i.e. they do not encode the pleasantness of somatosensory stimuli. In an fMRI investigation in humans, it was found that activations in the somatosensory cortex and ventral posterior insula were correlated with the intensity ratings but not the pleasantness ratings of thermal stimuli, which were warm (41°C), cold (12°C) stimuli, and combinations of warm and cold stimuli, applied to the hand (see Fig. 4.31d-f) (Rolls, Grabenhorst & Parris 2008b). In contrast, the mid-orbitofrontal and pregenual cingulate cortex and a region to which they project, the ventral striatum, had activations that correlated with the subjective pleasantness ratings made to thermal stimuli (Fig. 4.31a-c) (Rolls et al. 2008b).

4.9 Effects of emotion on cognitive processing and memory

The analyses above of the neural mechanisms of emotion have been concerned primarily with how stimuli are decoded to produce emotional states, and with how these states can influence behaviour. In addition, current mood state can affect the cognitive evaluation of events or memories (Blaney 1986, Robinson, Watkins & Harmon-Jones 2013). For example, happy memories are more likely to be recalled when happy. Another example is that when people are in a depressed mood, they tend to recall memories that were stored when they were depressed. The recall of depressing memories when depressed can have the effect of perpetuating the depression, and this may be a factor with relevance to the aetiology and treatment of depression. Effectively in humans an attractor state may be set up between the cognitive and mood systems, which activate each other (Rolls & Stringer 2001), and tend to perpetuate the depressed state.

A normal function of the effects of mood state on memory recall might be to facilitate continuity in the interpretation of the reinforcing value of events in the environment, or in the interpretation of an individual's behaviour by others, or simply to keep behaviour motivated to a particular goal. Another possibility is that the effects of mood on memory do not have adaptive value, but are a consequence of having a general cortical architecture with backprojections (Rolls 2016c). According to the latter hypothesis, the selection pressure is great for leaving the general architecture operational, rather than trying to find a genetic way to switch off backprojections just for the projections of mood systems back to perceptual systems (Rolls & Stringer 2000).

How does mood affect memory?

It is suggested that whenever memories are stored, part of the context is stored with the memory. This is very likely to happen in associative neuronal networks such as those in the hippocampus (Rolls 1989, Rolls 2000d, Rolls 1990b, Rolls 1996, Treves & Rolls 1994, Rolls & Treves 1998, Rolls, Stringer & Trappenberg 2002, Rolls 2004a, Rolls & Kesner 2006, Rolls & Xiang 2006, Rolls 2016c, Rolls 2010b, Rolls 2013c, Rolls 2015d, Kesner & Rolls 2015, Rolls 2018). The CA3 part of the hippocampus may operate as a single autoassociative memory capable of linking together almost arbitrary co-occurrences of inputs, including inputs about emotional state that reach the entorhinal cortex from, for example, the amygdala. Recall of a memory occurs best in such networks when the input key to the memory is nearest to the original input pattern of activity that was stored (Rolls & Treves 1990, Treves & Rolls 1991, Treves & Rolls 1992, Treves & Rolls 1994, Rolls, Treves, Foster & Perez-Vicente 1997b, Rolls & Treves 1998, Rolls 2016c). It thus follows that a memory of, for example, a happy episode is recalled best when in a happy mood state. This is a special case of a general theory of how context is stored with a memory, and of how context influences recall (Treves & Rolls 1994, Rolls 1996, Rolls 2016c, Rolls 2018). The recall itself from the hippocampus is likely to use the highly developed backprojections from the hippocampus to the neocortex (Treves & Rolls 1994, Rolls 1996, Rolls 2016c, Rolls 2018). The effect of emotional state on cognitive processing and memory is thus suggested to be a particular case of a more general way in which context can affect the storage and retrieval of memories, or can affect cognitive processing.

There is now direct evidence that the hippocampus, which is implicated in the memory for past episodes (Rolls & Treves 1998, Rolls 1999b, Rolls et al. 2002, Rolls 2016c, Rolls 2010b, Rolls 2018), contains neurons in primates that respond to combinations of spatial information and reward information (Rolls & Xiang 2005), as described next. The ability to form associations between events including where they occur and what is present is a fundamental property of episodic memory (Treves & Rolls 1994, Rolls 1996, Rolls &

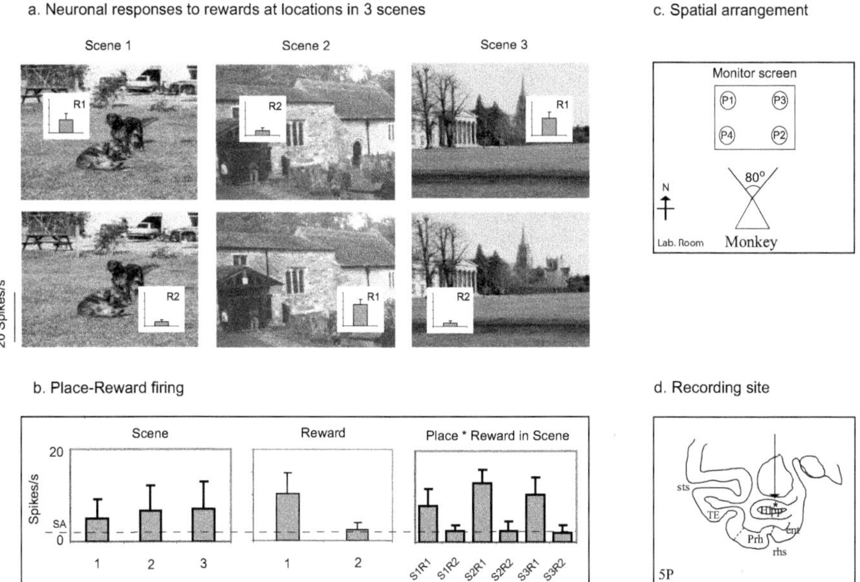

Fig. 4.32 A hippocampal neuron that encoded the particular rewards available at different locations in different scenes. On each trial the monkey could touch a circled location in the scene, and, depending on the location, received either a preferred juice reward or a less preferred juice reward. (a) Firing rate inserts to show the firing in 3 different scenes (S1–S3) of the locations associated with reward 1 (R1, preferred) and reward 2 (R2, less preferred). The mean responses $\pm$ s.e.m. are shown. SA, spontaneous firing rate. (b) The firing rates sorted by scene, by reward (1 vs 2), and by scene–reward combinations (e.g. scene 1 reward 1 = S1R1). (c) The spatial arrangement on the screen of the 4 spatial locations (P1–P4). (d) The recording site of the neuron. ent, entorhinal cortex; Hipp, hippocampal pyramidal cell field CA3/CA1 and dentate gyrus; Prh, perirhinal cortex; rhs, rhinal sulcus; sts, superior temporal sulcus; TE, inferior temporal visual cortex. (Reproduced from E. T. Rolls, and J. Z. Xiang, Reward–spatial view representations and learning in the primate hippocampus, *The Journal of Neuroscience* 25, pp. 6167–6174. doi.org/10.1523/JNEUROSCI.1481-05.2005. Copyright © 2005, The Society for Neuroscience.)

Kesner 2006, Rolls 2016c, Rolls 2010b, Rolls 2018, Kesner & Rolls 2015), and this neurophysiological evidence shows that reward-related information, relevant to affect and mood, is associated with other events in the representations in the primate hippocampus (Rolls 2015d). The primate anterior hippocampus (which corresponds to the rodent ventral hippocampus) receives inputs from brain regions involved in reward processing such as the amygdala and orbitofrontal cortex via the entorhinal and perirhinal cortex (Amaral et al. 1992, Suzuki & Amaral 1994, Pitkanen, Kelly & Amaral 2002, Stefanacci, Suzuki & Amaral 1996, Ongur & Price 2000, Price 2006).

To investigate how this affective input may be incorporated into primate hippocampal function, Rolls & Xiang (2005) recorded neuronal activity while macaques performed a reward–place association task in which each spatial scene shown on a video monitor had one location that if touched yielded a preferred fruit juice reward, and a second location that yielded a less preferred juice reward. Each scene had different locations for the different rewards. An example of a hippocampal neuron recorded in this task is shown in Fig. 4.32. The neuron responded more to the location in each scene at which the preferred reward was available.

Of 409 neurons analysed, 16% responded more to the location of the preferred reward in different scenes, and 4% to the location of the less preferred reward (Rolls & Xiang

2005). When the locations of the preferred rewards in the scenes were reversed, 70% of 50 neurons tested reversed the location to which they responded, showing that the reward–place associations could be altered by new learning in a few trials. The majority (80%) of these 50 reward–place neurons tested did not respond to object–reward associations in a visual discrimination object–reward association task. Thus the primate hippocampus contains a representation of the reward associations of places 'out there' being viewed, and this is a way in which affective information can be stored as part of an episodic memory, and how the current mood state may influence the retrieval of episodic memories. There is consistent evidence that rewards available in a spatial environment can influence the responsiveness of rodent place neurons (Hölscher, Jacob & Mallot 2003, Tabuchi, Mulder & Wiener 2003) which respond to the place where the animal is located, not to the view of a place 'out there' (Rolls 1999b, De Araujo, Rolls & Stringer 2001).

This discovery of reward–spatial view neurons built on findings that some hippocampal neurons in primates respond to the place at which the monkey is looking. These spatial view neurons (Rolls, Robertson & Georges-François 1997a, Rolls, Treves, Robertson, Georges-François & Panzeri 1998b, Robertson, Rolls & Georges-François 1998, Rolls 1999b, Rolls & Xiang 2006, Rolls 2010b, Rolls & Wirth 2018) code for particular locations at which the monkey is looking in allocentric (world-based rather than egocentric) space, and do not encode the place where the monkey is located (Georges-François, Rolls & Robertson 1999, Rolls, Treves, Robertson, Georges-François & Panzeri 1998b, Rolls & Wirth 2018). Part of the interest of spatial view cells is that they could provide the spatial representation required to enable primates to perform object–place memory, for example remembering where they saw a person or object, which is an example of an episodic memory. Consistent with this, some hippocampal neurons respond in object–place memory tasks to combinations of the object being shown and where it is being shown in space (Rolls, Miyashita, Cahusac, Kesner, Niki, Feigenbaum & Bach 1989a, Rolls, Xiang & Franco 2005b, Rolls & Wirth 2018).

Thus the primate hippocampus contains a representation of places 'out there', and can combine this information by associative learning not only with which object is present at the viewed location (Rolls, Xiang & Franco 2005b, Rolls & Xiang 2006), but also with which reward is present at the viewed location (Rolls & Xiang 2005).

The general principle here then is that the hippocampus may store information about where emotion-related (e.g. rewarding) events happened; may take part in the recall of emotions when particular places are seen again; is part of a hippocampus-related limbic system that is largely independent of limbic structures involved in emotion (Rolls 2015d); and may provide a system in which the current mood can influence which memories are recalled (Rolls & Xiang 2006, Rolls 2016c, Rolls 2010b, Rolls & Wirth 2018).

4.10 Summary of brain systems involved in emotion

Some of the fundamental architectural and design principles of the brain for sensory, reward, and punishment information processing relevant to emotion in primates *including humans* include the following:

1. For primary reinforcers, the reward value encoding may occur after several stages of processing, as in the primate taste system in which reward is decoded only after the primary taste cortex. The architectural principle here is that in primates there is one main taste information-processing stream in the brain, via the thalamus to the primary taste cortex, and the information about the identity of the taste is not biased with modulation by how good the taste is before this. Thus the taste representation in the primary taste cortex can be used for purposes that are not reward-dependent. For example, it may be important to learn about a particular taste, even if one is not hungry. Even for the primary reinforcers of pleasant touch and pain, although there are different peripheral nerve fibres for pain and touch, it appears that the affective component in primates involves especially the activation of higher cortical areas such as the orbitofrontal cortex, as shown by functional neuroimaging studies and by the effects of damage to the orbitofrontal cortex.

2. For potential secondary reinforcers, analysis is to the stage of invariant object identification in structures such as the inferior temporal visual cortex (Tier 1 in Fig. 4.2) before reward and punisher associations are learned. The reason for this is to enable correct generalization to other instances of the same or similar objects, when a reward or punisher has been associated with as little as one instance (e.g. one view of an object) previously.

3. The representation of the object provided at the end of 'what' processing streams (e.g. the inferior temporal visual cortex) is (appropriately) in a form which is ideal as an input to pattern associators which allow the associations with primary reinforcers to be learned at the next stage of processing. The representations are appropriately encoded in that they can be decoded by dot product decoding of the type that is very neuronally plausible; are distributed so allowing excellent generalization and graceful degradation; have relatively independent information conveyed by different neurons in the ensemble thus allowing very high capacity; and allow much of the information to be read off very quickly, in periods of 20–50 ms.

4. Especially in primates, the visual processing in emotional and social behaviour requires sophisticated representation of individuals using face identity, and for this there are many neurons devoted to face processing. In addition, there is a separate system that encodes face expression, gesture, movement, and view, as all are important in social behaviour, for interpreting whether a particular individual, with his or her own reinforcement associations, is producing threats or appeasements.

5. After mainly unimodal processing to the object level, sensory systems then project into convergence zones. Those especially important for reward and punishment value, and therefore for emotion and motivation, are the orbitofrontal cortex and amygdala (in Tier 2), where primary reinforcers are represented in terms of their value. These parts of the brain appear to be especially important in emotion and motivation not only because they are the parts of the brain where in primates the primary (unlearned) reward or punisher value of stimuli is represented, but also because they are the parts of the brain that perform pattern-association learning between potential secondary reinforcers and primary reinforcers to compute expected value. They are thus the parts of the brain involved in learning the emotional and motivational value of stimuli.

6. The value and expected value representations in the orbitofrontal cortex take into account 'risk', i.e. the probability of obtaining a reward outcome, reward magnitude, the temporal discounting of reward value, and the 'intrinsic costs' of stimuli i.e. whether there are positive and negative components, to represent the economic value of stimuli (Rolls 2014b, Grabenhorst & Rolls 2011). The value representations are on a common scale, but are not converted into a common single currency, in that different single neurons respond to different rewarding and punishing stimuli. Further evidence that the orbitofrontal cortex provides a value representation is that orbitofrontal cortex neuronal responses and activations selectively decrease to zero during devaluation experiments such as feeding to satiety. The value representations are of stimuli, and actions and responses made are not clearly represented in the orbitofrontal cortex.

7. The activations in the orbitofrontal cortex are linearly related to the subjective value, the subjective consciously reported affective pleasantness or unpleasantness of stimuli, and these representations thus drive the subjective experience of *pleasure* in the explicit system, which is considered further in Chapter 10.

8. The orbitofrontal cortex represents the value of stimuli on a continuous scale. For decisions between stimuli of different value, there is evidence that a more anterior region identified as the *medial prefrontal cortex area 10 is involved in the choice decision-making mechanism*, and that decision confidence is represented in medial area 10, as described further in Chapter 8.

9. The orbitofrontal cortex is involved in the rapid, one-trial, rule-based, reversal of the value assigned to a stimulus and of emotional behaviour when the instrumental reinforcement contingencies change. This very rapid reversal may be implemented by switching a rule, and is probably one of the developments made possible by the great development of the granular prefrontal cortex including the granular orbitofrontal cortex areas that appear not to be present in rodents. The rapid reversal which is provided by the orbitofrontal cortex much more than the amygdala may be facilitated by the recurrent collateral connections between neurons in the orbitofrontal cortex, which provide for a short-term memory of the current rule. The orbitofrontal cortex thus allows flexibility of emotional behaviour, and rapid sensitivity to the changes in the reinforcers being received. This is very important in primates (including humans), in which it is important in social situations to change behaviour rapidly to what may be subtle cues, such as changes in face expression.

10. Cognitive inputs and states that are decoded as reinforcing and thus lead to emotions are represented in the orbitofrontal cortex. An example is monetary reward or loss. Modulation by cognition of the reinforcement or subjective affective value of stimuli also is expressed in the orbitofrontal cortex. An example is the modulating effect that a word can have on the pleasantness vs unpleasantness value of a test odour, taste, flavour, or touch which is represented in the orbitofrontal cortex.

11. Damage to the orbitofrontal cortex in humans can affect subjective emotional states, can impair emotional behaviour (producing for example some disinhibition and uncooperativeness), can be associated with personality changes including increased impulsiveness, and can impair the ability to identify correctly face and voice expressions.

12. The outputs of the amygdala are involved in many Pavlovian (classically conditioned) effects of stimuli on behaviour, including the elicitation of autonomic responses, and via the ventral striatum of Pavlovian effects on instrumental behaviour, such as Pavlovian-instrumental transfer (PIT).

13. The outputs of the orbitofrontal cortex may be used in structures such as the anterior cingulate cortex for action–outcome learning. As part of this, the pregenual part of the anterior cingulate cortex provides a representation, received from the orbitofrontal cortex, of positive value; and the anterodorsal part of the anterior cingulate cortex provides a representation of negative value. Damage to these anterior cingulate cortex regions does alter emotional behaviour, for example to face expressions, and does alter the subjective experience of emotion. In implementing action–outcome learning, which depends on the value of the goal, the cingulate cortex takes into account the costs of actions required to obtain the rewards (which have been termed extrinsic costs (Grabenhorst & Rolls 2011, Rolls 2014b)).

14. The outputs of the orbitofrontal cortex, amygdala, and anterior cingulate cortex are used in the basal ganglia for stimulus–response (habit) learning (see further Section 6.3).

15. The outputs of the orbitofrontal cortex, amygdala, and anterior cingulate cortex are used, in part via the insula, hypothalamus and brainstem, in autonomic responses to emotion-provoking stimuli that prepare the body. Activations in the anterior insula to emotion-provoking stimuli may reflect the use of these outputs of the orbitofrontal cortex, amygdala, and anterior cingulate cortex in the elicitation of autonomic including visceral, heart-rate, etc. responses.

16. A separate route to action is provided by an explicit, language-based system, for humans can sometimes state verbally what action they should have taken to a reinforcer, even though after orbitofrontal cortex damage they may not have made the appropriate choice when reinforcement contingencies change.

17. A subcallosal anterior cingulate cortex region is implicated in depression, in that it is activated by sadness induction, in that neurons in it respond to negative stimuli, and in that treatments for depression may alter activity in this region, as described in Chapter 9. Deep brain stimulation for depression in a nearby area may activate the reward value system that extends from the orbitofrontal cortex through the pregenual cingulate cortex to medial prefrontal cortex area 10.

18. In non-primates including rodents, the design principles may involve less sophisticated design features, partly because the stimuli being processed are simpler. For example, view-invariant object recognition is less developed in non-primates, with the recognition that is possible being based more on physical similarity in terms of texture, colour, simple features, etc. It may be because there is less sophisticated cortical processing of visual stimuli that other sensory systems are also organized more simply, with, for example, some (approximately 30%) modulation of taste processing by hunger early in sensory processing in rodents (Rolls & Scott 2003), and even connectivity of the taste system that allows brainstem taste processing to gain direct access to the amygdala without cortical processing. Further, while it is appropriate usually to have emotional responses to well-processed objects or individuals (e.g. the sight of a particular person), there are instances, such as a loud noise or a pure tone associated with punishment, where it may be possible to tap off a sensory representation early in sensory information processing that can be used to produce emotional responses. This may occur, for example, in rodents, where the subcortical auditory system provides afferents to the amygdala. Another important difference from rodents may be the use of rules that can be rapidly reversed by switching attractor network states, using mechanisms especially developed in the granular prefrontal including orbitofrontal cortical areas of primates and humans (Rolls 2016c).

5 Food reward value, pleasure, appetite, hunger, and over-eating

5.1 Overview

Food tastes pleasant when we are hungry, and is a reward. The representations of affective value in the relevant brain system are important, for they control how much we eat, and influence whether we overeat. Moreover, we can analyse in the neural systems that control food intake how reward value and its subjective correlate affective / emotional value or pleasantness are determined, and how different rewards are represented.

The reward value of food (measured by how hard we will work for the food, and whether we choose it), and its subjective complement, the rated affective pleasantness of food, is decoded in primates including humans only after several stages of analysis.

First the representation of the taste of the food (its identity and intensity) is made explicit in neuronal firing in the primary taste cortex. Similarly, for vision, objects are represented in the inferior temporal visual cortex, but only as objects, and not in terms of their reward or affective value.

Only later, in the orbitofrontal cortex, is the reward value made explicit in the representation, for it is here that satiety signals modulate the responses of the taste, olfactory, flavour, and sight of food neurons.

Thus in the control of food intake, the reward value or pleasantness is crucial to the design of how food intake is controlled, and the reward value is represented only in specialized cortical areas.

The orbitofrontal cortex is moreover where multimodal representations of food are built, which include taste, texture, olfactory, and visual components. Moreover, different neurons respond to different combinations of all the properties, and this provides a mechanism for the sensory-specific satiety described below.

The actual satiety signals are complex, and include gastric distension, gut satiety signals, plasma glucose, and hormones such as leptin.

Sensory-specific satiety is an important principle in the control of food reward. It describes the fact that the pleasantness and reward value of food decrease for a particular food eaten to satiety, but may remain high for other foods not eaten in the meal. This has biological utility, in encouraging the selection of a range of foods with different nutrients. I discovered this while recording from hypothalamic neurons, and then showed that it is computed in the orbitofrontal cortex, for the taste, smell, texture, flavour, and sight of food. Sensory-specific satiety is the most important factor influencing the amount of food eaten in a meal. Because of sensory-specific satiety, the availability of a wide variety of food can increase the amount of food eaten.

My theory is that sensory-specific satiety applies to all reward systems, because it has adaptive value in encouraging animals (including humans) to switch their behaviour to another reward after some time, helping to ensure that many different rewards are chosen, which is in the interest of reproductive success. In contrast, sensory-specific satiety applies to no punishment system, for here it is adaptive to avoid or escape from the punisher.

The primate orbitofrontal cortex is more closely related to the changing affective value of food than the amygdala, in that the orbitofrontal cortex shows responses that decrease to zero as the reward value and subjective pleasantness decrease to zero with satiety, and in that the orbitofrontal cortex tracks (and probably computes) the changing food reward value of stimuli as they are altered by stimulus–reinforcer association learning and reversal.

The outputs of the orbitofrontal cortex reach brain regions such as the cingulate cortex and striatum, where behavioural responses to food may be initiated in order to make the orbitofrontal cortex reward neurons fire, as the firing of orbitofrontal cortex neurons represents a goal for behaviour. At the same time, outputs from the orbitofrontal cortex, cingulate cortex, and amygdala, in part via the insula and hypothalamus, may provide for appropriate autonomic and endocrine responses to food to be produced, including the release of hormones such as insulin.

In modern times, the palatability and availability of food has increased greatly, but the satiety mechanisms remain those that have evolved over hundreds of thousands of years. A consequence is that the enhanced activity in the food reward system may tend to override the satiety signals, contributing to over-eating and the obesity epidemic. Ways to counteract these obesogenic effects are described.

5.2 The control signals for hunger and satiety

5.2.1 Reward vs satiety signals

The reward value of food is produced by its taste, smell, flavour, texture and sight. This is shown by sham feeding experiments, in which food drains from the stomach so that no food is absorbed, and the food is still rewarding. Placing food in the stomach or intestine is much less rewarding, although tastes can become conditioned to food delivered to the intestine.

Satiety, but little reward, is produced by factors such as stomach distension, food entering the intestine, absorbed food then entering the blood stream, and hormones that are released. The evidence for these fundamental points, and for how neurons in the hypothalamus are influenced by the satiety signals, is described elsewhere (Rolls 2014b, Kim, Seeley & Sandoval 2018).

Here the focus is on the brain systems that make food rewarding and subjectively pleasant (Rolls 2016e, Rolls 2014b).

5.2.2 Sensory-specific satiety

During experiments on brain mechanisms of reward and satiety, E. T. Rolls and colleagues observed in 1974 that if a lateral hypothalamic neuron had ceased to respond to a food on which the monkey had been fed to satiety (a discovery described in *The Brain and Reward* (Rolls 1975)), then the neuron might still respond to a different food (see example in Fig. 5.1). This occurred for neurons with responses associated with the taste (Rolls 1981b, Rolls 1981a, Rolls, Murzi, Yaxley, Thorpe & Simpson 1986) or sight (Rolls 1981b, Rolls & Rolls 1982b, Rolls, Murzi, Yaxley, Thorpe & Simpson 1986) of food. Corresponding to this neuronal specificity

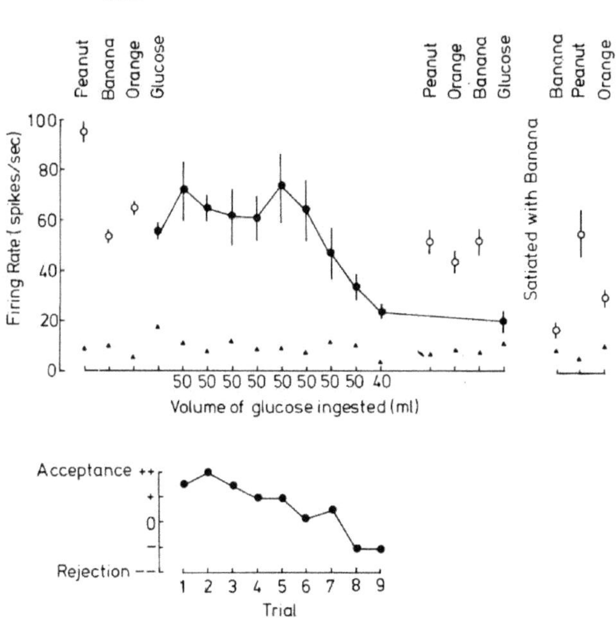

Fig. 5.1 The effect of feeding the monkey to satiety with 20% glucose solution on the responses of a lateral hypothalamic neuron to the sight the glucose (filled circles) and to the sight of other foods (open circles). After the monkey had fed to satiety with glucose, the neuron responded much less to the sight of glucose, but still responded to the other foods. The mean responses of the neuron (± s.e.m.) are shown to the stimuli at different stages of the experiment. The satiety of the monkey, shown below, was measured by whether he accepted or rejected the glucose. After satiety with glucose, a second satiety experiment was performed in which banana was fed to satiety, and after this, the responses of the neuron decreased to the sight of the banana, but remained to the sight of peanut and orange, for which he still had an appetite. (Reprinted from *Brain Research*, 368, E. T. Rolls, E. Murzi, S. Yaxley, S. J. Thorpe and S. Simpson, Sensory-specific satiety: food-specific reduction in responsiveness of ventral forebrain neurons after feeding in the monkey, pp. 79–86. doi.org/10.1016/0006-8993(86)91044-9. Copyright © 1986 Published by Elsevier B.V.)

of the effects of feeding to satiety, the monkey rejected the food on which he had been fed to satiety, but accepted other foods that he had not been fed. I well remember the occasion on which we discovered sensory-specific satiety in 1974 when we were recording from a lateral hypothalamic neuron in the monkey that responded to the sight of glucose (fed to the monkey from a syringe) and other foods. We fed the monkey to satiety with glucose, and observed the neuronal response to the glucose fall to zero, as illustrated for one such neuron in Fig. 5.1. I then showed the monkey a peanut, and heard a large response of the neuron, which was confirmed by the high firing rate printed out by the PDP11 computer. I was disconcerted at first because the monkey was supposed to be satiated, having drunk as much glucose as it wanted. However, I had the presence of mind to offer the peanut to the monkey, and found that the monkey reached out for the peanut, and avidly consumed it. I realized that something interesting was happening in terms of the brain mechanisms that implement satiety, and repeated the observations a number of times, confirming that the lateral hypothalamic neuron did not respond to the sight of the glucose and that the monkey did not accept the glucose, whereas the neuron did respond vigorously to the sight of the peanut, which the monkey avidly reached for and ate. The fact that quantitative firing rates were being printed out quantitatively helped to impress on me the fact that this was a strong effect, which we

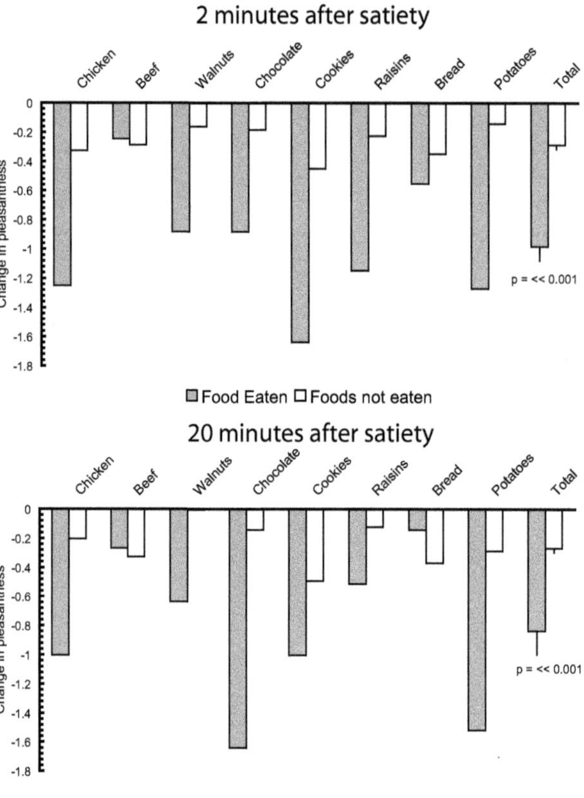

Fig. 5.2 Sensory-specific satiety for the flavour of a food. The change in the pleasantness of the flavour of food after eating one to satiety. For each food, the change of pleasantness after eating that food to satiety is shown (food eaten), compared to the average change of pleasantness of the other foods not eaten in the meal. The ratings are on a scale from +2 very pleasant to –2 very unpleasant, and the change of pleasantness rating from before until after eating one of the foods to satiety is shown. The ratings were made by a group of participants 2 min and 20 min after eating one of the foods to satiety for lunch. (Reprinted from *Physiology and Behavior*, 27 (1), Barbara J. Rolls, Edmund T. Rolls, Edward A. Rowe, and Kevin Sweeney, Sensory specific satiety in man, pp. 137–142. doi.org/10.1016/0031-9384(81)90310-3. Copyright © 1981 Published by Elsevier Inc.)

termed sensory-specific satiety. The neurophysiological finding was published for example in Rolls (1981b) and Rolls et al. (1986). This is now described as a devaluation procedure, and provides evidence that these, and orbitofrontal cortex neurons which provide inputs to the lateral hypothalamus, encode **value**.

I lectured on the result to my Oxford undergraduate class, and proposed an experiment to explore the effect in humans. The experiment was performed as an undergraduate practical (with Barbara Rolls as a co-organizer) in which humans rated the pleasantness and intensity of 6 foods, and then ate one of the foods to satiety. Whichever food was eaten to satiety showed a large decrease in the pleasantness rating, whereas other foods that had not been eaten to satiety showed a much smaller decrease, or in some cases even a small increase in pleasantness (e.g. for a sweet food after a savory food had been eaten to satiety), as shown in Fig. 5.2. The result was published by Rolls, Rolls, Rowe & Sweeney (1981a), and led to a series of other investigations on sensory-specific satiety described below.

We performed further experiments to determine whether satiety in humans is specific to

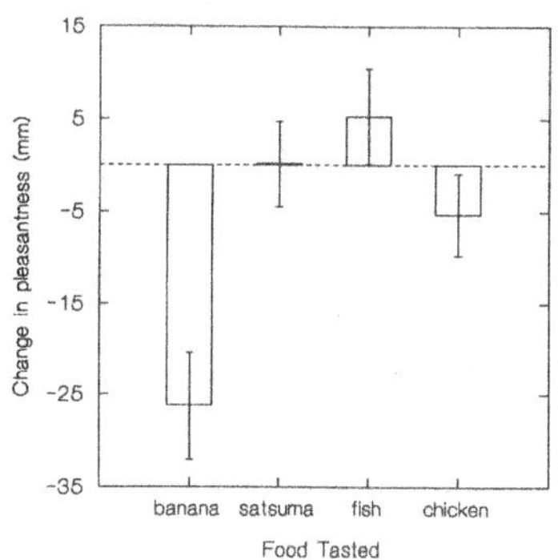

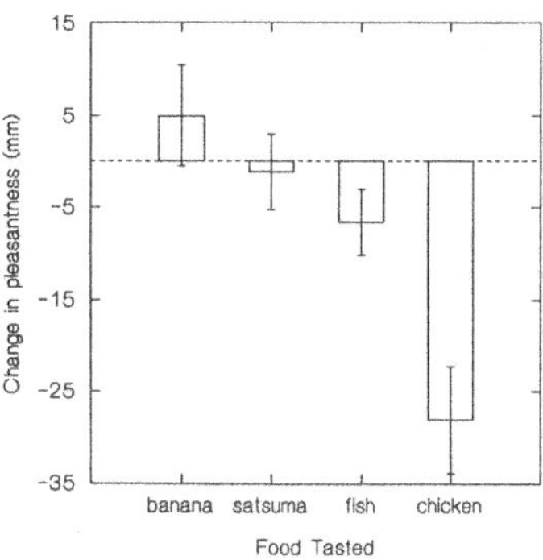

Fig. 5.3 Sensory-specific satiety for the flavour of a food: the changes in the pleasantness of the taste of four different foods after eating banana (left) or chicken (right) to satiety are shown. The change is shown as mm difference (± the standard error of the mean, s.e.m.) on a 100 mm visual analogue rating scale marked at one end 'very pleasant' and at the other end 'very unpleasant'. The decrease of pleasantness of the taste of a food was greater for the food eaten to satiety. (Reprinted from *Physiology and Behavior*, 61 (3), Edmund T. Rolls and Juliet H. Rolls, Olfactory Sensory-Specific Satiety in Humans, pp. 461–473. doi.org/10.1016/S0031-9384(96)00464-7. Copyright © 1997 Elsevier Science Inc. All rights reserved.)

foods eaten. These experiments were performed as a result of the neurophysiological and behavioural observations showing the specificity of satiety in the monkey (Rolls 1981b, Rolls 1981a, Rolls, Murzi, Yaxley, Thorpe & Simpson 1986), and the experiment illustrated in Fig. 5.2 In the further experiments, it was found that the pleasantness of the taste (Rolls et al. 1981a) and smell (Rolls & Rolls 1997) of food eaten to satiety decreased more than for foods that had not been eaten. The results of an experiment of this type are shown in Fig. 5.3.

One implication of this finding is that if one food is eaten to satiety, appetite reduction for other foods is often incomplete, and this should mean that in humans also at least some of the other foods will be eaten. This was confirmed by an experiment in which either sausages or cheese with crackers were eaten for lunch. The liking for the food eaten decreased more than for the food not eaten and, when an unexpected second course was offered, more was eaten if a subject had not been given that food in the first course than if he had been given that food in the first course (98% vs 40% of the first course intake eaten in the second courses, Rolls, Rolls, Rowe & Sweeney (1981a)).

A further implication of these findings is that if a variety of foods is available, the total amount consumed will be more than when only one food is offered repeatedly. This prediction was confirmed in a study in which humans ate more when offered a variety of sandwich fillings than one filling or a variety of types of yoghurt which differed in taste, texture, and colour (Rolls, Rowe, Rolls, Kingston, Megson & Gunary 1981b). It has also been confirmed in a study in which humans were offered a relatively normal meal of four courses, and it was found that the change of food at each course significantly enhanced intake (Rolls, Van Duijenvoorde & Rolls 1984a). Because sensory factors such as similarity of colour, shape, flavour, and texture are usually more important than metabolic equivalence in terms of energy, protein, carbohydrate, and fat content in influencing how foods interact in this type of satiety, it has been termed 'sensory-specific satiety' (Rolls & Rolls 1977, Rolls & Rolls 1982b, Rolls, Rolls, Rowe & Sweeney 1981a, Rolls, Rowe, Rolls, Kingston, Megson & Gunary 1981b, Rolls, Rowe & Rolls 1982a, Rolls, Rowe & Rolls 1982b, Rolls & Rolls 1997, Rolls 1999a, Rolls 2005).

It should be noted that sensory-specific satiety is distinct from alliesthesia, in that alliesthesia is a change in the pleasantness of sensory inputs produced by internal signals (such as glucose in the gut) (Cabanac & Duclaux 1970, Cabanac 1971, Cabanac & Fantino 1977), whereas sensory-specific satiety is a change in the pleasantness of sensory inputs which is accounted for at least partly by the external sensory stimulation received (such as the taste of a particular food), in that as shown above it is at least partly specific to the external sensory stimulation received. Further evidence for the sensory-driven nature of sensory-specific satiety is that it can be produced just by tasting or even smelling a food for a few minutes, without swallowing any of it (Rolls & Rolls 1997).

The parallel between these studies of feeding in humans and of the neurophysiology of hypothalamic neurons in the monkey has been extended by the observations that in humans, sensory-specific satiety occurs for the sight (Rolls, Rowe & Rolls 1982a) and smell (Rolls & Rolls 1997) as well as for the taste and even texture (Rolls, Rowe & Rolls 1982a) of food.

It is a general finding with sensory-specific satiety that the decrease is pleasantness is much greater than any decrease in intensity of the food eaten to satiety. Indeed, Rolls, Rolls & Rowe (1983b) specifically addressed this using different concentrations of glucose and salt (NaCl), and showed that the subjective intensity but much less the subjective pleasantness of the tastes was related to the concentrations. Conversely, feeding to satiety produced a much greater decrease in pleasantness than in intensity. The neurophysiological basis for this is that processing as far as the primary taste cortex (Rolls, Scott, Sienkiewicz & Yaxley 1988, Yaxley, Rolls & Sienkiewicz 1988, Grabenhorst & Rolls 2008), the primary olfactory cortex (Rolls, Kringelbach & De Araujo 2003c), and the inferior temporal visual cortex is related to the identity and intensity of the stimulus (Rolls, Judge & Sanghera 1977); whereas in the orbitofrontal cortex it is the pleasantness of the taste (Rolls, Sienkiewicz & Yaxley 1989b, Grabenhorst & Rolls 2008) (Fig. 4.21), smell, and sight of food which is represented (Critchley & Rolls 1996c, Rolls, Kringelbach & De Araujo 2003c, De Araujo, Rolls, Kringelbach, McGlone & Phillips 2003c, Kringelbach, O'Doherty, Rolls & Andrews 2003, De Araujo, Rolls, Velazco, Margot & Cayeux 2005). The adaptive value of this is that it is important that we do not go 'blind' to the taste or sight of food after we have eaten it to satiety, for it is important to be able to learn about the food (e.g. where food has been seen), even when we are not hungry.

It should be noticed that this decrease in the pleasantness of the sensory stimulation produced by a food only occurs if the sensory stimulation is repeated for several minutes. It has the adaptive value of changing the behaviour after a significant amount of that behaviour has been performed. In contrast, the reward value of sensory stimulation may increase over the first short period (of the order of a minute). This is called *incentive motivation* (and the 'salted-nut phenomenon' by Hebb (1949)). It has the adaptive value that once a behaviour has been initiated, it will tend to continue for at least a little while. This is much more adaptive than continually switching behaviour, which has at least some cost in terms of efficiency, and might have a high cost if the different rewards are located far apart.

The enhanced eating when a variety of foods is available, as a result of the operation of sensory-specific satiety, may have been advantageous in evolution in ensuring that different foods with important different nutrients were consumed, but today in humans, when a wide variety of foods is readily available, it may be a factor which can lead to overeating and obesity. In a test of this in the rat, it was found that variety itself can lead to obesity (Rolls, Van Duijenvoorde & Rowe 1983a, Rolls & Hetherington 1989).

Advances in understanding the neurophysiological mechanisms of sensory-specific satiety are being made in analyses of information processing in the taste and olfactory systems, as described below.

In addition to the sensory-specific satiety described above which operates primarily during the meal (see above) and during the post-meal period (Rolls, Van Duijenvoorde & Rolls 1984a), there is also evidence for a long-term form of sensory-specific satiety (Rolls & de Waal 1985). This was shown in a study in an Ethiopian refugee camp, in which it was found that refugees who had been in the camp for 6 months found the taste of their three regular foods less pleasant than that of three comparable foods which they had not been eating. The effect was a long-term form of sensory-specific satiety in that it was not found in refugees who had been in the camp and had been eating the same (regular) foods for two days (Rolls & de Waal 1985). It is suggested that it is important to recognize the operation of long-term sensory-specific satiety in conditions such as these, for it may enhance malnutrition if the regular foods become less acceptable and so are rejected, exchanged for other less nutritionally effective foods or goods, or are inadequately prepared. It may be advantageous in these circumstances to attempt to minimize the operation of long-term sensory-specific satiety by providing some variety, perhaps even with spices (Rolls & de Waal 1985).

5.2.3 Conditioned appetite and satiety

If we eat food containing much energy (e.g. rich in fat) for a few days, we gradually eat less of it. If we eat food containing little energy, we gradually, over days, ingest more of it. This regulation involves learning, learning to associate the sight, taste, smell, texture, etc., of the food with the energy that is released from it in the hours after it is eaten. This form of learning was demonstrated by Booth (1985) who, after several days of offering sandwiches with different energy content and flavours, on a test day offered subjects medium-energy sandwiches (so that the subjects could not select by the amount of energy in the food). The subjects ate few of the sandwiches if they had the flavour of the high-energy sandwiches eaten previously, and many of the sandwiches if they had the flavour of the low-energy sandwiches eaten previously.

5.3 The brain control of eating and reward

5.3.1 Brain mechanisms for taste reward value

5.3.1.1 Taste processing up to and including the primary taste cortex of primates is related to the identity of the tastant, and not to its reward value

Given that there are neurons in the hypothalamus that can respond to the taste (and/or sight) of foods but not of non-foods, and that modulation of this sensory input by motivation is seen when recordings are made from these hypothalamic neurons (Rolls 2014b, Rolls 2016e), it may be asked whether these are special properties of hypothalamic neurons which they show because they are specially involved in the control of motivational responses, or whether this degree of specificity and type of modulation are general properties that are evident throughout sensory systems.

Evidence has now been obtained for primates on the tuning of neurons in the gustatory pathways, and on whether responsiveness at different stages is influenced by motivation, as follows. These investigations on the gustatory pathways have also been able to show where flavour, that is a combination of taste and olfactory input, is computed in the primate brain. The gustatory and olfactory pathways, and some of their onward connections, are shown in Fig. 4.2.

The first central synapse of the gustatory system is in the rostral part of the nucleus of the solitary tract (Beckstead & Norgren 1979, Beckstead, Morse & Norgren 1980, Rolls 2015b).

At this stage of processing in primates, there is no decrease in the neuronal response to taste stimuli when they feed themselves to normal self-induced satiety (Yaxley, Rolls, Sienkiewicz & Scott 1985).

In the primate primary gustatory cortex in the frontal operculum and insula, neurons are more finely tuned to gustatory stimuli than in the nucleus of the solitary tract, with some neurons responding primarily, for example, to sweet, and much less to salt, bitter, or sour stimuli (Scott, Yaxley, Sienkiewicz & Rolls 1986, Yaxley, Rolls & Sienkiewicz 1990). However, here also, hunger does not influence the magnitude of neuronal responses to gustatory stimuli (Rolls, Scott, Sienkiewicz & Yaxley 1988, Yaxley, Rolls & Sienkiewicz 1988). Consistent with this, activations in the human insular primary taste cortex are linearly related to the subjective intensity of the taste and not to the pleasantness rating (Fig. 4.21 (Grabenhorst & Rolls 2008)). Further, activations in the human insular primary taste cortex are related to the concentration of the tastant, for example monosodium glutamate (Grabenhorst, Rolls & Bilderbeck 2008a).

5.3.1.2 Taste and taste-related processing in the orbitofrontal (secondary taste) cortex, including umami taste, astringency, fat, viscosity, temperature and capsaicin

A secondary cortical taste area has been discovered in the caudolateral orbitofrontal taste cortex of the primate in which gustatory neurons can be even more finely tuned to particular taste stimuli (Rolls, Yaxley & Sienkiewicz 1990, Rolls & Treves 1990, Rolls, Sienkiewicz & Yaxley 1989b, Verhagen, Rolls & Kadohisa 2003, Rolls, Verhagen & Kadohisa 2003e, Kadohisa, Rolls & Verhagen 2004, Kadohisa, Rolls & Verhagen 2005b, Rolls, Critchley, Verhagen & Kadohisa 2010a) (see Fig. 4.10). In addition to representations of the 'prototypical' taste stimuli sweet, salt, bitter, and sour, different neurons in this region respond to other taste and taste-related stimuli that provide information about the reward value of a potential food (Rolls 2006b, Kadohisa, Rolls & Verhagen 2005b, Rolls 2016e). One example of this additional taste information is a set of neurons that respond to umami taste, as described next.

Umami taste. An important food taste which appears to be different from that produced by sweet, salt, bitter, or sour is the taste of protein. At least part of this taste is captured by the Japanese word 'umami', which is a taste common to a diversity of food sources including fish, meats, mushrooms, cheese, some vegetables such as tomatoes, and human mothers' milk. Within these food sources, it is glutamates and 5′ nucleotides, sometimes in a synergistic combination, that create the umami taste (Ikeda 1909, Yamaguchi 1967, Yamaguchi & Kimizuka 1979, Kawamura & Kare 1992). Monosodium L-glutamate (MSG), and the 5′ nucleotides guanosine 5′-monophosphate (GMP), and inosine 5′-monophosphate (IMP), are examples of umami stimuli.

To investigate the neural encoding of glutamate in the primate, recordings were made from taste-responsive neurons in the primary taste cortex and adjoining orbitofrontal cortex taste area in macaques. Single neurons were found that were tuned to respond best to monosodium glutamate (umami taste), just as other cells were found with best responses to glucose (sweet), sodium chloride (salty), HCl (sour), and quinine HCl (bitter) (Baylis & Rolls 1991, Rolls et al. 1996b).

There is now clear evidence that there are taste receptors on the tongue specialized for umami taste (Chaudhari, Landin & Roper 2000, Zhao, Zhang, Hoon, Chandrashekar, Erlenbach, Ryba & Zucker 2003, Lin, Ogura & Kinnamon 2003, Chandrashekar, Hoon, Ryba & Zuker 2006, Chaudhari & Roper 2010, Haid, Widmayer, Voigt, Chaudhari, Boehm & Breer 2013).

In addition, the umami tastants monosodium glutamate and inosine monophosphate

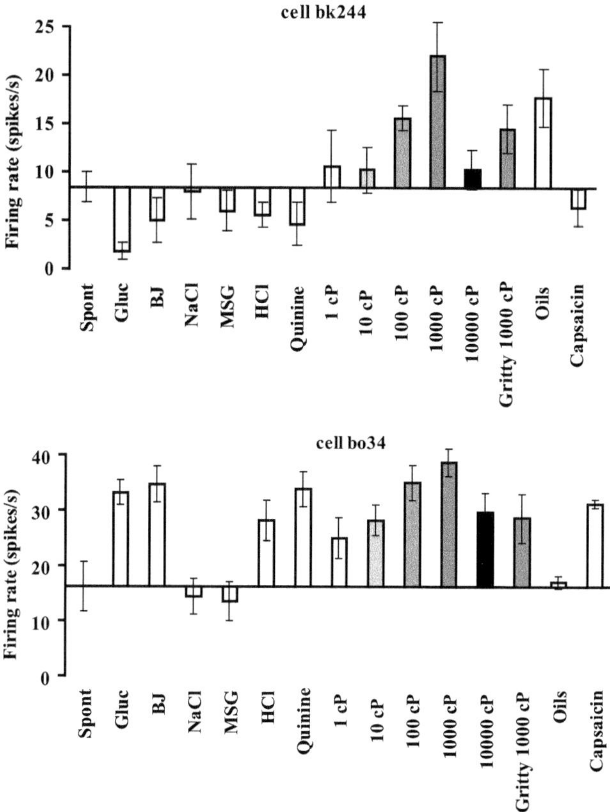

Fig. 5.4 Above. Firing rates (mean $\pm$ s.e.m.) of orbitofrontal cortex viscosity-sensitive neuron bk244 which did not have taste responses. The firing rates are shown to the viscosity series (carboxymethylcellulose in the range 1–10,000 centiPoise), to the gritty stimulus (carboxymethylcellulose with Fillite microspheres), to the taste stimuli 1 M glucose (Gluc), 0.1 M NaCl, 0.1 M MSG , 0.01 M HCl and 0.001 M QuinineHCl, and to fruit juice (BJ). Spont = spontaneous firing rate. Below. Firing rates (mean $\pm$ s.e.m.) of viscosity-sensitive neuron bo34 which had no response to the oils (mineral oil, vegetable oil, safflower oil and coconut oil, which have viscosities which are all close to 50 cP). The neuron did not respond to the gritty stimulus in a way that was unexpected given the viscosity of the stimulus, was taste tuned, and did respond to capsaicin. (Reproduced from *Journal of Neurophysiology*, 90 (6), Representations of the texture of food in the primate orbitofrontal cortex: neurons responding to viscosity, grittiness, and capsaicin, E. T. Rolls, J. V. Verhagen, and M. Kadohisa, pp. 3711–3724,)

activate the human primary taste cortex in the insula/operculum, the secondary taste cortex in the orbitofrontal cortex, and the cingulate cortex (De Araujo, Kringelbach, Rolls & Hobden 2003a).

This evidence shows that umami taste, an indicator of the presence of protein, is implemented by neurons in the primary and secondary taste cortex that are tuned to umami stimuli. Umami is a component of many foods which helps to make them taste pleasant, especially when the umami taste is paired with a consonant savoury odour (Rolls, Critchley, Browning & Hernadi 1998a, McCabe & Rolls 2007, Rolls 2009a).

Food texture: viscosity. Another important type of input to the same region of the orbitofrontal cortex that is concerned with detecting the reward value of a potential food is an input produced by the texture of food in the mouth. We have shown for example that single neurons influenced by taste in this region can in some cases have their responses modulated by the texture of the food (Rolls 2011e). This was shown in experiments in which the texture of food was manipulated by the addition of methyl cellulose or gelatine, or by puréeing a semi-solid food (Rolls 2011e). We have been able to show that some of these neurons respond to the viscosity of the food in the mouth, as altered parametrically using the standard food thickening agent carboxymethylcellulose made up in viscosities of 1–10,000 cPoise (Rolls, Verhagen & Kadohisa 2003e). (10,000 cP is approximately the viscosity of toothpaste.) Some of these neurons are unimodal, responding just to texture and not to taste (see Fig. 5.4 upper). Others respond to different combinations of texture and taste, as illustrated in Fig. 5.4 (lower). These recordings provide unique evidence about the texture channels that convey information from the mouth to the cortex, for they show that the system can potentially have responses to texture separately from the other sensory attributes of food, as well as to particular combinations of taste, texture, and other sensory properties of food.

The somatosensory inputs may reach the orbitofrontal cortex via the primary taste cortex in the rostral insula and adjoining frontal operculum, which we have shown does project into this region (Baylis, Rolls & Baylis 1994), and which also contains a representation of the viscosity of what is in the mouth (Verhagen, Kadohisa & Rolls 2004). A number of parts of the insula are known to receive somatosensory inputs (Mesulam & Mufson 1982a, Mesulam & Mufson 1982b, Mufson & Mesulam 1982). The texture of food is an important cue about the quality of the food, for example about the ripeness of fruit.

These findings have been extended to the human, with the finding with fMRI that the activation of the primary taste cortex and the subjective rating of the thickness is proportional to the logarithm of the viscosity of the stimulus in the mouth (De Araujo & Rolls 2004, Kadohisa, Rolls & Verhagen 2005b).

Food texture: fat. Texture in the mouth is also an important indicator of whether fat is present in the food, which is important not only as a high value energy source, but also as a potential source of essential fatty acids. In the orbitofrontal cortex, Rolls, Critchley, Browning, Hernadi & Lenard (1999a) have found a population of neurons that responds when fat is in the mouth. An example of such a neuron is shown in Fig. 5.5. This neuron had no response to taste, but some other neurons had convergence of fat texture and taste inputs. The fat-related responses of these neurons are produced at least in part by the texture of the food rather than by chemical receptors sensitive to certain chemicals, in that such neurons typically respond not only to foods such as cream and milk containing fat, but also to paraffin oil (which is a pure hydrocarbon) and to silicone oil (which contains $(Si(CH_3)_2O)_n$).

Some of the fat-related neurons do though have multimodal convergent inputs from the chemical senses, in that in addition to taste inputs some of these neurons respond to the odour associated with a fat, such as the odour of cream (Rolls, Critchley, Browning, Hernadi & Lenard 1999a). The texture-related responses of these oral fat-sensitive neurons are independent of the viscosity of what is in the mouth and of fatty acids in the mouth (Verhagen, Rolls & Kadohisa 2003), so that fat in food can be detected orally by a specialized fat/oil texture channel (Rolls 2011e). Similar neurons have been recorded in the pregenual cingulate cortex (Rolls 2008b).

This type of discovery can be made only at the single neuron level, and paves the way for further studies of the transducing mechanism, understanding of which could be important in the design of foods with pleasant textures that do not bring with them high caloric content with its implications for obesity (Rolls 2011e, Rolls et al. 2018c).

These findings have been extended to the human, with the finding with fMRI that activation of the orbitofrontal cortex and perigenual cingulate cortex is produced by the texture of fat in the mouth (De Araujo & Rolls 2004). Moreover, activations in the orbitofrontal cortex and

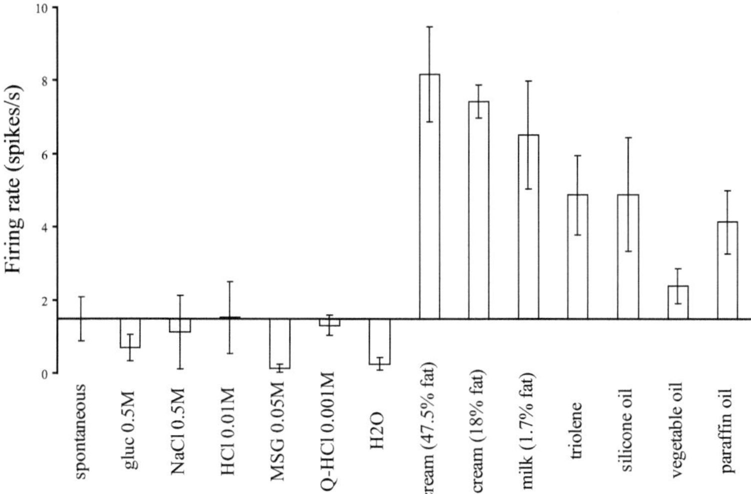

Fig. 5.5 A neuron in the primate orbitofrontal cortex responding to the texture of fat in the mouth. The neuron increased its firing rate to cream (double and single cream, with the fat proportions shown), and responded to texture rather than the chemical structure of the fat in that it also responded to 0.5 ml of silicone oil ($(Si(CH_3)_2O)_n$) or paraffin oil (hydrocarbon). The neuron did not have a taste input. Gluc, glucose; NaCl, salt; HCl, sour; Q-HCl, quinine, bitter. The spontaneous firing rate of the cell is also shown. (Reproduced from *Journal of Neuroscience*, 19 (4), Responses to the sensory properties of fat of neurons in the primate orbitofrontal cortex, E. T. Rolls, H. D. Critchley, A. S. Browning, A. Hernadi, and L. Lenard, pp. 1532–1540, © 1999, The Society for Neuroscience.)

pregenual cingulate cortex are correlated with the pleasantness of fat texture in the mouth (Grabenhorst, Rolls, Parris & D'Souza 2010b).

5.3.1.3 The reward value of taste is represented in the orbitofrontal cortex

In the primate orbitofrontal cortex, it is found that the responses of taste neurons to the particular food with which a monkey is fed to satiety decrease to zero (Rolls, Sienkiewicz & Yaxley 1989b). An example is shown in Fig. 4.6. This neuron reduced its responses to the taste of glucose during the course of feeding as much glucose as the monkey wanted to drink. When the monkey was fully satiated, and did not want to drink any more glucose, the neuron no longer responded to the taste of glucose. Thus the responses of these neurons decrease to zero when the reward value of the food decreases to zero. Interestingly the neuron still responded to other foods, and the monkey chose to eat these other foods. Thus the modulation of the responses of these orbitofrontal cortex taste neurons occurs in a sensory-specific way, and they represent *reward outcome value*.

Another example is that some orbitofrontal cortex neurons decrease their response to the fatty texture of cream when fed to satiety with cream, but still respond to the taste of glucose after feeding to satiety with cream (Rolls, Critchley, Browning, Hernadi & Lenard 1999a). This indicates sensory-specific satiety for the reward value of the texture of cream in the mouth, and also provides evidence that absolute value and not relative value is represented in the orbitofrontal cortex (Grabenhorst & Rolls 2009, Rolls 2014b).

The orbitofrontal cortex is the first stage of the primate taste system in which this modulation of the responses of neurons to the taste of food is affected by hunger, in that this modulation is not found in the nucleus of the solitary tract, or in the frontal opercular or insular primary gustatory cortices (Yaxley, Rolls, Sienkiewicz & Scott 1985, Rolls, Scott,

Sienkiewicz & Yaxley 1988, Yaxley, Rolls & Sienkiewicz 1988). It is of course only when hungry that the taste of food is rewarding. This is an indication that the responses of these orbitofrontal cortex taste neurons reflect the reward value of food. The firing of these orbitofrontal neurons may actually implement the reward value of a food. The hypothesis is that primates work to obtain firing of these reward value neurons, by eating food when they are hungry.

The situation appears to be the same in humans, in whom fMRI investigations show that sensory-specific satiety for food is represented in the orbitofrontal cortex (Kringelbach, O'Doherty, Rolls & Andrews 2003) (see Fig. 4.11 on page 72); that activations in the orbitofrontal cortex and pregenual cingulate cortex are linearly correlated with the subjective pleasantness value of taste (Grabenhorst & Rolls 2008, Rolls 2012c); and in that activations in the insular primary taste cortex are linearly correlated with the subjective intensity of taste (Grabenhorst & Rolls 2008) (Fig. 4.22).

These findings lead to the following proposed neuronal mechanism for sensory-specific satiety (see also Rolls & Treves (1990)). Neurons in the orbitofrontal cortex respond to different combinations or food-related inputs, as illustrated in Fig. 5.4. If then it is a property that the synapses that convey input to these neurons adapt (i.e. decrease their efficacy) over the time course of a typical meal, then the neuron will stop responding to that food, but will still respond to other foods. For this mechanism to operate efficiently, the neurons that provide the inputs have to be rather selective, which they are. Further details are provided by Rolls (2014b).

5.3.1.4 Taste processing in rodents

There are major differences in the neural processing of taste in rodents and primates (Rolls & Scott 2003, Small & Scott 2009, Scott & Small 2009, Rolls 2014b, Rolls 2015b, Rolls 2016b). In rodents (and also in primates) taste information is conveyed by cranial nerves 7, 9 and 10 to the rostral part of the nucleus of the solitary tract (NTS) (Norgren 1990, Norgren & Leonard 1971, Norgren & Leonard 1973). However, although in primates the NTS projects to the taste thalamus and thus to the cortex (Fig. 4.2), in rodents the majority of NTS taste neurons responding to stimulation of the taste receptors of the anterior tongue project to the ipsilateral medial aspect of the pontine parabrachial nucleus (PbN), the rodent 'pontine taste area' (Small & Scott 2009, Cho, Li & Smith 2002). The remainder project to adjacent regions of the medulla. From the PbN the rodent gustatory pathway bifurcates into two pathways; 1) a ventral 'affective' projection to the hypothalamus, central gray, ventral striatum, bed nucleus of the stria terminalis and amygdala and 2) a dorsal 'sensory' pathway, which first synapses in the thalamus and then the agranular and dysgranular insular gustatory cortex (Norgren 1990, Norgren & Leonard 1971, Norgren 1974, Norgren 1976, Kosar, Grill & Norgren 1986). These regions, in turn, project back to the PbN to "sculpt the gustatory code" and guide complex feeding behaviours (Norgren 1990, Norgren 1976, Li & Cho 2006, Li, Cho & Smith 2002, Lundy & Norgren 2004, Di Lorenzo 1990, Scott & Small 2009, Small & Scott 2009).

It may be noted that there is strong evidence to indicate that the PbN gustatory relay is absent in the human and the nonhuman primate (Small & Scott 2009, Scott & Small 2009). First, second-order gustatory projections that arise from rostral NTS appear not to synapse in the PbN and instead join the central tegmental tract and project directly to the taste thalamus in primates (Beckstead, Morse & Norgren 1980, Pritchard, Hamilton & Norgren 1989). Second, despite several attempts, no one has successfully isolated taste responses in the monkey PbN (Norgren (1990); Small & Scott (2009) who cite Ralph Norgren, personal communication and Tom Pritchard, personal communication). Third, in monkeys the projection arising from the PbN does not terminate in the region of ventral basal thalamus that contains gustatory responsive neurons (Pritchard et al. 1989).

A further difference of rodent taste processing from that of primates is that physical and chemical signals of satiety have been shown to reduce the taste responsiveness of neurons in the nucleus in the solitary tract, and the pontine taste area, of the rat, with decreases in the order of 30%, as follows (Rolls & Scott 2003, Scott & Small 2009). Gastric distension by air or with 0.3 M NaCl suppress responses in the NTS, with the greatest effect on glucose (Gleen & Erickson 1976). Intravenous infusions of 0.5 g/kg glucose (Giza & Scott 1983), 0.5 U/kg insulin (Giza & Scott 1987a), and 40 μg/kg glucagon (Giza, Deems, Vanderweele & Scott 1993) all cause reductions in taste responsiveness to glucose in the NTS. The intraduodenal infusion of lipids causes a decline in taste responsiveness in the PBN, with the bulk of the suppression borne by glucose cells (Hajnal, Takenouchi & Norgren 1999). The loss of signal that would otherwise be evoked by hedonically positive tastes implies that the pleasure that sustains feeding is reduced, making termination of a meal more likely (Giza, Scott & Vanderweele 1992). Further, if taste activity in NTS is affected by the rat's nutritional state, then intensity judgements in rats should change with satiety. There is evidence that they do. Rats with conditioned aversions to 1.0 M glucose show decreasing acceptance of glucose solutions as their concentrations approach 1.0 M. This acceptance gradient can be compared between euglycemic rats and those made hyperglycemic through intravenous injections (Scott & Giza 1987). Hyperglycemic rats showed greater acceptance at all concentrations from 0.6 to 2.0 M glucose, indicating that they perceived these stimuli to be less intense than did conditioned rats with no glucose load (Giza & Scott 1987b).

The implication is that taste, and the closely related olfactory and visual processing that contribute to food reward value and expected value, are much more difficult to understand in rodents than in primates, partly because there is less segregation of 'what' (identity and intensity) from hedonic processing in rodents, partly because of the more serial hierarchical processing in primates (Fig. 4.2), and partly because in primates there has been great development of the granular orbitofrontal cortex which may help to support the rule-based switching of behaviour important for rapidly reversing stimulus-reward associations and behaviour (Section 1.3). Taste and flavour processing in the brain, and how reward value is decoded, appear to follow different principles in rodents, and primates including humans (Rolls 2016b, Rolls 2017c).

5.3.2 Convergence between taste and olfactory processing to represent flavour

We have discovered that there are regions in the orbitofrontal cortex of primates where the sensory modalities of taste, vision, and olfaction converge; and that in many cases the neurons have corresponding sensitivities across modalities which are built by associative learning (Rolls & Baylis 1994, Critchley & Rolls 1996b, Rolls, Critchley, Mason & Wakeman 1996a).

It appears to be in these orbitofrontal cortex areas that flavour representations are built, where flavour is taken to mean a representation that is evoked best by a combination of gustatory and olfactory input. This orbitofrontal region does appear to be an important region for convergence, for there is only a very low proportion of bimodal taste and olfactory neurons in the primary taste cortex (Rolls & Baylis 1994), and in general primary taste cortex neurons do not respond to olfactory or visual stimuli even if they are associated with the taste of food (Verhagen, Kadohisa & Rolls 2004).

To investigate where flavour is formed in humans by olfactory and taste convergence, De Araujo, Rolls, Kringelbach, McGlone & Phillips (2003c) performed an fMRI investigation with unimodal taste (sucrose), unimodal olfactory (strawberry odour), and a mixture of both. They found that a part of the human insular taste cortex was unimodal for taste, and that both olfactory and taste stimuli activated the orbitofrontal cortex and its posterior extension into the agranular insula. Moreover, supralinear additivity of the olfactory and taste components was found in a part of the orbitofrontal cortex. Further, the consonance and pleasantness subjective ratings of the olfactory and taste mixtures (which included some non-consonant mixtures such as sucrose and savory odour) were correlated with activations in the medial orbitofrontal cortex.

In an investigation to analyse what makes umami delicious, we found with fMRI that a combination of glutamate taste with a savory odour (vegetable) produced much greater activation of the medial orbitofrontal cortex and pregenual cingulate cortex than the sum of the activations by the taste and olfactory components presented separately (McCabe & Rolls 2007). Supralinear effects were much less (and significantly less) evident for sodium chloride and vegetable odour. Further, activations in these brain regions were correlated with the pleasantness and fullness of the flavor, and with the consonance of the taste and olfactory components. Supralinear effects of glutamate taste and savory odour were not found in the insular primary taste cortex. We thus proposed that glutamate acts by the nonlinear effects it can produce when combined with a consonant odour in multimodal cortical taste-olfactory convergence regions far beyond the taste receptors to produce a delicious flavour of umami (McCabe & Rolls 2007, Rolls 2009a).

Thus the processing that it is possible to analyse in detail at the neuronal level in primates appears to provide a good model for how taste and odour combine to produce pleasant flavour in humans (Rolls 2011f, Rolls 2012c, Rolls 2014b, Rolls 2016e). Further, the anterior insular taste cortex does not normally respond to odour (though if a taste was being recalled by an odour this might happen), though areas just anterior to the anterior insular taste cortex do combine odour and taste, including what may be an agranular area of the insula.

5.3.3 Brain mechanisms for the reward produced by the odour of food

A schematic diagram of the olfactory pathways in primates is shown in Fig. 4.2 on page 52. There are direct connections from the olfactory bulb to the primary olfactory cortex, pyriform cortex, and from there a connection to a caudal part of the mid (in terms of medial and lateral) orbitofrontal cortex, area 13a, which in turn has onward projections to the lateral orbitofrontal cortex area which we have shown is secondary taste cortex, and to more rostral parts of the orbitofrontal cortex (area 11) (Price et al. 1991, Carmichael & Price 1994, Carmichael et al. 1994, Ongur & Price 2000, Price 2006) (see Fig. 4.2).

There is evidence that in the olfactory bulb, a coding principle is that in many cases each glomerulus (of which there are approximately 1000) is tuned to respond to its own characteristic hydrocarbon chain length of odourant (Mori, Mataga & Imamura 1992, Imamura, Mataga & Mori 1992, Mori, Nagao & Yoshihara 1999, Mori & Sakano 2011).

Is this same coding principle, based on simple physico-chemical properties, used later on in the (primate) olfactory system, or do other principles operate? We have shown that 35% of the olfactory neurons in the orbitofrontal cortex responded on the basis of the taste reward association of the odourants (Critchley & Rolls 1996b). Moreover, Rolls, Critchley, Mason & Wakeman (1996a) found that 68% of the odour-responsive orbitofrontal cortex neurons analysed modified their responses following the changes in the taste reward associations of the odourants during an odour-taste discrimination reversal task.

These findings demonstrate directly a coding principle in primate olfaction whereby the responses of some orbitofrontal cortex olfactory neurons are modified by and depend upon the taste with which the odour is associated. This modification is likely to be important for setting the motivational or reward value of olfactory stimuli for feeding and other rewarded behaviour. It was of interest however that this modification was less complete, and much slower, than the modifications found for orbitofrontal cortex visual neurons during visual-taste reversal (Rolls, Critchley, Mason & Wakeman 1996a). This relative inflexibility of olfactory responses is consistent with the need for some stability in odour–taste associations to facilitate the formation and perception of flavours (Rolls 2011f).

It has also been possible to investigate whether the olfactory representation in the orbitofrontal cortex is affected by hunger and reflects reward value in this way too. In satiety devaluation experiments, Critchley & Rolls (1996c) have been able to show that the responses of some olfactory neurons to a food odour are reduced when the monkey is fed to satiety with a food (e.g. fruit juice) with that odour. In particular, seven of nine olfactory neurons that were responsive to the odours of foods, such as blackcurrant juice, were found to reduce their responses to the odour of the satiating food. The decrease was typically at least partly specific to the odour of the food that had been eaten to satiety, potentially providing part of the basis for sensory-specific satiety (Fig. 4.6).

In humans, it has been shown that the modulation of the pleasantness of odour by satiety is represented in the orbitofrontal cortex, in that there is a sensory-specific reduction of the fMRI BOLD signal in the orbitofrontal cortex to the odour of a food eaten to satiety, but not to the odour of another food not eaten in a meal (O'Doherty, Rolls, Francis, Bowtell, McGlone, Kobal, Renner & Ahne 2000). In addition, there is evidence in humans that the primary olfactory cortical areas (including the pyriform cortex and cortico-medial amygdala region) represent the identity and intensity of olfactory stimuli, in that in a functional magnetic resonance imaging (fMRI) investigation, activation of these regions was correlated with the subjective intensity ratings but not the subjective pleasantness ratings of six odours (Rolls, Kringelbach & De Araujo 2003c). In contrast, the reward value of odours is represented in the human medial orbitofrontal cortex, in that activation here was correlated with the pleasantness but not intensity ratings of six odours (Rolls, Kringelbach & De Araujo 2003c) (cf. Anderson et al. (2003)), and are increased by paying attention to pleasantness but not intensity (Rolls, Grabenhorst, Margot, da Silva & Velazco 2008a).

5.3.4 The responses of orbitofrontal cortex taste and olfactory neurons to the sight of food: expected value neurons

Many of the neurons with visual responses in this region also show olfactory or taste responses (Rolls & Baylis 1994), reverse rapidly in visual discrimination reversal (Rolls, Critchley, Mason & Wakeman 1996a), and only respond to the sight of food if hunger is present (Critchley & Rolls 1996c), and therefore encode expected reward value. This part of the orbitofrontal cortex thus seems to implement mechanisms that can flexibly alter the neuronal responses to visual stimuli depending on the reward (e.g. the taste) associated with the visual stimulus (Thorpe, Rolls & Maddison 1983, Rolls 2000b, Rolls 2004b, Rolls 2014b). This enables prediction of the taste associated with ingestion of what is seen, and this representation of expected value is important of food selection.

The convergence of visual information onto neurons in this region not only enables associations to be learned between the sight of a food and its taste and smell, but also may provide the neural basis for the well-known effect which the sight of a food has on its perceived taste (see Section 4.5.3.6).

5.3.5 Functions of the amygdala in feeding

We have seen in Section 4.6.4 that lesions of the amygdala can result in increased selection of non-food items. The neuronal recordings in the primate amygdala described in Section 4.6.5 show that different populations of amygdala neurons can respond to the taste, smell, oral texture, temperature, and sight of food (Sanghera, Rolls & Roper-Hall 1979, Ono, Nishino, Sasaki, Fukuda & Muramoto 1980, Ono, Tamura, Nishijo, Nakamura & Tabuchi 1989, Nishijo, Ono & Nishino 1988, Ono & Nishijo 1992, Scott, Karadi, Oomura, Nishino, Plata-Salaman, Lenard, Giza & Aou 1993, Kadohisa, Rolls & Verhagen 2005a) (see example in Fig. 4.27). A comparison between brain areas shows that the amygdala emphasizes the representation of oral texture (Kadohisa, Rolls & Verhagen 2005b, Kadohisa, Rolls & Verhagen 2005a).

The visual representation of foods by amygdala neurons is not completely specific to foods (in that some food-related neurons respond to non-foods or novel stimuli, reversal of neuronal responses when the reward contingencies reverse are not as clear and fast as in the orbitofrontal cortex, and nor are the effects of devaluation by feeding to satiety (Section 4.6.5).

These findings thus suggest that the amygdala could be involved in a somewhat inflexible circuit by which visual stimuli are associated with reinforcement. Neuronal responses here do not code uniquely for whether a visual stimulus is associated with reinforcement, partly because the neurons do not reverse rapidly, and partly because the neurons can respond to relatively novel stimuli, which monkeys frequently pick up and place in their mouths for further exploration. The amygdala may thus be a somewhat slow and inflexible system, compared with the orbitofrontal cortex which has developed greatly in primates, in learning about which visual stimuli have the taste and smell of food (Rolls 2014b).

5.3.6 Functions of the orbitofrontal cortex in eating

All the evidence summarized in the earlier parts of Section 5.3 and in Chapter 4 show that the orbitofrontal cortex has representations related to the affective value or pleasantness of food.

This is complemented by evidence that damage to the orbitofrontal cortex alters food preferences, in that monkeys with damage to the orbitofrontal cortex select and eat foods that are normally rejected (Butter et al. 1969, Baylis & Gaffan 1991). Their food choice behaviour is very similar to that of monkeys with amygdala lesions (Baylis & Gaffan 1991). Lesions of the orbitofrontal cortex also lead to a failure to correct feeding responses when these become inappropriate. Examples of the situations in which these abnormalities in feeding responses are found include: (a) extinction, in that feeding responses continue to be made to the previously reinforced stimulus; (b) reversals of visual discriminations, in that the monkeys make responses to the previously reinforced stimulus or object; (c) Go/Nogo tasks, in that responses are made to the stimulus that is not associated with food reward; and (d) passive avoidance, in that feeding responses are made even when they are punished (Butter 1969, Iversen & Mishkin 1970, Jones & Mishkin 1972, Tanaka 1973, Rosenkilde 1979, Murray & Izquierdo 2007, Fuster 2008) (see Section 4.4.1). Further, lesions of orbitofrontal cortex areas 11/13 disrupt the rapid updating of food object value during selective satiation (Rudebeck & Murray 2011). Changes in the orbitofrontal cortex may be related to some of the changes in eating habits in frontotemporal dementia, in which there may be escalating desire for sweet food coupled with reduced satiety, which is often followed by weight gain (Piguet 2011).

The more rapid reversal of neuronal responses in the orbitofrontal cortex, and in a region to which it projects, the basal forebrain (Thorpe, Rolls & Maddison 1983, Wilson & Rolls 1990b, Wilson & Rolls 1990c), than in the amygdala suggest that the orbitofrontal cortex is more involved than the amygdala in the rapid readjustments of behavioural responses made to stimuli when their reinforcement value is repeatedly changing, as in discrimination reversal tasks (Thorpe, Rolls & Maddison 1983, Rolls 1999a, Deco & Rolls 2005a). The ability to flexibly alter responses to stimuli based on their changing reinforcement associations is important in motivated behaviour (such as feeding) and in emotional behaviour, and it is this flexibility which it is suggested the orbitofrontal cortex adds to a more basic capacity that the amygdala implements for stimulus–reinforcement learning.

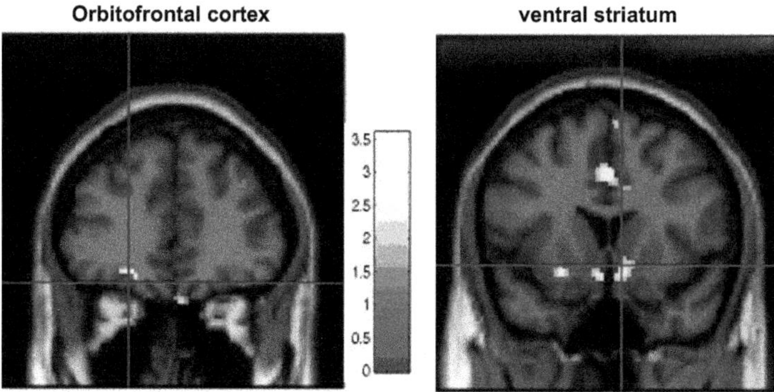

Fig. 5.6 The sight of chocolate produced more activation of mid and medial parts of the orbitofrontal cortex in chocolate cravers than non-cravers (e.g. [-28 42 -10] at the crosshairs), and in the ventral striatum ([-4 16 -12]). (Reproduced from Edmund T. Rolls and Ciara McCabe, Enhanced affective brain representations of chocolate in cravers vs. non-cravers, *European Journal of Neuroscience*, 26 (4) pp. 1067–1076, Copyright © 2007, John Wiley and Sons.)

The great development of the orbitofrontal cortex in primates, yet the similarity of its connections to those of the amygdala (see Fig. 4.25), and its connections with the amygdala, lead to the suggestion that in evolution, and as part of continuing corticalization of functions, the orbitofrontal cortex has come to be placed hierarchically above the amygdala, and is especially important when rapid readjustment of stimulus–reinforcement associations is required (Rolls 1990a, Rolls 2014b, Rolls 2017c). This suggestion is also consistent with the indication that whereas in rodents subcortical structures such as the amygdala and hypothalamus have access to taste information from the precortical taste system, the same does not occur in primates; and that some precortical processing of taste in relation to the control of feeding occurs in rodents (see above and Scott & Giza (1992) and Rolls & Scott (2003)). In contrast, there is great development and importance of cortical processing of taste in primates, and it is very appropriate that the orbitofrontal cortex area just described is found just medial to the secondary taste cortex, which is in primates in the caudolateral orbitofrontal cortex. It appears that close to this orbitofrontal taste cortex the orbitofrontal cortical area just described develops, and receives inputs from the visual association cortex (inferior temporal cortex), the olfactory (pyriform) cortex, and probably from the somatosensory cortex, so that reward associations between these different modalities can be determined rapidly.

An interesting topic for the future is whether the satiety signals summarized in Sections 5.2 and by Rolls (2014b) also gain access to the orbitofrontal cortex, and the details of how they modulate there the taste, olfactory and visual neuronal responses to food.

5.3.7 Output pathways for feeding

The orbitofrontal cortex projects to the anterior cingulate cortex, and this provides an output for feeding where action–outcome learning is being or has been performed and the actions are goal-dependent (Section 4.7) (see Fig. 4.2). The orbitofrontal cortex and amygdala project to the striatum, and this basal ganglia route provides an output for feeding, especially for stimulus-response habit controlled feeding (Section 6.3). Autonomic and endocrine functions involved in the control of feeding can be influenced by the hypothalamic and related output connections of the orbitofrontal cortex, amygdala, and anterior cingulate cortex described in Chapter 4.

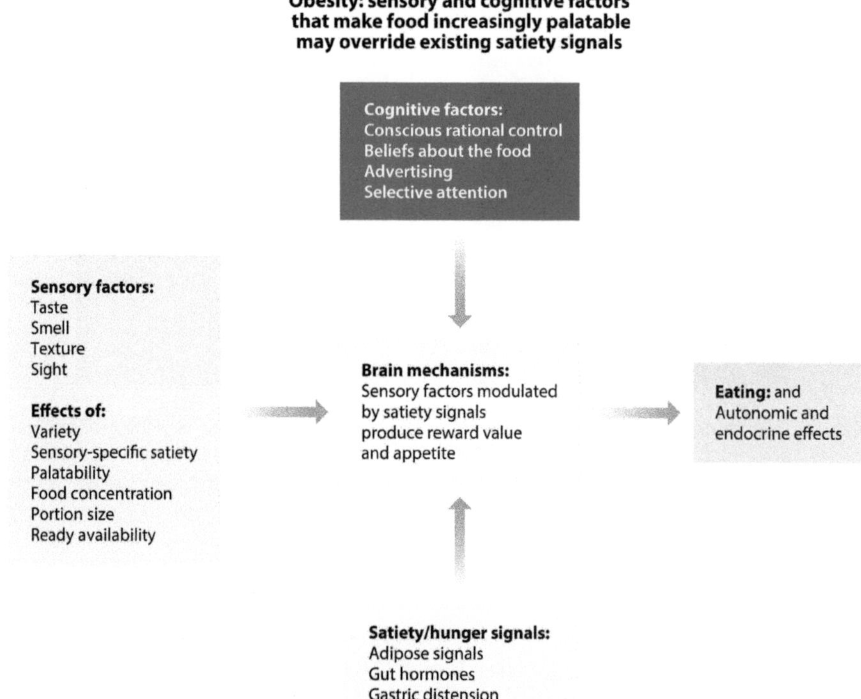

Fig. 5.7 Schematic diagram to show how sensory factors interact in the orbitofrontal cortex with satiety signals to produce the hedonic, rewarding value of food, which leads to appetite and eating. Cognitive and attentional factors directly modulate the reward system in the brain. (After Edmund T. Rolls, Reward Systems in the Brain and Nutrition, *Annual Review of Nutrition*, 36, pp. 435 – 470.)

5.4 Obesity and the reward value of food

I conclude this chapter on the brain mechanisms involved in affective responses to food, and appetite control, by considering some of the disturbances in these systems that may contribute to obesity and other eating disorders.

Understanding the mechanisms that control appetite is becoming an increasingly important issue, given the increasing incidence of obesity. Obesity affects approximately one third of adults in the United States (with an additional one third falling into the overweight category). In the UK, there has been a three-fold increase since 1980 to a figure of 20% defined by a Body Mass Index > 30, and there is a realization that it is associated with major health risks (with 1000 deaths each week in the UK attributable to obesity). It is important to understand and thereby be able to minimize and treat obesity because many diseases are associated with a body weight that is much above normal. These diseases include hypertension, cardiovascular disease, hypercholesterolaemia, and gall bladder disease; and in addition obesity is associated with some deficits in reproductive function (e.g. ovulatory failure), and with an excess mortality from certain types of cancer (Schwartz & Porte 2005, O'Rahilly 2009, Guyenet & Schwartz 2012).

There are many factors that can cause or contribute to obesity in humans (Schwartz & Porte 2005, O'Rahilly 2009, Guyenet & Schwartz 2012, Rolls 2007b, Rolls 2011b, Rolls 2012c). Rapid progress is being made in understanding many of these factors at present with the aim of leading to better ways to minimize and treat obesity. These factors include the following (Rolls 2012c, Rolls 2014b, Rolls 2016e):

5.4.1 Genetic factors

Genetic factors are of some importance, with some of the variance in weight and resting metabolic rate in a population of humans attributable to inheritance (Barsh & Schwartz 2002, O'Rahilly 2009, Farooqi & O'Rahilly 2017). A small proportion of cases of obesity can be related to dysfunctions of the peptide systems in the hypothalamus, with for example 4% of obese people having deficient (MC4) receptors for melanocyte stimulating hormone (Barsh, Farooqi & O'Rahilly 2000, Cummings & Schwartz 2003, Horvath 2005, O'Rahilly 2009). Cases of obesity that can be related to changes in the leptin system are rare (O'Rahilly 2009, Farooqi & O'Rahilly 2017). Further, obese people generally have high levels of leptin, so leptin production is not the problem, and instead leptin resistance (i.e. insensitivity) may be somewhat related to obesity, with the resistance perhaps related in part to smaller effects of leptin on arcuate nucleus NPY/AGRP neurons (Munzberg & Myers 2005). However, although there are similarities in fatness within families, these are as strong between spouses as they are between parents and children, so that these similarities cannot be attributed to genetic influences, but presumably reflect the effect of family attitudes to food and weight.

Further, the 'obesity epidemic' that has occurred since 1990 cannot be attributed to genetic changes, for which the time scale is far too short, but instead to factors such as the increased palatability, variety, and availability of food which are some of the crucial drivers of food intake and the amount of food that is eaten in our changed modern environment (Rolls 2014b, Rolls 2007b, Rolls 2011b, Rolls 2012c, Heitmann, Westerterp, Loos, Sorensen, O'Dea, Mc Lean, Jensen, Eisenmann, Speakman, Simpson, Reed & Westerterp-Plantenga 2012) and that are described below. Consistent with this view, food intake has increased in the United States by 20% since 1980 (Guyenet & Schwartz 2012). This view (Rolls 2014b, Rolls 2016e, Rolls 2007b, Rolls 2010d, Rolls 2011b, Rolls 2012c) is becoming increasingly accepted (O'Rahilly 2009).

5.4.2 Brain processing of the sensory properties and pleasantness of food

The way in which the sensory factors produced by the taste, smell, texture and sight of food interact in the brain with satiety signals (such as gastric distension and satiety-related hormones) to determine the pleasantness and palatability of food, and therefore whether and how much food will be eaten, is described above in this chapter. The concept is that convergence of sensory inputs produced by the taste, smell, texture and sight of food occurs in the orbitofrontal cortex to build a representation of food flavour. The orbitofrontal cortex is where the pleasantness and palatability of food are represented, as shown by the discoveries that these representations of food value are only activated if appetite is present and the food is chosen, and correlate with the subjective pleasantness of the food flavour. The orbitofrontal cortex representation of whether food is pleasant (which takes into account any satiety signals present) then drives brain areas such as the striatum and cingulate cortex that then lead to eating behaviour.

The fundamental concept this leads to about some of the major causes of obesity is that, over the last 30 years, sensory stimulation produced by the taste, smell, texture and appearance of food, as well as its availability, have increased dramatically, yet the satiety signals produced by stomach distension, satiety hormones etc. summarized in Section 5.2 have remained essentially unchanged. The consequence is that the effect on the brain's control system for appetite is to lead to a net average increase in the reward value and palatability of food which over-rides the satiety signals, and contributes to the tendency to be overstimulated by food and to overeat (Rolls 2014b, Rolls 2007b, Rolls 2011b, Rolls 2012c, Rolls 2016e).

In this scenario, it is important to understand much better the rules used by the brain to produce the representation of the pleasantness of food and how the system is modulated by eating and satiety. This understanding, and how the sensory factors can be designed and controlled so as not to override satiety signals, are important research areas in the understanding, prevention, and treatment of obesity. Advances in understanding the receptors that encode the taste, olfactory, fat texture (Rolls 2011e) and other properties of food, and the processing in the brain of these properties (Rolls 2014b, Rolls 2007b, Rolls 2011b, Rolls 2012c, Rolls 2016e), are also important in providing the potential to produce highly palatable food that is at the same time nutritious and healthy.

An important aspect of this hypothesis is that different humans may have reward systems that are especially strongly driven by the sensory and cognitive factors that make food highly palatable. In a test of this, we showed that activation to the sight and flavor of chocolate in the orbitofrontal and pregenual cingulate cortex were much higher in chocolate cravers than non-cravers (Rolls & McCabe 2007). In more detail, the sight of chocolate produced more activation in chocolate cravers than non-cravers in the medial orbitofrontal cortex and ventral striatum (Fig. 5.6). For cravers vs non-cravers, a combination of a picture of chocolate with chocolate in the mouth produced a greater effect than the sum of the components (i.e. supralinearity) in the medial orbitofrontal cortex and pregenual cingulate cortex. Furthermore, the pleasantness ratings of the chocolate and chocolate-related stimuli had higher positive correlations with the fMRI signals in the pregenual cingulate cortex and medial orbitofrontal cortex in the cravers than in the non-cravers. Thus there are differences between cravers and non-cravers in their responses to the reward components of a craved food in the orbitofrontal and pregenual cingulate cortex and a region to which they project the ventral striatum that is implicated in addiction (see Chapter 6), and in some of these regions the differences are related to the subjective pleasantness rating value of the craved food (Rolls & McCabe 2007). It was of interest that there were no differences between the cravers and the non-cravers in the activations in the taste insula to the chocolate, so that the differences found were in the tuning of the reward system and not of the purely sensory system (Rolls & McCabe 2007). Individual differences in brain responses to images of food have also been described by Beaver, Lawrence, Ditzhuijzen, Davis, Woods & Calder (2006).

The concept that individual differences in responsiveness to food reward are reflected in brain activations in regions related to the control food intake (Rolls 2014b, Rolls 2007b, Rolls 2011b, Rolls 2012c) may provide a way for understanding and helping to control food intake. In this context, we should remember from Chapters 2 and 3 that individual differences in the reward systems are to be expected given that variation in these systems is an important part of the process of evolution by natural selection. Research in this area with the aim of understanding the relation between the activation of different brain systems by food, and obesity, is developing rapidly (Volkow, Wang, Tomasi & Baler 2013).

5.4.3 Food palatability

A factor in obesity is food palatability, which with modern methods of food production can now be greater than would have been the case during the evolution of our feeding control systems. These brain systems evolved so that internal signals from for example gastric distension and glucose utilization could act to decrease the pleasantness of the sensations produced by feeding sufficiently by the end of a meal to stop further eating. However, the greater palatability of modern food may mean that this balance is altered, so that there is a tendency for the greater palatability of food to be insufficiently decreased by a standard amount of food eaten, so that extra food is eaten in a meal (Rolls 2014b, Rolls 2012c, Rolls 2016e) (see Fig. 5.7).

5.4.4 Sensory-specific satiety

Sensory-specific satiety is the decrease in the appetite for a particular food as it is eaten in a meal, without a decrease in the appetite for different foods, as shown above in Chapters 4 and 5. It is an important factor influencing how much of each food is eaten in a meal, and its evolutionary significance may be to encourage eating of a range of different foods, and thus obtaining a range of nutrients. As a result of sensory-specific satiety, if a wide variety of foods is available, overeating in a meal can occur. Given that it is now possible to make available a very wide range of food flavours, textures, and appearances, and that such foods are readily available, this variety effect may be a factor in promoting excess food intake.

5.4.5 Fixed meal times, and the availability of food

Another factor that could contribute to obesity is fixed meal times, in that the normal control of food intake by alterations in inter-meal interval is not readily available in humans, and food may be eaten at a meal-time even if hunger is not present (Rolls 2014b). Even more than this, because of the high and easy availability of food (in the home and workplace) and stimulation by advertising, there is a tendency to start eating again when satiety signals after a previous meal have decreased only a little, and the consequence is that the system again becomes overloaded.

5.4.6 Food saliency, and portion size

Making food salient, for example by placing it on display, may increase food selection particularly in the obese (Schachter 1971, Rodin 1976, Cornell, Rodin & Weingarten 1989), and portion size is a factor, with more being eaten if a large portion of food is presented (Rolls 2012a), though whether this is a factor that can lead to obesity and not just alter test meal size is not yet clear. The driving effects of visual and other stimuli, including the effects of advertising, on the brain systems that are activated by food reward may be different in different individuals, and may contribute to obesity.

5.4.7 Energy density of food

Although gastric emptying rate is slower for high energy density foods, this does not fully compensate for the energy density of the food (Hunt & Stubbs 1975, Hunt 1980). The implication is that eating energy dense foods (e.g. high fat foods) may not allow gastric distension to contribute sufficiently to satiety. Partly at least because of this, the energy density of foods is an important factor that influences how much energy is consumed in a meal (Rolls 2012a). Indeed, it is notable that obese people tend to eat foods with high energy density, and to visit restaurants with high energy density (e.g. high fat) foods. It is also a matter of clinical experience that gastric emptying is faster in obese than in thin individuals, so that gastric distension may play a less effective role in contributing to satiety in the obese. It is also important to remember that the flavour of a food can be conditioned to its energy density, leading over a few days to more eating of low than high energy dense foods, in the phenomena known as conditioned appetite and conditioned satiety (Booth 1985).

5.4.8 Eating rate

A factor related to the above is eating rate, which is typically fast in the obese, and may provide insufficient time for the full effect of satiety signals as food reaches the intestine to operate.

5.4.9 Stress

Another potential factor is stress, which can induce eating and could contribute to a tendency to obesity. (In a rat model of this, mild stress in the presence of food can lead to overeating and obesity. This overeating is reduced by antianxiety drugs.)

5.4.10 Food craving

Binge eating has some parallels to addiction. In one rodent model of binge eating, access to sucrose for several hours each day can lead to binge-like consumption of the sucrose over a period of days (Berner, Bocarsly, Hoebel & Avena 2011). The binge-eating is associated with the release of dopamine. This model brings binge eating close to an addictive process, at least in this model, in that after the binge-eating has become a habit, sucrose withdrawal decreases dopamine release in the ventral striatum (a part of the brain involved in addiction to drugs such as amphetamine), altered binding of dopamine to its receptors in the ventral striatum is produced, and signs of withdrawal from an addiction occur including teeth chattering. In withdrawal, the animals are also hypersensitive to the effects of amphetamine. Another rat model is being used to investigate the binge eating of fat, and whether the reinforcing cues associated with this can be reduced by the GABA-B receptor agonist baclofen (Berner et al. 2011). In humans, there is some overlap of the brain systems activated by food and by cues related to addiction (Volkow et al. 2013).

5.4.11 Energy output

If energy intake is greater than energy output, body weight increases. Energy output is thus an important factor in the equation. However, studies in humans show that although exercise has health benefits, it does not have very significant effects on body weight gain and adiposity in the obese or those who become obese (Wilks, Besson, Lindroos & Ekelund 2011, Thomas, Bouchard, Church, Slentz, Kraus, Redman, Martin, Silva, Vossen, Westerterp & Heymsfield 2012). These findings help to emphasize the importance of understanding the factors that lead to overeating, including factors such as increased responsiveness of the reward system for food in some individuals, and the effects described here that contribute to reward signals produced in modern society being greater than the satiety signals, which have not changed from those in our evolutionary history (Heitmann et al. 2012).

5.4.12 Cognitive factors, and attention

As shown above, cognitive factors, such as preconceptions about the nature of a particular food or odour, can reach down into the olfactory and taste reward value systems in the orbitofrontal cortex that control the palatability of food to influence how pleasant an olfactory, taste, or flavor stimulus is (De Araujo, Rolls, Velazco, Margot & Cayeux 2005, Grabenhorst, Rolls & Bilderbeck 2008a). This has implications for further ways in which food intake can be controlled by cognitive factors, and this needs further investigation. For example, the cognitive factors that have been investigated in these studies are descriptors of the reward value of the food, such as 'rich and delicious'. But it could be that cognitive descriptions of the consequences of eating a particular food, such as 'this food tends to increase body weight', 'this food tends to alter your body shape towards fatness', 'this food tends to make you less attractive', 'this food will reduce the risk of a particular disease', etc., could also modulate the reward value of the food as it is represented in the orbitofrontal cortex. If so, these further types of cognitive modulation could be emphasized in the prevention and treatment of obesity.

In addition, attention to the affective properties of food modulates processing of the reward value of food in the orbitofrontal cortex (Rolls, Grabenhorst, Margot, da Silva & Velazco 2008a, Grabenhorst & Rolls 2008, Ge, Feng, Grabenhorst & Rolls 2012, Luo, Ge, Grabenhorst, Feng & Rolls 2013), and this again suggests that how attention is directed may be important in the extent to which food over-stimulates food intake. Not drawing attention to the reward properties of food, or drawing attention to other properties such as its nutritional value and energy content, could reduce the activation of the brain's reward system by the food, and could be another useful way to help prevent and treat obesity.

5.4.13 Weight gain in women at midlife

Weight gain may occur in women at midlife (Kapoor, Collazo-Clavell & Faubion 2017). Several factors may be involved, including decreased physical activity, and the decreased metabolism associated with the decrease of lean body mass. The menopause itself may not be associated with the weight gain, because the increase of body fat is compensated by a decrease in lean body mass. But the decrease in estrogen at the menopause does tend to be associated with an increase in visceral fat distribution (Kapoor et al. 2017). A Mediterranean diet may help with weight loss, and decreases cardiovascular disease risk. This diet emphasizes plant-based foods, including fruits, vegetables, whole grains, nuts, and legumes, and moderation in fat intake (Kapoor et al. 2017).

5.4.14 Compliance with information about risk factors for obesity

It is important to develop better ways to provide information that will be effective in the long term in decreasing food intake while maintaining a healthy diet, and in promoting an increase in energy expenditure by for example encouraging exercise. In this respect, the individual differences in the brain's response to the reward value of a food, found for example in our study with chocolate cravers and non-cravers (Rolls & McCabe 2007), is one type of factor that may influence whether an individual can comply. But there are individual differences in other factors that may influence compliance, such as impulsiveness, and the orbitofrontal cortex is implicated in this (Berlin, Rolls & Kischka 2004, Berlin, Rolls & Iversen 2005, Robbins, Gillan, Smith, de Wit & Ersche 2012). It is important to better understand possible individual differences in the ability for an individual to stop, and be influenced by the reasoning system with its long-term interests in comparison to the immediate rewards specified by genes (Chapter 10). It could also be that substances such as alcohol shift this balance, making an individual temporarily or possibly in the long term more impulsive and less under control of the reasoning executive system (Crews & Boettiger 2009), and therefore more likely to eat, and to eat unhealthily. These effects of alcohol on impulsiveness may be complemented by hormonal processes (Barson, Karatayev, Chang, Johnson, Bocarsly, Hoebel & Leibowitz 2009). Understanding these processes, and enabling individuals to benefit from this understanding, may also be useful in the prevention and treatment of obesity.

Overall, I suggest that understanding of all the above processes, and their use in combination rather than purely individually, may provide new avenues to the control of overeating and body weight (Rolls 2012c, Rolls 2014b, Rolls 2016e). I have outlined a number of factors that may tend to promote overeating and obesity in our modern society, for example by increasing the impact of reward signals on the brain's appetite control system, or by making it difficult for individuals to resist the increased hedonic value of food. It is possible that any one of these, or a few in combination, could produce overeating and obesity. In these circumstances, to prevent and treat obesity it is unlikely to be sufficient to reduce and focus on or test just one or a few of these factors. As there are many factors, there may always be others that apply and that tend to promote overeating and obesity. The conclusion I therefore reach is that to prevent and treat obesity, it may be important to address all of the above factors together, given that any one, or a few, could tend to lead to overeating and obesity.

6 Pharmacology of emotion, reward, and addiction; the basal ganglia

6.1 Overview of the pharmacology of emotion

The psychomotor drugs of addiction such as amphetamine and cocaine have their effects through dopamine mechanisms that influence the ventral striatum, a part of the basal ganglia, the operation of which is described in Section 6.3.

Dopamine is released from a relatively small number of neurons whose cell bodies are located in the brainstem but which have extensive connections with the basal ganglia and the frontal and temporal cortex. Some dopamine neurons fire when the reward received is greater than expected. They may be involved is the slow training of habit, stimulus-response, systems in the basal ganglia. Because they respond when the reward is greater than expected, but not just to reward value, they appear to play a less direct role in emotion than the orbitofrontal cortex, where neurons do encode reward value, and where the activations are correlated with subjective pleasure.

Other dopamine neurons respond to aversive stimuli. This raises the question of whether the dopamine system is more of a 'Go' system than a system just for rewards that are better than expected. Consistent with this, it is the dopamine system that degenerates in Parkinson's disease in which the initiation of movements is impaired.

The issue of where dopamine neurons receive their inputs from is a surprisingly little addressed question, but it is suggested that possible pathways originate in the orbitofrontal cortex and amygdala and influence the brainstem dopamine (and serotonin) neurons via pathways such as the ventral striatum and habenula.

Drugs such as morphine act on opiate receptors in the brain to reduce pain, and can therefore be reinforcing. In the brain, endogenous opiates such as enkephalin may be released by some types of sensory stimulation to control pain.

Many antianxiety drugs including the benzodiazepines act to increase inhibition in some brain areas produced by the inhibitory transmitter GABA (gamma-amino-butyric acid).

Cannabis sativa derivatives (marijuana, hashish etc.) contain substances such as Δ^9-tetra-hydro-cannabinol (Δ^9-THC) that activate a brain cannabinoid receptor (CB1) to influence pain, memory, and cognitive function.

The pharmacology of drugs that influence depression including drugs that influence serotonin neurons is described in Chapter 9.

6.2 Dopamine systems in the brain

Dopamine is involved in reward systems in the brain with major dopamine inputs to the orbitofrontal cortex; in addiction; and in the functions of the basal ganglia considered in

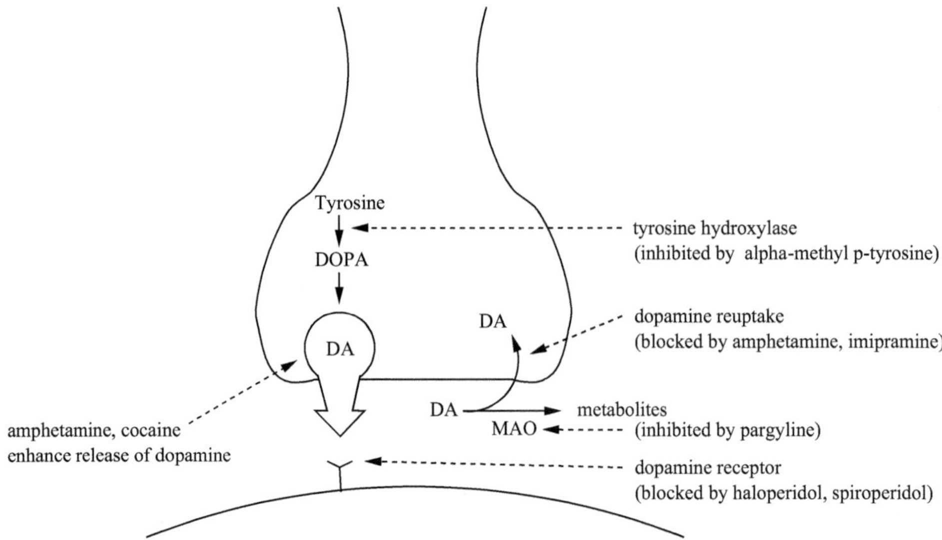

Fig. 6.1 Schematic diagram showing how pharmacological agents affect a dopaminergic synapse. The presynaptic terminal above is shown separated by the synaptic cleft from the postsynaptic cell below. DOPA, dihydroxyphenylalanine; DA, dopamine; MAO, monoamine oxidase.

Section 6.3 which provide one set of outputs from the orbitofrontal cortex, cingulate cortex, and amygdala. We therefore start with an introduction to some of the pharmacology of the dopamine systems in the brain.

6.2.1 Dopamine pharmacology

Dopamine is normally released from the presynaptic membrane in vesicles when an action potential occurs. The released dopamine travels across the synaptic cleft to activate dopamine receptors (of which there are several types) in the postsynaptic membrane. The pharmacological agents haloperidol, spiroperidol, and pimozide block the DA receptors in the postsynaptic membrane. The drug amphetamine enhances the release of DA from the presynaptic membrane (Fig. 6.1) (Iversen, Iversen, Bloom & Roth 2009).

After dopamine is released into the synapse, and some of it activates the postsynaptic receptors, the remaining dopamine is removed from the synapse quickly by a number of mechanisms. One is reuptake into the presynaptic terminal. This process involves dopamine transporter (DAT), and is blocked by amphetamine and by cocaine, which both thus increase the concentration of dopamine in the synapse. Another mechanism for removing DA from the synapse is by monoamine oxidase (MAO), which destroys the DA. MAO is present in the synapse, and also in the presynaptic mechanism. MAO inhibitors (MAOI) thus also increase the concentration of DA in the synapse (and also of NA in noradrenergic synapses, and 5-hydroxytryptamine (5-HT, serotonin) in serotonergic synapses). Another mechanism is diffusion out of the synaptic cleft.

6.2.2 Dopamine pathways

The dopaminergic neurons' pathways have been traced using histofluorescence and other techniques (Dahlström & Fuxe 1965, Ungerstedt 1971, Bjorklund & Lindvall 1986, Cooper, Bloom & Roth 2003, Haber 2016). The mesostriatal dopamine projection (see Fig. 6.2)

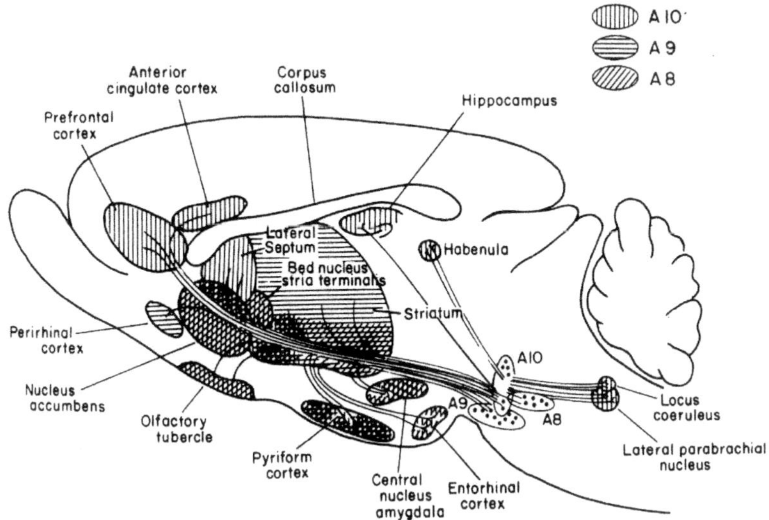

Fig. 6.2 Schematic diagram illustrating the distribution of the main central neuronal pathways containing dopamine. The stippled regions indicate the major nerve-terminal areas and their cell groups of origin. The cell groups in this figure are named according to the nomenclature of Dahlstrom and Fuxe (1965). The A9 cell group in the substantia nigra pars compacta is one of the main DA-containing cell groups, and gives rise mainly to the nigro-striatal dopamine pathway terminating in the striatum. The A10 cell group in the ventral tegmental area is the other main DA-containing cell groups, and gives rise mainly to the meso-limbic DA pathway which terminates in the nucleus accumbens and the olfactory tubercle (together known as the ventral striatum), and the meso-cortical DA pathway which terminates in prefrontal, anterior cingulate, and some other cortical areas. Reproduced from *The Biochemical Basis of Neuropharmacology*, 8th edition, by Jack R. Cooper, Floyd E. Bloom, and Robert H. Roth, p. 227, Figure 9.1a © Oxford University Press, 2004. Reproduced by permission of Oxford University Press.

originates mainly (but not exclusively) from the A9 dopamine cell group in the substantia nigra, pars compacta, and projects to the (dorsal or neo-) striatum, in particular the caudate nucleus and putamen. The mesolimbic dopamine system originates mainly from the A10 cell group, and projects to the nucleus accumbens and olfactory tubercle, which together constitute the ventral striatum (see Fig. 6.2). In addition there is a mesocortical dopamine system projecting mainly from the A10 neurons to the frontal cortex, but especially in primates also to other cortical areas, including parts of the temporal cortex.

6.2.3 Self-administration of dopaminergic substances, and addiction

In this section evidence is summarized that a major class of drug, the psychomotor stimulants such as amphetamine and cocaine and both of which stimulate the release of dopamine, can produce their reward by acting on a dopaminergic mechanism in the nucleus accumbens (part of the ventral striatum) (Everitt & Robbins 2013, Koob & Volkow 2016), which receives a dopaminergic input from the A10 cell group in the ventral tegmental area. These drugs are addictive, and understanding their mode of action in the brain helps to clarify how these drugs produce their effects. Some of the evidence is as follows:

1. Amphetamine (which increases the release of dopamine and noradrenaline) is self-administered intravenously by humans, monkeys, rats, etc.
2. Amphetamine self-injection intravenously is blocked by dopamine receptor blockers such as pimozide and spiroperidol. The implication is that the psychomotor stimulants produce their reward by causing the release of dopamine which acts on dopamine receptors. The

receptor blocker at first increases the rate at which the animal will work for the intravenous injection. The reason for this is that with each lever press for amphetamine, less reward is produced than without the receptor blockade, so the animal works more to obtain the same net amount of reward. This is typical of what happens with low rate operant response behaviour when the magnitude of the reward is reduced. The rate increase is a good control which shows that the dopamine receptor blockade at the doses used does not produce its reward-reducing effect by interfering with motor responses.

3. Apomorphine (which activates D2 dopamine receptors) is self-administered intravenously.
4. Intravenous self-administration of indirect DA agonists such as D-amphetamine and cocaine is much decreased by 6-OHDA lesions of the nucleus accumbens.
5. Rats will learn to self-administer very small quantities of amphetamine to the nucleus accumbens. This effect is abolished by 6-OHDA lesions of the meso-limbic dopamine pathway.

In rodents early on in cocaine self-administration the behaviour is under control of an action–outcome system in the nucleus accumbens core and dorsomedial striatum, whereas a dorsolateral striatum-dependent stimulus-response, habit, process controls the behaviour after repeated self-administration over several weeks (Everitt, Belin, Economidou, Pelloux, Dalley & Robbins 2008, Everitt & Robbins 2013).

When humans receive amphetamine, some of the main brain areas that are activated are the medial orbitofrontal cortex, and the rostral part of the anterior cingulate cortex, as well as the ventral striatum (Voellm, De Araujo, Cowen, Rolls, Kringelbach, Smith, Jezzard, Heal & Matthews 2004). This indicates that at least part of the reward and pleasure produced by the psychomotor stimulants may be being produced by activation of the medial orbitofrontal and anterior cingulate cortex, both of which receive dopamine inputs, and in both of which there are neurons and activations produced by natural rewards. Consistently, the orbitofrontal cortex as well as the areas to which it projects such as the ventral striatum are activated in cocaine (another psychomotor stimulant) addicts by exposure to drug-related conditioned stimuli associated with the cocaine (Volkow et al. 2013). Also consistent with the role of the orbitofrontal cortex in the reward value of psychomotor stimulants, amphetamine is self-administered to the orbitofrontal cortex by monkeys (Phillips, Mora & Rolls 1981).

The (Pavlovian) conditioned cues that support addiction and may lead to relapse to addiction by Pavlovian-instrumental transfer (Cardinal et al. 2002) may operate in part via the orbitofrontal cortex, for Childress et al. (1999) have shown that cocaine-related cues shown visually in a video to addicts activate the orbitofrontal cortex, and also parts of the anterior cingulate and medial prefrontal cortex.

However, dopamine does not appear to implement the rewarding effects of other drugs, including opiates, nicotine, and cannabis, and the evidence that dopamine implements the addictive effects even of stimulant drugs in humans needs re-evaluation (Nutt, Lingford-Hughes, Erritzoe & Stokes 2015).

6.2.4 Behaviours associated with the release of dopamine

The functional role of dopamine can be investigated by determining what factors influence its release. It has been found that the preparatory behaviours for feeding, including foraging for food, food hoarding, and performing instrumental responses to obtain food and other reinforcers, are more associated with dopamine release than is the consummatory behaviour of feeding itself (Phillips, Vacca & Ahn 2008, Phillips, Pfaus & Blaha 1991). Dopamine may also be released in relation to movement and incentive motivation (Phillips et al. 2008).

Although the majority of the studies have focused on rewarded behaviour, there is also extensive evidence that dopamine can be released by stimuli that are aversive or stressful (Bromberg-Martin, Matsumoto & Hikosaka 2010). For example, Rada, Mark & Hoebel

(1998) showed that dopamine was released in the nucleus accumbens when rats worked to escape from aversive hypothalamic stimulation.

6.2.5 Dopamine neurons and reward prediction error

There is extensive evidence that dopamine neurons may signal positive reward prediction error, that is, can respond when a reward is unexpectedly obtained, or when the reward obtained is greater than predicted, or when a stimulus predicting reward is given (Schultz 2013, Glimcher 2011b, Schultz 2016b, Schultz 2016a). The phasic response of the dopamine neurons has an initial non-selective component, and is followed with a latency that may be as long as 200 ms by a second component that is increased firing if the reward is greater and expected, and a decrease of the very low spontaneous rate if the reward is less that expected. However, the evidence for this interpretation is not fully consistent, in that some dopamine neurons respond to aversive stimuli, some to rewarding and aversive stimuli, and others to stimuli that may be salient in other ways, for example novel stimuli (Matsumoto & Hikosaka 2009a, Bromberg-Martin et al. 2010). Further, some of the positive reward prediction error neurons also increase their firing to a bitter taste in low concentrations (Schultz 2016b), even though a bitter taste can not be a positive reward prediction error. A further complication is that the tonic, sustained, firing of the dopamine neurons has been related to reward uncertainty (Fiorillo, Tobler & Schultz 2003). Another complication is that some dopamine neurons are related to habit-based rewards, and do not signal normal positive reward prediction error (Kim, Ghazizadeh & Hikosaka 2015).

These dopamine neurons are thus very different from the reward encoding neurons in the orbitofrontal cortex which respond to the value of the outcomes, and of activations in the orbitofrontal cortex, which are linearly relate to the subjective affective value of tastes, flavours etc, and are thus closely related to emotional value, as described in Chapters 4 and 5 including Section 4.3. The difference is that the dopamine neurons respond to a better than expected outcome, not to the value of the outcome. Further, the dopamine neurons may stop responding to the primary (unlearned) reinforcer or outcome quite rapidly as the task is learned, and instead respond only to the earliest indication that a trial of the task is about to begin (Schultz, Romo, Ljunberg, Mirenowicz, Hollerman & Dickinson 1995). **Thus dopamine neurons could not convey information about a primary reward obtained and is subjective affective value if the trial is successful. They are thus unlike, and could not perform the functions of, the outcome value neurons in the orbitofrontal cortex described in Chapter 4**.

These dopamine neurons are also very different from the orbitofrontal cortex negative reward prediction error neurons, which have strong increased firing when the reward outcome is *lower* than expected (as illustrated in Fig. 4.16, Thorpe, Rolls & Maddison (1983)).

Another difficulty is the issue of where dopamine neurons receive their inputs from, given that the necessary signals for the computation of positive reward prediction error, namely expected value, and outcome value, are not a feature of midbrain neurons. This is a surprisingly little addressed question (Schultz 2013, Schultz 2016b, Schultz 2016a). However, I have suggested that possible pathways originate in the orbitofrontal cortex and amygdala and influence the brainstem dopamine (and serotonin) neurons via pathways such as the ventral striatum and habenula (Rolls 2017b), as considered in Section 9.7.1 and Fig. 9.14.

Despite these difficulties, the dopamine positive reward prediction error hypothesis has been built into models of learning in which the error signal is used to train synaptic connections in dopamine pathway recipient regions (such as presumably the striatum) (Waelti et al. 2001, Dayan & Abbott 2001, Schultz 2013, Glimcher 2011b). The error would be used in a reinforcement learning system to implement temporal difference learning (both of which are described by Dayan & Abbott (2001) and Rolls (2014b).) A possible effect of the dopamine to implement temporal difference learning would be for dopamine release to act via D1 receptors in the striatum to facilitate long-term synaptic potentiation (LTP) of the cortical glutamatergic excitatory inputs onto striatal neurons (see Schultz (2013)). This form of slow learning might help the striatum to learn stimulus-response habits (see Section 6.3). Consistently, we (Rolls et al. 2008e), and many others (Garrison, Erdeniz & Done 2013), have found that activations in the ventral striatum are correlated with temporal difference reward/punishment prediction errors in a number of tasks.

Overall, although there is much evidence that some dopamine neurons encode a reward prediction error signal, there are difficulties with the hypothesis, and an alternative hypothesis is that overall the dopamine neurons together reflect the effects of many salient stimuli, and that dopamine release has the important function of turning on behaviour to such salient stimuli by facilitating information transmission through the basal ganglia and other brain regions. These possibilities are further discussed by Rolls (2014b).

6.3 The basal ganglia as an output system for emotional and motivational behaviour

6.3.1 Overview of the basal ganglia

The basal ganglia are evolutionarily old subcortical structures that provide a route for emotion-related parts of the brain, including the orbitofrontal cortex, amygdala, and anterior cingulate cortex, to produce habit-related stimulus-response behaviours (Fig. 4.3).

More generally, the striatum, which consists of the caudate nucleus, putamen, and ventral striatum / nucleus accumbens, receive from the nearest part of the cerebral cortex, and then converge further to a second stage of processing in the globus pallidus and substantia nigra (Figs. 6.3 and 6.4).

The principle of operation of both the striatum, and globus pallidus / substantia nigra is that the neurons directly inhibit each other, using the inhibitory transmitter GABA (gamma-amino-butyric acid). This is a simple and safe way to select outputs, with the two stage convergence (cortex to striatum; striatum to pallidum / substantia nigra) helping to make this possible by limiting the number of inputs to neurons at any stage of processing to $\approx$ 10,000.

The dopamine inputs to the striatum may facilitate the appropriate mappings from input to output in this system.

Interestingly, the outputs of the basal ganglia are not directed down towards the brainstem motor areas, but instead project via the thalamus back up to the cortex, including motor cortical areas, but also other cortical areas (Fig. 6.3). The basal ganglia may thus be a more general system for allowing competition between the outputs of different cortical areas, to select mapping to a few outputs, to ensure consistency in the execution of movements.

In Parkinson's disease, the dopamine neurons gradually degenerate, and the linkage between cortical inputs and movements starts to fail.

Fuller evidence on the operation of the basal ganglia is provided elsewhere (Rolls 2014b, Rolls 2016c).

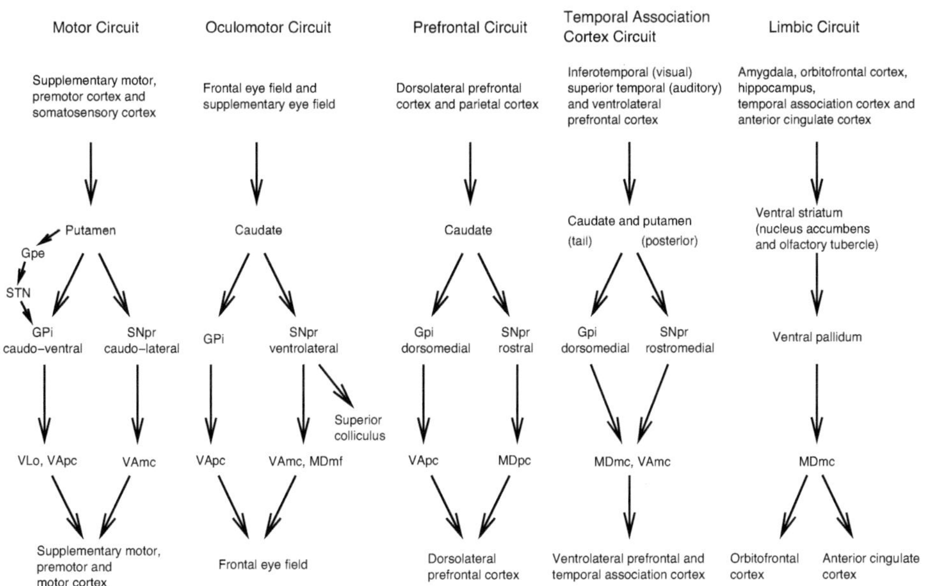

Fig. 6.3 A synthesis of some of the anatomical studies (see text) of the connections of the basal ganglia. GPe, Globus Pallidus, external segment; GPi, Globus Pallidus, internal segment; MD, nucleus medialis dorsalis; SNpr, Substantia Nigra, pars reticulata; VAmc, n. ventralis anterior pars magnocellularis of the thalamus; VApc, n. ventralis anterior pars compacta; VLo, n. ventralis lateralis pars oralis; VLm, n. ventralis pars medialis. An indirect pathway from the striatum via the external segment of the globus pallidus and the subthalamic nucleus (STN) to the internal segment of the globus pallidus is present for the first four circuits (left to right in the figure) of the basal ganglia.

6.3.2 Systems-level architecture of the basal ganglia

The point-to-point connectivity of the basal ganglia as shown by experimental anterograde and retrograde neuroanatomical path tracing techniques in the primate is indicated in Figs. 6.3 and 6.4. The general connectivity is for cortical or limbic inputs to reach the striatum, which then projects to the globus pallidus and substantia nigra pars reticulata, which in turn project via the thalamus back to the cerebral cortex (DeLong & Wichmann 2010, Gerfen & Surmeier 2011, Buot & Yelnik 2012, Haber 2016). Within this overall scheme, there is a set of at least partially segregated parallel processing streams, as illustrated in Figs. 6.3 and 6.4 (Rolls & Johnstone 1992, Rolls 2014b, Rolls 2016c, Haber 2016, Bostan, Dum & Strick 2018). Of especial interest in the context of reward mechanisms in the brain, limbic and related structures such as the amygdala, orbitofrontal cortex, and hippocampus project to the ventral striatum (which includes the nucleus accumbens), which has connections through the ventral pallidum to the mediodorsal nucleus of the thalamus and thus to the prefrontal and cingulate cortices (Buot & Yelnik 2012, Julian, Keinath, Frazzetta & Epstein 2018). It is notable that the projections from the amygdala and orbitofrontal cortex are not restricted to the nucleus accumbens, but also occur to the adjacent ventral part of the head of the caudate nucleus (Amaral & Price 1984, Seleman & Goldman-Rakic 1985).

At striatal neurons of the direct pathway (from the striatum directly to the globus pallidus internal segment), dopamine has excitatory effects via the D1 receptor by eliciting or prolonging glutamate excitatory inputs. At striatal neurons in the indirect pathway (from the striatum via the external segment of the globus pallidus via the subthalamic nucleus to the internal segment of the globus pallidus, see Fig. 6.3), D2 receptor activation has inhibitory effects by reducing glutamate release and prolonging membrane down states (hyperpolarization). Both

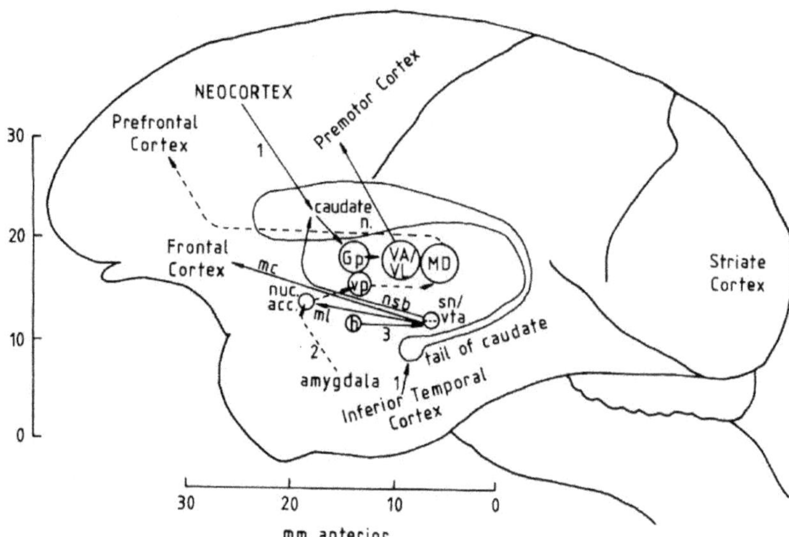

Fig. 6.4 Some of the striatal and connected regions in which the activity of single neurons is described shown on a lateral view of the brain of the macaque monkey. Gp, globus pallidus; h, hypothalamus; sn, substantia nigra, pars compacta (A9 cell group), which gives rise to the nigrostriatal dopaminergic pathway, or nigrostriatal bundle (nsb); vta, ventral tegmental area, containing the A10 cell group, which gives rise to the mesocortical dopamine pathway (mc) projecting to the frontal and cingulate cortices and to the mesolimbic dopamine pathway (ml), which projects to the nucleus accumbens (nuc acc). There is a route from the nucleus accumbens to the ventral pallidum (vp) which then projects to the mediodorsal nucleus of the thalamus (MD) which in turn projects to the prefrontal cortex. Correspondingly, the globus pallidus projects via the ventral anterior and ventrolateral (VA/VL) thalamic nuclei to cortical areas such as the premotor cortex.

effects of dopamine tend to promote behavioural output (Gerfen & Surmeier 2011).

6.3.3 Neuronal activity in different parts of the striatum

We will focus first on neuronal activity in the **ventral striatum**, because it is particularly relevant to the processing of rewards by the basal ganglia. We again focus on neuronal research in monkeys, because the inputs from the orbitofrontal cortex are so different to those in rodents. Some neurons in the macaque ventral striatum respond to rewarding visual stimuli in a visual discrimination task, but the responses are less clear than of neurons in the orbitofrontal cortex that projects into the ventral striatum. Other ventral striatal neurons responded to faces; to novel visual stimuli; to other visual stimuli; in relation to somatosensory stimulation and movement; or to cues that signalled the start of a task (Rolls & Williams 1987, Williams, Rolls, Leonard & Stern 1993).

Neurons in the **tail of the caudate nucleus** and adjoining putamen which receive from the inferior temporal visual cortex and the prestriate cortex (Kemp & Powell 1970, Saint-Cyr, Ungerleider & Desimone 1990) respond to visual stimuli, but habituate quite rapidly (Caan, Perrett & Rolls 1984). These neurons may be involved in detecting and orienting to new visual stimuli.

Neurons in the **Postero-ventral putamen**, which receives from the inferior temporal visual cortex and the prefrontal cortex (Goldman & Nauta 1977, Van Hoesen, Yeterian & Lavizzo-Mourey 1981) had responses in a visual short-term memory task (delayed match-to-

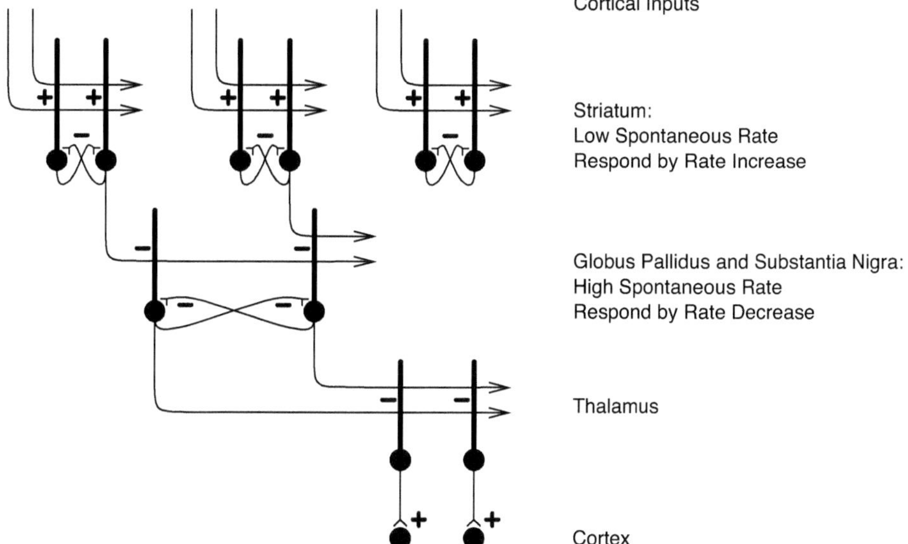

Fig. 6.5 Simple hypothesis of basal ganglia network architecture. A key aspect is that in both the striatum, and in the globus pallidus and substantia nigra pars reticulata, there are direct inhibitory connections (–) between the principal neurons, as shown. These synapses use GABA as a transmitter. Excitatory inputs to the striatum are shown as +. (Reproduced from *Neural Networks and Brain Function* by Edmund T. Rolls and Alessandro Treves, p. 220, Figure 9.14 © Edmund T. Rolls and Alessandro Treves, 1998. Reproduced by permission of Oxford University Press and The Authors.)

sample) task, responding for example in the delay period (Johnstone & Rolls 1990, Rolls & Johnstone 1992). They reflect the activity in the cortical areas that project into this part of the striatum.

Neurons in the **head of the caudate nucleus**, which receives from the prefrontal cortex (Kemp & Powell 1970, Haber 2016) had activity to many environmental stimuli, and frequently to cues that a task was about to start (Rolls, Thorpe & Maddison 1983c). These neurons may be involved in the preparation for movement.

The activity of many neurons in the anterior **putamen**, which receives from motor and somatosensory cortical areas, is related to movements (Rolls, Thorpe, Boytim, Szabo & Perrett 1984b, DeLong & Wichmann 2010). There is a somatotopic organization of neurons in the putamen, with separate areas containing neurons responding to arm, leg, or orofacial movements. Some of these neurons respond only to active movements, and others to active and to passive movements. Many of these neurons respond in relation to mouth movements such as licking. Similar neurons are found in the substantia nigra, pars reticulata, to which the putamen projects (Mora, Mogenson & Rolls 1977).

This evidence, and much other evidence on the dendritic arrangements within the basal ganglia (Percheron, Yelnik & François 1984a, Percheron, Yelnik & François 1984b, Percheron, Yelnik, François, Fenelon & Talbi 1994, Yelnik 2002, Buot & Yelnik 2012), have been put together to formulate a hypothesis about the operation of the basal ganglia, with is sketched in Fig. 6.5 (Rolls 2014b, Rolls 2016c). The hypothesis is that the basal ganglia with multistage convergence, with learning of associated inputs onto striatal neurons, and mutual inhibition between the neurons provides a mechanism for selecting a few outputs to drive behaviour. In the context of reinforcing stimuli, this provides a basis for stimuli for any cortical area to be linked associatively, perhaps with the facilitation of dopamine, to link the stimuli to responses.

6.4 Opiate reward systems, analgesia, and food reward

Electrical stimulation of some regions of the brain can lead to analgesia in animals ranging from rats to humans and can be equivalent in its pain-reducing properties to large doses of morphine (Liebeskind & Paul 1977). These analgesic effects can last for hours after only seconds of stimulation. The analgesia is often for only part of the body, so that a strong pinch to one side but not to the other might be ignored. This shows that the stimulation-produced analgesia is not simply some general interference with the animal's ability to respond to stimulation. The effective stimulation sites are in the medial brainstem, and extend from the rostral medulla (nucleus raphe magnus), through the midbrain central grey matter, towards the hypothalamus. As described by Rolls (2005), at some sites both analgesia and self-stimulation are found, and at other sites the stimulation is aversive but is followed by analgesia. It has been shown that naloxone, a specific morphine antagonist, reverses, at least partly, stimulation-produced analgesia in both the rat and in humans (Adams 1976, Akil, Mayer & Liebeskind 1976). The endogenous morphine-like peptide enkephalin (Hughes 1975, Hughes, Smith, Kosterlitz, Fothergill, Morgan & Morris 1975) injected intraventricularly yields analgesia (Beluzzi, Grant, Garsky, Sarantakis, Wise & Stein 1976), and central grey matter stimulation releases this substance or a peptide similar to it (Liebeskind, Giesler & Urca 1985). Further, there are stereospecific opiate-binding sites in the central grey matter, and elsewhere in the brain (Kuhar, Pert & Snyder 1973, Snyder 2004) which mediate the many effects of opioids including pain relief and some types of reward and addiction including that to alcohol (Terenius & Johansson 2010). These findings raise the possibility that stimulation-produced analgesia is effective because it causes the release of a naturally occurring morphine-like substance which acts on opiate receptors in the central grey matter and elsewhere to provide analgesia. The function of this pain-reduction may be, after injury and the initial behavioural reaction to it to prevent further injury, to reduce the on-going effects of continuing severe pain, which could otherwise impair the animal's ability to cope well behaviourally with other needs.

At some of these analgesia-producing sites the electrical stimulation can produce reward (see Koob & Le Moal (1997)). The reward at these sites might be related to the pain-reducing effect of the release of opiates, which can itself be pleasurable and positively reinforcing. However, it is also known that endogenous opiates can be released by behaviours such as grooming (Dunbar 1996), and this may be part of the mechanism by which grooming produces pleasure and relaxation, for blockade of opiate receptors with naloxone greatly reduces grooming interactions.

6.5 Pharmacology of anxiety in relation to brain systems involved in emotion

One class of antianxiety drug, the benzodiazepines, bind to 'benzodiazepine receptors' in the brain, increasing the frequency of opening of the $GABA_A$ (γ-aminobutyric acid) receptor-activated chloride channels. The influx of chloride through these channels produces hyper-polarization of neurons, and thus a decrease in firing (Cooper, Bloom & Roth 2003, Iversen, Iversen, Bloom & Roth 2009). Barbiturates, which have antianxiety properties, prolong the opening of the same chloride channels. Indeed, many antianxiety treatments facilitate GABA actions, with $GABA_A$ receptors being relevant (Nemeroff 2003). Current guidelines do not recommend benzodiazepines as first-line treatments due to their potential side effects. Selective serotonin reuptake inhibitors and selective serotonin norepinephrine reuptake inhibitors are recommended with psychotherapy as first-line treatments (Thibaut 2017).

Given that GABA is the most widespread inhibitory transmitter in the brain, these findings leave open, of course, where the antianxiety drugs work. One early suggestion is that they influence the hippocampus (Gray 1987). However, there is almost no evidence linking the hippocampus to emotion, and instead the evidence indicates that it is involved in memory, often when this has a spatial aspect (including a spatial context), or is episodic, about a particular past event or episode (Rolls 2016c, Kesner & Rolls 2015). Indeed, fornix section, which produces many of the effects of hippocampal and related damage on memory, has no effects on stimulus–reinforcement association learning or reversal (Gaffan, Saunders, Gaffan, Harrison, Shields & Owen 1984, Jones & Mishkin 1972). Further, Rawlins, Winocur & Gray (1983) showed that damage to the hippocampus of rats did not abolish the antianxiety effects of the antianxiety drug chlordiazepoxide in an animal model of anxiety. However, it is possible that if in anxiety states particular episodic memories are retrieved, then the hippocampus may play a role in this memory-related aspect of anxiety.

Evidence is now being sought about the brain states in a number of different clinical anxiety syndromes (Cannistraro & Rauch 2003):

In *post-traumatic stress disorder* (PTSD) there is some evidence for hyperresponsivity of the amygdala, and deficient activation of the ventral/medial prefrontal cortex and hippocampus (Cannistraro & Rauch 2003). It is hypothesized that the low activation of the ventral/medial prefrontal cortex may contribute to difficulty in reversing the learning that led to the anxiety.

In *specific phobias*, there may be abnormal activation produced by phobia-producing stimuli in phobics relative to controls of areas afferent to the amygdala such as the insula (perhaps because tactile imagery is activating somatosensory regions), but not of the amygdala itself; and also abnormal activation of the dorsolateral prefrontal cortex and hippocampus, perhaps related to mnemonic processes being activated during the phobic processing (Cannistraro & Rauch 2003).

In *social phobias* (anxiety states associated with social situations) there may be increased amygdala activation by faces (Cannistraro & Rauch 2003).

In *panic disorder*, there may be increased activation in regions such as the cingulate and orbitofrontal cortex and the hippocampus (Cannistraro & Rauch 2003).

In *obsessive–compulsive disorders* (OCD) there is evidence from PET studies of increased activity in the orbitofrontal cortex, anterior cingulate cortex, and striatum, and activations in these regions are greater in the symptomatic compared to the control neutral state (Cannistraro & Rauch 2003).

In *generalized anxiety disorder* (GAD) cognitive behaviour therapy is frequently used, sometimes in combination with a wide range of types of pharmacological treatment (Hoge, Ivkovic & Fricchione 2012).

As in the case of antidepressant drugs, it may be hoped that future studies will be able to link the effects of antianxiety drugs more closely to areas of the brain known to be involved in emotion, as this may help in the development of better treatments for anxiety, whether by drugs or by other forms of treatment (Farb & Ratner 2014).

6.6 Cannabinoids

Cannabis sativa derivatives (marijuana, hashish etc.) contain substances such as Δ^9-tetrahydro-cannabinol (Δ^9-THC) that activate a brain cannabinoid receptor (CB1) to influence pain, memory, and cognitive function (Wilson & Nicoll 2002). The brain produces its own (endogenous) cannabinoids such as anandamide, and these may act retrogradely across synapses to influence the release of other transmitters (Wilson & Nicoll 2002). Cannabinoid receptors are widespread in the brain, but those in the hippocampus and neocortex may be related to effects of cannabinoids on memory and cognition, and receptors in the brainstem (e.g. the periaqueductal gray and rostral ventromedial medulla) and spinal cord to effects on pain (Wilson & Nicoll 2002). CB1 receptor agonists produce hyperalgesia, consistent with the hypothesis that endogenous cannabinoids normally regulate nociception. Cannabinoids can also increase appetite and body weight (Di Marzo & Matias 2005). Cannabinoids may have some therapeutic uses in for example the treatment of pain (Abrams 2018).

7 Sexual behaviour, reward, and brain function

7.1 Introduction

There have been many advances recently in understanding and theorizing about the different patterns of sexual behaviour and why they have evolved (Buss 2015). The main aim of this Chapter is to describe some of these advances, and some of the basic brain mechanisms involved. An aim that arises is to link much of the recent research on sociobiology, evolutionary psychology and the Darwinian adaptive approaches to different types of sexual behaviour (Buss 2015), to new ideas about how these behaviours could be produced by the sculpting during evolution of systems that are sensitive to different types of reward, and how these processes may be implemented in the brain. That approach is taken here, and is developed further elsewhere with specific hypotheses about the reward systems that are likely to be involved (Rolls 2014b).

Before embarking on describing the research in this area, I would like to warn the reader that some of the strategies used by animals in their aims to reproduce may seem somewhat shocking. But I would like to make it clear that humans, although their emotional systems may be influenced by such processes, are not bound to follow what the genes may encourage for sexual behaviour, because humans, and perhaps closely related animals, have, in addition, a reasoning system that enables humans to choose on rational bases what behaviours are appropriate. This reasoning system, and how it enables choices to be made that may not be encouraged by gene-related behavioural strategies, is described in Chapter 10.

The selection processes that lead to the development of some aspects of sexual behaviour are related to the adaptive value of the function being performed. For example, being healthy and strong enables a male to survive long enough to reproduce, and to fight off competitors for females. Reward systems built by genes that favour these characteristics evolve by what we can call **natural selection**, in a use of the term that is close to that of Darwin (1859, 1871). A distinguishing concept here is that the body survives long enough and is healthy enough to reproduce, and when natural selection is used in its narrow sense here it implies 'survival selection'.

However, Darwin (1871) also recognized that evolution can occur by **sexual selection**, when what is being selected for has no inherent adaptive or survival value for the individual, but is attractive to potential mates (inter-sexual selection), or helps individuals of the same sex to compete better with each other (intra-sexual selection, for e.g. male–male competition). The most cited example is the peacock's large 'tail', which does not have survival value for the peacock (and indeed it is somewhat of a handicap to have a very long tail), but, because it is attractive to the peahen, becomes prevalent in the population. It turns out that sexual selection may lead to all sorts of behaviours being selected, which have in common that they make the bearer attractive to the opposite sex of the species, and are thus useful in courtship, but which would normally be considered as non-sexual types of behaviour, such as kindness and humour (Miller 2000). Thus in this chapter we also consider the reward and punishment systems that may be built by sexual selection (see Section 7.7).

There will be primary reinforcers to consider specified by genes, and then in addition the possibility of learning associations between previously neutral stimuli and these primary reinforcers. A major emphasis in this book is that reward and punishment systems are built to guide behaviour efficiently and appropriately for the specifying genes, and in this chapter I show how sexual selection as well as natural ('survival') selection is involved in this process. Insofar as the states elicited by rewards and punishers are emotional states (see Chapters 2 and 3), this chapter thus extends the understanding of emotion to systems shaped by sexual selection.

The intentional stance is adopted in much writing about sociobiology and evolutionary psychology, and is sometimes used here, but should not be taken literally. It is used just as a shorthand. An example is that it might be said that genes are selfish. But this does not mean at all that genes think about whether to be selfish, and then take the decision. Instead it is just shorthand for a statement along the lines 'genes produce behaviour that operates in the context of natural selection to maximize the number of copies of the gene in the next generations'. Much of the behaviour produced is implicit or unconscious, and when the intentional stance is used as a descriptive tool, it should not be taken to mean that there is usually any explicit or conscious processing involved in the behavioural outcome.

Some of the points may seem 'obvious' once they have been made, if the reader is a neo-Darwinian used to the approach taken in evolutionary biology. However, a potential problem of sociobiology is that its stories do seem plausible, given Darwinism – but many stories are plausible. So we must be careful to seek evidence too, not just plausibility; and we need to know how much of the variance of behaviour is accounted for by each sociobiological account of a type of behaviour. In the long term, once sociobiological hypotheses have been presented, they must be tested.

One of the themes developed elsewhere (Rolls 2014b) is how the underlying physiology of reward is related to the sexual behaviour shown by different types of women, and different types of men. One of the key ideas is that reward systems become tuned to biological functions that they serve.

We now turn to consider what sex reward value systems have been set up by evolution.

7.2 Mate selection, attractiveness, and love

What factors are decoded by our brains to influence mate attractiveness (reward value) and selection? Many factors are involved in mate selection, and they are not necessarily the same for selection of a short-term vs a long-term partner. The selection of a long-term partner in species with long-term relatively monogamous relationships is influenced for example by parental investment, which is a major evolutionary adaptive factor in promoting long-term relationships. Thus in humans, males choose females because human males do make a parental investment; and females compete for males. Indeed, the selection of a long-term partner in humans is mutual, and this tends to reduce sex differences in partner choice. Consistent with this, David Buss has shown that in contrast, human sex differences in mate selection are more evident in short-term mating (Buss 1989, Buss 2016, Buss 2015).

Species with shared parental investment are primarily those where two parents can help the offspring to survive better than one, and this includes many birds (where one bird must sit on the eggs to incubate them, while the other finds food), and humans (where the human infant is born so immature that care of the offspring for a number of years could, when humans were evolving, make it more likely that the offspring, containing the father's genes, would survive, and then reproduce). Most other mammals are not good models of human pair mate selection and pair bonding, because there is generally less advantage to joint care of the young, and the female, who has made the major investment of the gestation period for the baby, and breast feeding it post-partum (for the whole of which period she will remain relatively infertile), generally assumes most of the responsibility for bringing up her young[3]. In most mammals, females will maximize their reproductive success, given the cost of gestation and lactation, by focussing on the successful rearing of offspring. In contrast, male mammals do not invest by gestation and lactation in their offspring, and the most effective way for males to influence their reproductive success is to maximize the number of fertilizations they achieve, and this is a major factor in mammalian mate selection. This tendency is tempered in humans by the advantage of male investment in the offspring, to help the immature offspring to survive sufficiently long that the chances of their reproductive success is high.

[3]Some male mammals do take part in child care e.g. gibbons; but it is striking that among the great apes, humans do stand out in terms of males contributing to bringing up the children. For example, among the great apes, chimpanzees are very promiscuous, and gorillas have a harem system.

7.2.1 Female preferences

Factors that influence female selection of male mates include the following across a range of species (including humans (Buss 2015, Buss 2016, Motta-Mena & Puts 2017)).

1. Athleticism. The ability to compete well in mate selection (including being healthy and strong) is attractive, as this will be useful for her genes when present in her male offspring. Athleticism may be attractive (rewarding) also as an indicator of protection from male marauding (single females are at risk in some species of abuse, and forced copulation, which circumvents female mate choice), from predators, and as an indicator of hunting competency (meat was important in human evolution (Aiello & Wheeler 1995), although the hunt may also have been co-opted by sexual selection as a mating ritual giving the males a chance to show off). Consistent with these points, Buss & Schmitt (1993) showed that women show a strong preference for tall, strong, athletic men.

2. Resources, power and wealth. In species with shared parental investment (which include many birds and humans), having power and wealth may be attractive to the female, because they are indicators of resources that may be provided for her young. Women should desire men who show willingness to invest resources in his partner. Women place a greater premium on income or financial prospects than men (Buss 1989). Further, in a cross-cultural study of 37 cultures with 10,047 participants, it was found that irrespective of cultural/political/social background, women consistently placed more value on financial resources (100% more) than men (Buss 1989, Buss 2016, Buss 2015). Women value a man's love as an indicator of resource commitment.

3. Status. Both now and historically, status hierarchies are found in many cultures (and species, for example monkeys' dominance hierarchies, and chickens' pecking order). Status correlates with the control of resources (e.g. alpha male chimpanzees take precedence in feeding), and therefore acts as a good cue for women. Women should therefore find men of high status attractive (e.g. rock stars, politicians, and tribal rulers), and these men should be able to attract the most attractive partners (Betzig 1986). Consistent with this, Buss (1989) showed cross-culturally that women regard high social status as more valuable than do men; and Udry & Eckland (1984) showed that attractive women marry men of high status.

4. Age. Status and higher income are generally only achieved with age, and therefore women should generally find older men attractive. Buss (1989) showed cross-culturally that women prefer older men (3.42 years older on average; and marriage records from 27 countries showed that the average age difference was 2.99 years).

5. Ambition and industriousness, which may be good predictors of future occupational status and income, are attractive. Valued characteristics include those that show a male will work to improve their lot in terms of resources or in terms of rising up in social status. Cross-culturally, women rated ambition/industriousness as highly desirable (Buss 1989).

6. Testosterone-dependent features may also be attractive. These features include a strong (longer and broader) jaw, a broad chin, strong cheekbones, defined eyebrow ridges, a forward central face, and a lengthened lower face (secondary sexual characteristics which are a result of pubertal hormone levels). High testosterone levels are immuno-suppressing, so these features may be indicators of immuno-competence (and thus honest indicators of fitness). The attractiveness of these masculinized features increases with increased likelihood of conception across the menstrual cycle (Penton-Voak, Perrett, Castles, Kobayashi, Burt, Murray & Minamisawa 1999, Johnston, Hagel, Franklin, Fink & Grammer 2001). The implication is that the neural mechanism controlling perception of attractiveness must be sensitive to oestrogen/progesterone levels in women.

Another feature thought to depend on prenatal testosterone levels is the 2nd/4th digit ratio. A low ratio reflects a testosterone-rich uterine environment. It has been found that low ratios correlate with female ratings of male dominance and masculinity, although the relationship to attractiveness ratings was less clear (Swaddle & Reierson 2002).

7. Symmetry (in both males and females) may be attractive, in that it may reflect good development in utero, a non-harmful birth, adequate nutrition, and lack of disease and parasitic infections. Fluctuating asymmetry (FA) reflects the degree to which individuals deviate from perfect symmetry on bilateral features (e.g. in humans, both ears, both feet, both hands and arms; in other species, bilateral fins, bilateral tail feathers). Greater asymmetry may reflect deviations in developmental design resulting from the disruptive effects of environmental or genetic abnormalities, and in some species is associated with lower fecundity, slower growth, and poorer survival. A low fluctuating asymmetry may thus be a sign of reproductive fitness (Gangestad & Simpson 2000). In a number of bird species, attractive (symmetric) males employ a strategy of investing more in extra-pair mating than in paternal care, and maximize their reproductive success in this way (Moller & Thornhill 1998). In humans, more symmetrical men reported more lifetime partners ($r=0.38$), and more extra-pair partners; and women's choice of extra-pair partners was predicted by male symmetry (see Gangestad & Simpson (2000)). Moreover, women rate men as more attractive if they have high symmetry (low FA). Intellectual ability (which may be attractive to women) is also correlated with symmetry (Gangestad & Thornhill 1999). A further type of evidence here is that the frequency of human female orgasm (which probably results in high sperm retention) correlates with low fluctuating asymmetry (FA) (i.e. being symmetrical) in male partners (Thornhill, Gangestad & Comer 1995).

8. Dependability and faithfulness may be attractive, particularly where there is paternal investment in bringing up the young, as these characteristics may indicate stability of resources (Buss et al. 1990). Emotionally unstable men may also inflict costs on women, and thus women rate emotional stability and maturity as important. For example, jealousy might lead to abuse.

9. Risk-taking by men may be attractive to women, perhaps because it is a form of competitive advertising: surviving the risk may be an honest indicator of high quality genes (Barrett et al. 2002).

10. Sexually selected characteristics. Characteristics that may not be adaptive in terms of the survival of the male, but that may be attractive because of inter-sexual sexual selection, are common in birds, perhaps less common in most mammals, though present in some primates (Kappeler & van Schaik 2004), and may be present in humans (see Section 7.7). An example of a sexually selected characteristic that may not increase the survival of the individual, but that may be attractive to females and thus increase the fitness of the male in terms of whether his genes are passed on to the next generation by reproduction, is the peacock's tail. These characteristics may in some cases be an honest indicator of health, in the sense that having a large gaudy tail may be a handicap.

11. Odour. The preference by women for the odour of symmetrical men is correlated with the probability of fertility of women as influenced by their cycle (Thornhill & Gangstad 1999).

It is important to note that physical factors such as high symmetry and that are indicators of genetic fitness may be especially attractive when women choose short-term partners, and that factors such as resources and faithfulness may be especially important when women choose long-term partners, in what may be termed a conditional mating strategy (Gangestad & Simpson 2000, Buss 2015). This conditionality means that the particular factors that influence preferences alter dynamically, and preferences will often depend on the prevailing circumstances, including the current opportunities and costs.

7.2.2 Male preferences

Males are not always indiscriminate. (In fact, males are probably rarely indiscriminate, in that producing sperm and performing sexual behaviour do have costs, including for example the risk of catching disease.) When a male chooses to invest (for example to produce offspring), there are preferences for the partner with whom they will make the investment. Accurate evaluation of female quality (reproductive value) is therefore important, and a male will need to look out for cues to this, and find these cues attractive (rewarding). The factors that influence female attractiveness to males include the following (Buss 2015, Buss 2016, Barrett et al. 2002).

1. Youth. As fertility and reproductive value in females is linked to age (reproductive value is higher when younger, and actual fertility in humans peaks in the twenties), males (unlike females) place a special premium on youth. It is not youth per se that men find attractive, but indicators of youth, for example neotenous traits such as blonde hair and wide eyes. An example of this preference is that Buss (1989) showed that male college students preferred an age difference on average of 2.5 years younger. Another indicator of youth might be a small body frame, and it is interesting that this might contribute to the small body frame of some women in this example of sexual dimorphism.

2. Beauty. Features that are most commonly described as the most attractive tend to be those that are oestrogen-dependent, e.g. full lips and cheeks, and short lower facial features. (Oestrogen caps the growth of certain facial bones.) Like testosterone, oestrogen also affects the immune system, and its effects might be seen as 'honest indicators' of genetic fitness.

In a cross-cultural study, people of different races agreed in their ratings of the attractiveness of faces of Asian, Hispanic, black, and white women (Cunningham, Roberts, Barbee & Druen 1995). In meta-analyses of 11 studies, Langlois, Kalakanis, Rubenstein, Larson, Hallam & Smoot (2000) demonstrated that (a) raters agree about who is and is not attractive, both within and across cultures; (b) attractive children and adults are judged and treated more positively than unattractive children and adults, even by those who know them; and (c) attractive children and adults exhibit more positive behaviours and traits than unattractive children and adults. In an fMRI study, it was found that attractive faces produce more activation of the human medial orbitofrontal cortex than unattractive faces (O'Doherty et al. 2003).

Further, small babies were even shown to gaze for longer at slides of the more attractive woman when shown pairs of pictures of women that differed in attractiveness (Langlois, Roggman, Casey & Ritter 1987, Langlois, Ritter, Roggman & Vaughn 1991). In another study, 12-month-olds interacted with a stranger. The infants showed more positive affective tone, less withdrawal, and more play involvement with a stranger who wore a professionally constructed attractive than unattractive mask; and played longer with an attractive than an unattractive doll (Langlois, Roggman & Reiser-Danner 1990). These results extend and amplify earlier findings showing that young infants exhibit visual preferences for attractive over unattractive faces. Both visual and behavioural preferences for attractiveness are evidently exhibited much earlier in life than was previously supposed.

Women appear to spend more time on fashion and enhancing beauty than men. Why should this be, when in most mammals it is men who may be gaudy to help in their competition for females, given that females make the larger investment in offspring? In humans, there is of course value to investment by males in their offspring, so women may benefit by attracting a male who will invest time and resources in bring up children together. But nevertheless, women do seem to invest more in bearing and then raising children, so why is the imbalance so marked, with women apparently competing by paying attention to their own beauty and fashion? Perhaps the answer is that males who are willing to make major investments of time and resources in raising the children of a partner are a somewhat limiting resource (as other factors may make it advantageous genetically for men not to invest all their resources in one partner), and because women are competing to obtain and maintain this scarce resource, being beautiful and fashionable is important to women. Faithful men may be a limited resource because there are alternative strategies that may have a low cost, whereas women are essentially committed to a considerable investment in their offspring. These factors lead to greater variability in men's strategies, and thus contribute to making men who invest in their offspring a more limited resource than women who invest in their offspring.

3. Body fat. The face is not the only cue to a woman's reproductive capacity. Although the ideal body weight varies significantly with culture (in cultures with scarcity, obesity is attractive, and relates to status), the ideal distribution of body fat seems to be a universal standard, as measured by the waist-to-hip ratio (which cancels out effects of actual body weight). Consistently, across cultures, men preferred an average ratio of 0.7 (small waist/bigger hips) when rating female figures (line drawings and photographic images) for attractiveness (Singh & Young 1995). Thornhill & Grammer (1999) also found high correlations between rating of attractiveness of nude females by men of different ethnicity. Long-term health risks (diabetes, hypertension, coronary disease, and stroke) are also associated with a high waist-to-hip ratio, which may therefore be an 'honest indicator' of fitness.

4. Fidelity. The desire for fidelity in females is most obviously related to her concealed ovulation (see next paragraph and Section 7.6), and therefore the degree of paternity certainty that males may suffer. Males therefore place a premium on a woman's sexual history. Virginity was a requisite for marriage both historically (before the arrival of contraceptives) and cross-culturally (in non-Westernized societies where virginity is still highly valued) (Buss 1989). Nowadays, female monogamy in previous relationships is a sought after characteristic in future long-term partners (Buss & Schmitt 1993). (Presumably with simple genetic methods now available for identifying the father of a child (Baker & Shackelford 2017), the rational thought system (see Chapter 10) might place less value on fidelity with respect to paternity issues as paternity can be established genetically, yet the implicit emotional system may still place high value on fidelity, as during evolution, fidelity was valued as an indicator of paternity probability.) The modern rational emphasis might be especially placed on valuing fidelity because this may indicate less risk of sexually transmitted disease, and perhaps the emotional value of fidelity will be a help in this respect.

5. Attractiveness and the time of ovulation. Although ovulation in some primates and in humans is concealed (perhaps so that males may be uncertain who the father is of a baby, and thus not threaten infanticide – see Sections 7.6 and 7.3), it would be a premium for men to pick up other cues to ovulation, and find women highly desirable at these times. Possible cues include an increased body temperature reflected in the warm glow of vascularized skin (vandenBerghe & Frost 1986), and pheromonal cues. Indeed, male raters judged the odours of T-shirts worn during the follicular phase as more pleasant and sexy than odours from T-shirts worn during the luteal phase (Singh & Bronstad 2001). In macaques, male interest in females increases during the fertile period, and alpha males more often mate guard females during the fertile phase of the cycle, with possible cues related to the high levels of oestrogen at the time of ovulation (Engelhardt, Pfeifer, Heistermann, Niemitz, Van Hoof & Jodges 2004). Women generally do not know when they are ovulating (and in this sense ovulation may be double blind), but there is a possibility that ovulation could unconsciously affect female behaviour (Section 7.6). In fact, Event-Related Potentials (ERPs) were found to be greater to sexual stimuli in ovulating women, and these could reflect increased affective processing of the stimuli (Krug, Plihal, Fehm & Born 2000). This in turn might affect outward behaviour of the female, helping her to attract a mate at this time.

In most species, females invest heavily in the offspring in terms of providing the eggs and providing the care (from gestation until weaning, and far beyond weaning in the case of humans). Females are therefore a 'limited resource' for males allowing the females to be the choosier sex during mate choice. This leads therefore to strong levels of male intra-sexual selection, resulting in males typically being the larger and/or more flamboyant sex (an example is the male mandrill's brightly coloured face in comparison to the dull one of the female's). If the sex roles become somewhat reversed, however, this can alter. Dramatic female ornamentation can be seen in the pipefish (a relative of the seahorse). Male pipefish overwhelmingly find the larger, most ornamented females the most attractive (Berglund & Rosenqvist 2001). This stems from the fact that the males of these species have evolved a brood pouch (which, in some species, is vascularized) into which the female can oviposit her eggs. Moreover, the size of the (male) brood pouch (which determines how many embryos a male can store) is also another limiting factor that females compete over. This accounts for why the males are the choosier sex and why females compete in pipefish. Female competition is also found in the spotted sandpiper – a bird with an unusual polyandrous breeding system (i.e. a breeding system with one female with multiple males) (Oring 1986). Here, females arrive on the breeding ground first and must attract males to it. The females must defend from other females the territory that contains the individual territories of their male consorts. The males then provide the important resource of incubating the clutch on their own, and therefore become unavailable as mates. This often leads to a chronic shortage of available males, and thus, female competition is intense, and displays are extremely vigorous and occasionally lead to physical combat. Similar polyandrous tactics are also seen in the jacana (Jenni & Collier 1972).

In humans, male investment in caring for the offspring means that male choice has a strong effect on intra-sexual selection in women. Female cosmetic use and designer clothing could be seen as weapons in this competition, and perhaps are reflected in extreme female self-grooming behaviour such as cosmetic surgery, or pathological disorders such as anorexia, bulimia and body dysmorphic disorder. The modern media, by bombarding people with images of beautiful women, may heighten intra-sexual selection even further, pushing women's competitive mating mechanisms to a major scale.

Finally in this section, we should note that in addition to the benefits of particular mate choices, the costs also need to be assessed, and may include the costs not only of sperm production and allocation (Edward, Stockley & Hosken 2015), but also of courtship, mate-guarding, risk of infection, and provision of resources.

7.2.3 Pair-bonding, and love

Attachment to a particular partner by pair bonding in a monogamous relationship, which in humans becomes manifest in love between pair-bonded parents, and which occurs in humans because of the advantage to the man of investing in his offspring, may have special mechanisms to facilitate it. Species in which attachment has been investigated include the prairie vole, which is a rodent (Young, Gobrogge, Liu & Wang 2011, Bosch & Young 2017). In monogamous species of prairie voles, mating can increase pair-bonding (as measured by partner preference). Oxytocin, a hormone released from the posterior pituitary, whose other actions include the milk let-down response, is released during mating. Exogenous administration of oxytocin facilitates pair bonding in both female and male prairie voles (Carter 1998). In female prairie voles, antagonists of oxytocin interfere with partner preference formation. In female prairie voles, the endogenous release of oxytocin is thus important in partner preference and attachment. Thus oxytocin has been thought of as the 'hormone of love'. Oxytocin gene knock-out mice fail to recognize familiar conspecifics after repeated social exposures, and injection of oxytocin in the medial amygdala restores social recognition (Ferguson, Aldag, Insel & Young 2001, Winslow & Insel 2004). In males, the effects of oxytocin are facilitated by vasopressin, another posterior pituitary hormone whose other effects include promoting the retention of water by the kidney. In the case of vasopressin, it has been possible to show that the vasopressin V1a receptor (V1aR) is expressed in higher concentration in the ventral forebrain of monogamous prairie voles than in promiscuous (i.e. polygamous) meadow voles, and that viral vector V1aR transfer into the forebrain of the meadow mouse increases its partner preference (i.e. makes it more like a monogamous prairie vole) (Lim, Wang, Olazabal, Ren, Terwilliger & Young 2004, Young & Wang 2004, Young et al. 2011). Thus a single gene may be important in influencing monogamy vs promiscuity in voles. Oxytocin in rodents can affect behaviour in other ways too, for example by facilitating penile erection, reducing the post-ejaculatory refractory period, facilitating receptivity and lordosis in females, and increasing the release of dopamine in the mesolimbic pathway (Argiolas & Melis 2013). Stress, or the administration of the hormone corticosterone which is released during stress, can facilitate the onset of new pair bonds (DeVries, DeVries, Taymans & Carter 1996).

Interestingly in relation to depression, in prairie voles loss of a partner results in multiple disruptions in oxytocin, and increased depressive-like behavior reminiscent of bereavement. Infusions of oxytocin into the striatum of prairie voles prevents the onset of depressive-like behavior following partner loss, and evoking endogenous oxytocin release using melanocortin agonists during neonatal social isolation rescues impairments in social bonding in adulthood (Bosch & Young 2017).

Are similar mechanisms at work in humans to promote pair-bonding and love? There is as yet no definitive evidence, but in humans, oxytocin is released by intercourse, and especially at the time of orgasm, in both women and men (Veening, de Jong, Waldinger, Korte & Olivier 2015).

Oxytocin can have many influences on social behaviour, including increasing trust in neuroeconomic games, and presumably between partners too (Churchland & Winkielman 2012). An interesting development is that there is now evidence from a social trust game that oxytocin reduces learning by reducing sensitivity to prediction error when feedback is received. In this sense, oxytocin may facilitate social behaviour by reducing sensitivity to negative feedback. Put another way, oxytocin may promote 'unjustified trust' in the face of likely betrayal (or, more generally, possible negative consequences). Oxytocin may also reduce sensitivity to reward feedback. The brain areas involved in these effects were the orbitofrontal cortex, amygdala, and habenula (Ide, Nedic, Wong, Strey, Lawson, Dickerson, Wald, La Camera & Mujica-Parodi 2018). I suggest that a possible evolutionary interpretation is that oxytocin enhances social stability by reducing sensitivity to non-rewards and to rewards, both of which might make a social relationship to a partner or kin less stable.

7.3 Parental attachment, care, and parent–offspring conflict

Many mammal females make strong attachments to their own offspring, and this is also facilitated in many species by oxytocin. One model is the sheep, in which vaginal-cervical stimulation and suckling, which release both oxytocin and endogenous opioids, facilitate maternal bonding (Keverne 1995, Keverne, Nevison & Martel 1997). Oxytocin injections can cause ewes to become attached to an unfamiliar lamb presented at the time oxytocin is released or injected, and oxytocin antagonists can block filial bonding in sheep. Perhaps oxytocin had an initial role in evolution in the milk let-down reflex, and then became appropriate as a hormone that might facilitate mother–infant attachment.

In humans the evidence is much more correlative, but oxytocin release during natural childbirth, and rapid placing of the baby to breast feed and release more oxytocin (Carter 2017), might facilitate maternal attachment to her baby. This provides an argument in favour (other things being equal) of natural childbirth. Prolactin, the female hormone that promotes milk production, may also influence maternal attachment. It is certainly a major factor in humans that bonding can change quite suddenly at the time that a child is born, with women having a strong tendency to shift their interests markedly towards the baby as soon as it is born (probably in part under hormonal influences), and this can result in relatively less attachment behaviour to the husband. Understanding the scientific basis for this, and stimulated by this understanding, counselling couples about how their affections and attachments may alter at the time of the birth of a child, may be and should be a very important benefit of this research. In men, oxytocin may also be involved in paternal behaviour (Veening et al. 2015).

Separation from the mother can cause distress (Harlow 1986, Bowlby 1969, Bowlby 1973, Bowlby 1980). In Harlow's studies in monkeys, factors that reduced the effects of separation from the mother included warm soft touch, and the presence of peers. In chicks some auditory signs of distress can be reduced by oxytocin, opioids, and prolactin (Panksepp, Nelson & Bekkedal 1997).

Another aspect of parental care is that there is competition between the mother and child, for example over weaning (Trivers 1974). The mother may wish to devote resources to preparing for her next offspring (by building herself up); and continuing to breast feed delays the onset of fertility and cycling. In contrast, it is to the offspring's genetic advantage to demand milk and attention. The infant's scream can be seen as part of trying to wring resources out of its mother, potentially to an extent that is unfavourable for the mother's genes (Buss 2015). In this context, it is relevant that the baby's genes are not the same as either of the parent's genes, and thus the interests of the children and parents are to this extent different. (The same applies to siblings who are not identical twins: their genes are different, and this might lead to some sibling rivalry and competition, though at the same time, they do have many genes in common, and this contributes to kin altruism.)

As described above, females generally have a greater investment in their offspring, and tend to provide more parental care and perhaps become more attached than fathers. This situation is not as extreme in humans as in most other mammals, because human offspring are born relatively immature, and a father who helps to rear the offspring can help to increase the reproductive fitness of his genes.

Lack of parental care in step-fathers is evident in many species, and can be as extreme as the infanticide by a male lion of the pups of another father, so that his new female may come into heat more quickly to have babies by him (Bertram 1975). Infanticide also occurs in non-human primates (Kappeler & van Schaik 2004). In humans, the statistics indicate that step-fathers are much more likely to harm children in the family than are genetic fathers (Hilton, Harris & Rice 2015).

7.4 Sperm competition and its consequences for sexual behaviour: a sociobiological approach

Monogamous primates well spread out over territory have small testes, for example gibbons and some tarsiers. Polygamous primates living in groups with several males in the group have large testes and frequent copulation, e.g. chimpanzees and monkeys (Baker & Shackelford 2017). The reason for this appears to be sperm warfare – in order to pass his genes on to the next population, a male in a polygamous society with competition between males needs to increase the probability that he will fertilize a female, and the best way to do this is to copulate often, and swamp the female with sperm, so that his sperm have a greater probability of getting to the egg to fertilize it. Therefore in polygamous groups with more than one male, males should have large testes, to produce large numbers of sperm and large quantities of seminal fluid[4]. The largest testis size in relation to body weight is found in chimpanzees, who live in multimale groups, are highly promiscuous, and have on average 13 partners per birth. Sperm competition can be seen as a form of non-combative, non-injurious, male-male intrasexual competition, which has evolved by intrasexual sexual selection (see Section 7.7). Not only testis size, but also seminal vesicle size, is large in species with frequent copulation. In monogamous societies, with little competition between sperm, the male should just pick a good partner, produce only enough sperm to fertilize an egg and not enough to compete with others' sperm, stay with her to bring up the children, and guard them because they are his genetic investment (Ridley 1993a).

What about humans? Despite being apparently mainly monogamous, they are intermediate in testis size and penis size – bigger than expected for a monogamous species (Baker & Shackelford 2017). Why? Maybe there is some sperm competition? Remember that although humans usually do pair, and are often apparently monogamous, humans do live in groups or colonies. Can we get hints from other animals that are paired, but also live in colonies?

A problem with comparing humans with most other primates in this respect is that in most primates (and indeed in most mammals), the main parental investment is by the female (in producing the egg, in carrying the foetus, and in feeding the baby until it can become independent). The male does not have to invest in his children for them to have a reasonable chance of surviving. For this reason, the typical pattern in mammals is that the female is choosy in order to obtain healthy and fit males, and to complement this the males compete for females. However, in humans, because the children must be reared for a number of years before they become independent, there is an advantage to paternal investment in helping to bring up the children, in that the paternal resources (e.g. food, shelter, and protection) can increase the chances of the male's genes surviving into the next generation to reproduce again. Part of the reason why investment by both parents is needed in humans is that because of the large final human brain size, at birth the brain is not fully developed, and for this reason the infant needs to be looked after, fed, protected, and helped for a considerable period while the infant's brain develops, favouring pair-bonding between the parents.

A more useful comparison can therefore be made with some birds, such as the swallow, which live in colonies but in which the male and the female pair, and both invest in bringing up the offspring, taking it in turns for example to bring food back to the nest. If checks are made in swallows using DNA techniques for determining paternity, it is found that actually approximately one third of a pair's young are not sired by the 'father', the male of the pair (Birkhead 2000). What happens is that the female mates sometimes with other males – she

[4]Competition between males is the key factor here, for in gorillas which have one male in a polygamous (or strictly polygynous, meaning multiple females) group the testis size is small. The term that describes a multi-male multi-female group is polygynandry, and it is in groups of this type that there are high levels of sperm competition, and the testes are large.

commits adultery. She probably does not do this just with a random male either – she may choose an 'attractive' male, in which the signals that attract her are signals that indicate health, strength, and fitness. One well known example of such a signal is the gaudy 'tail' of the male peacock. One argument is that, given that the tail is a real handicap in life, any male that can survive with such a large tail must be very healthy or fit. Another argument is that if his tail is very attractive indeed, then the female should choose him, because her sons with him would probably be attractive too, and also chosen by females[5]. (It is interesting that if a male were popular with females, then even if he had genes that were not better in terms of survival etc., it would be advantageous for a female to have offspring with him, as her sons would be more likely to be attractive to other females, and thus maximize her inclusive fitness. This is an example of Fisherian selection (Fisher 1958), see Section 7.7.)

In such a social system, such as that of the swallow, the wife needs a reliable husband with whom she mates (so that he thinks the offspring are his, which for the system to be stable they must be sometimes) to help provide resources for 'their' offspring. (Remember that a nest must be built, the eggs must be incubated, and the hungry young must be well fed to help them become fit offspring. Here fit means successfully passing on genes into the next generation – see Dawkins (1986b).) But the wife (or at least her genes) also benefits by obtaining as fit genes as possible, by sometimes cheating on her husband. To ensure that her husband does not find out and therefore leave her and stop caring for the young, she deceives the husband by committing her adultery as much as possible secretly, perhaps hiding behind a bush to mate with her lover. So the (swallow) wife maximizes care for her children using her husband, and maximizes her genetic potential by finding a lover with fit genes that are likely to be attractive in her sons to other females (see Ridley (1993a)).

Could anything like the situation just described for birds such as swallows also apply to humans? It appears that it might apply, at least in part, and that similar evolutionary factors might influence human sexual behaviour, and hence make obtaining particular stimuli in the environment rewarding to humans. We need to understand whether this is the case, in order to understand the rewards that drive sexual behaviour in humans.

One line of evidence already described is the large testis and penis size of men (Baker & Shackelford 2017). In humans, it has been shown that the number of sperm ejaculated is related to testis size (Simmons, Firman, Rhodes & Peters 2004, Baker & Shackelford 2017). In this context, it is if interest that human semen contains many hormones and other proteins, which might influence the woman's behaviour in some way, including possibly her mood, or whether she ovulates (Burch & Gallup 2006).

A second line is that some studies in humans of paternity using modern DNA tests suggest that in fact the woman's partner (e.g. husband) is not the father of about 15% of the children (Baker & Shackelford 2017). These data suggest that while sperm competition may not be a major factor in modern humans, it may be to some extent, and might have been much more important in our ancestors, and have shaped our behaviour to at least some extent. So the possible effects of sperm competition in influencing modern human behaviour are worth exploring further.

So might men produce large amounts of sperm, and have intercourse quite regularly, in order to increase the likelihood that the children produced are theirs, whether by their wife or by their mistress? When women choose men as their lovers, do they choose men who are likely to produce children who are fit, that is children good at passing on their genes, half of which originate from the woman? It appears that women might choose like this, as described below, and that this behaviour may even select genetically for certain characteristics in men,

[5] This is an example of the use of the intentional stance in the description, when no real propositional statement is likely to occur at all.

because the woman finds these characteristics rewarding during mate selection. Of course, if such a strategy were employed (presumably mainly unconsciously) all the time in women the system would break down (be unstable), because men would not trust their wives, and the men would not invest in making a home and bringing up their children[6]. So we would not expect this to be the only selective pressure on what women find attractive and rewarding as qualities in men. Pursuing this matter further, we might expect women to find reliability, stability, provision of a home, and help with bringing up her children to be rewarding when selecting a husband; and the likelihood of producing genetically fit children, especially sons who can themselves potentially have many children by a number of women, to be rewarding when selecting a lover (i.e. short-term mate).

A finding by Baker & Bellis (1995) indicates that men have evolved strategies to optimize the chances of their genes in this sperm selection process. One is that men were reported to ejaculate more sperm if they have not been for some time with the woman with whom they are having intercourse. An effect consistent with this is that a man who spends a greater (relative to a man who spends a lesser) proportion of time apart from the partner since the couple's last copulation report (a) that his partner is more attractive, (b) that other men find his partner more attractive, (c) greater interest in copulating with the partner, and (d) that his partner is more sexually interested in him (Shackelford, Le Blanc, Weekes-Shackelford, Bleske-Rechek, Euler & Hoier 2002, Shackelford & Goetz 2007). (This effect is not just dependent on the time since he has last inseminated his partner, but is related to the time the couple have been apart, so the effects may be interpreted as being related to possible insemination of the partner while away, and not just to sexual frustration (Shackelford et al. 2002).) The (evolutionary, adaptive) function of this may be for the man to increase the chances of his sperm in what could be a sperm war with the sperm of another man. The aim would be to outnumber the other sperm. Moreover, the man should do this as quickly as possible after returning from an absence, as time could be of the essence in determining which sperm get to the egg first if the woman has had intercourse with another man recently. The implication of this for reward mechanisms in men is that after an absence, having intercourse quite soon with the woman from whom the man has been absent should be very rewarding (and this is what is reported (Shackelford et al. 2002)). Possible neural mechanisms for this are considered by Rolls (2014b).

There is good evidence that processes of this type do occur in some species. For example, Pizzari, Cornwallis, Lovlie, Jakobsson & Birkhead (2003) found in domestic fowl that males show status-dependent investment in female according to the level of female promiscuity: they progressively reduce sperm investment in a particular female but, on encountering a new female, instantaneously increase their sperm investment; and they preferentially allocate sperm to females with large sexual ornaments signalling superior maternal investment. These results indicate that female promiscuity leads to the evolution of sophisticated male sexual behaviour.

In this context, it is relevant that a refractory period after ejaculation might be adaptive in men in part because of limited sperm resources, and the utility of competing with adequate sperm numbers when insemination does occur. In general, a second mating with the same female soon after a mating would be unlikely to increase the chances of reproductive success much, and it would be adaptive to be refractory with that female to conserve sperm for a possible second mating with a different female. Indeed, dominant males may release limited sperm because of their multiple matings, and this is a factor cited as accounting for females competing for the first mating with a high-ranking male (Wedell, Gage & Parker 2002). The

[6] In some tribes, brothers help to bring up their sisters' children, because these children share some of the mother's brother's genes. The brother and sister of course will share some of the same genes, so the behaviour of the brother is appropriate in terms of increasing the fitness of his genes in a promiscuous society.

refractoriness on this evolutionary adaptive value account should only hold for the female with whom the male has just mated, and the male should not be refractory for long if the opportunity for mating with another female arises. This is an example within sexual behaviour of sensory-specific satiety, and is known within the field of sexual behaviour as the Coolidge effect[7].

It even appears that there should be some reward value in having intercourse very soon with the woman after an absence, because the action of the glans penis, with its groove behind the head, may be to pull sperm already in the vagina out of it using repeated thrusting and pulling back (Baker & Bellis 1995) (at least in some ancestors (Birkhead 2000, Schilthuizen 2015, Barbaro & Shackelford 2015)). The potential advantage to this in the sperm warfare may be the biological function that, as a result of evolution, leads to thrusting and withdrawal of the penis during intercourse being rewarding (perhaps to both men and women). Further, after ejaculation, the vigorous thrusting should become less vigorous, and the penis should start to lose its erection, as otherwise the man might suck out his own sperm. This may be part of the adaptive value of the refractory period in men[8]. The thrusting and withdrawal of the penis during intercourse should occur especially vigorously (and should therefore have evolved to become especially rewarding) after an absence by the man. The possible advantage in the sperm warfare that shaped our evolution could also result in its being rewarding for a man to have intercourse with a woman if he has just seen her having intercourse with another man. (This could be part of the biological background of why some men find videos showing sex involving women rewarding.) However, large numbers of sperm from a previous man usually remain in the vagina for only up to 45 min after intercourse, after which a flowback of sperm and other fluids (the discharge of semen and other secretions) from the vagina may occur. Thus the evolutionary shaping of the glans penis, and the rewards produced by thrusting and withdrawing it and the shaft of the penis in the vagina, are likely to have adaptive value at least in our ancestors, and possibly in humans (Schilthuizen 2015, Barbaro & Shackelford 2015).

Another type of sperm competition that has implications for behaviour is that males may leave a plug behind in the vagina of a female after they have inseminated her, to make it difficult if another male mates with her for the second male's sperm to reach her eggs. This is a common practice in rodents, and occurs in many other animals including insects, snakes and lizards, and chimpanzees and bonobos. And it appears that something similar may happen in humans (and also in other primates in which there is sperm competition as there is not monogamy, including chimpanzees, and bonobos) (Schilthuizen 2015). In humans, the first part of the ejaculate contains mostly sperm from the epididymis (where the sperm mature and are stored) and seminal vesicles, together with the clear lubricant fluid from the Cowper's glands, and fluid from the prostate which contains an enzyme called transglutaminase 4, or TGM4. The later parts of the ejaculated fluid contain fewer sperm, but do contain semenogelin (a liquid protein) produced by the seminal vesicles. Once inside the vagina, the TGM4 enzyme works on the semenogelin and causes different molecules of semenogelin to cross-link, to create a tangled web which is a quite thick congealed mating plug. This mating plug acts as a barrier to new sperm; and it may also help to reduce sperm dumping by the woman, making the sperm that she has already received stay inside her (Schilthuizen 2015). The refractory period in men after ejaculation may be an adaptation to conserve sperm, for presumably if

[7] The story is that Calvin Coolidge and his wife were touring a farm when Mrs Coolidge asked the farmer whether the continuous and vigorous sexual activity among the flock of hens was the work of only one rooster. The reply was yes."You might point that out to Mr Coolidge", she said. The President then asked the farmer whether a different hen was involved each time. The answer, again, was yes. "You might point that out to Mrs Coolidge", he said.

[8] There might be no corresponding adaptive value of refractoriness in women, for whom the ability to have multiple orgasms might provide her with the opportunity to exercise choice, by helping her to have an orgasm after her partner had ejaculated, if she wished to increase the chances of him being the father, as described in Section 7.5.

his semen has congealed and left a plug in the woman, there would be little reproductive advantage to wanting to mate with her and ejaculate more sperm which would have little effect on reproductive success because of the plug that he had left in the woman.

7.5 Female cryptic choice and its consequences for sexual behaviour

We have seen in the preceding section that males may have hidden methods that may increase the chances of success of their sperm, and which are controlled by the information from the environment about benefits and costs of their sperm allocation, including to whom they are allocating their sperm.

It turns out that females in very many species in the animal kingdom also practice hidden, i.e. cryptic, methods of choice to influence who will be the father of their offspring. Again, the way in which the cryptic choice is made will be influenced by factors such as the potential reward value of having a particular male be the father of their offspring. It should be noted that these choices may be quite hidden, and may not be made consciously, but are nevertheless influenced by factors such as the resources that a male may provide, which might be food, protection, good genes, etc.

Cryptic female choice is the postcopulatory ability of females to favour the sperm of one male of the same species over another (Firman, Gasparini, Manier & Pizzari 2017). An example of female cryptic choice has been demonstrated by female red junglefowl, Gallus gallus, which reveal postcopulatory selection against the sperm of males that are related to them. In this case, the choice is based on major histocompatibility complex (MHC) similarity, which is part of the immune system. This selection is likely to give the offspring greater disease resistance, by selecting for a diverse immune system in the offspring because of fertilization by an unrelated male with different MHC genes. The effect of MHC similarity was lost following artificial insemination, suggesting that male phenotypic cues, for example the sight or smell of the male, might be required for females to select sperm differentially (Lovlie, Gillingham, Worley, Pizzari & Richardson 2013).

How is this choice made by females? One factor may be whether the female has an orgasm. In some female non-human primates (e.g. the Japanese macaque), orgasm is more likely to occur if the female is mating with a high-ranking male (Troisi & Carosi 1998), and it is possible that this serves as a reward for mating with high-ranking males, and at the same time promotes cryptic choice. It has also been reported that women desiring to become pregnant become more likely to have an orgasm with their partner, and indeed just after their partner ejaculates (Singh, Meyer, Zambarano & Hurlbert 1998).

But what is the mechanism by which a female orgasm might play a role in influencing whether she is fertilized by the male who is mating with her? Baker & Bellis (1995) investigated this in women. They reported that if a woman has no orgasm, or if she has an orgasm more than a minute before the man ejaculates, relatively little sperm is retained in the woman, and instead much of the sperm flows back out of the vagina and is lost. This is a low-retention orgasm. They also reported that if the woman has an orgasm less that a minute before him or up to 45 min after him, then much more of the sperm stays in the woman, and some of it appears to be sucked up by the cervix during and just following the later stages of her perceived orgasm. This is a high-retention orgasm.

Baker & Bellis (1995) then (using a questionnaire) found that in women who were faithful (having intercourse only with their husbands) about 55% of the orgasms were of the high-retention (i.e. most fertile) type. By contrast, in unfaithful women having intercourse with their husbands, only 45% of the copulations were high-retention, but 70% of the copulations with the lover were of the high-retention type. Moreover, the unfaithful women were having sex with their lovers at times of the month when they were most fertile, that is when they were just about to ovulate. Baker and Bellis suggested the women in this sample would be more than twice as likely to conceive during sex with their lover than with their partner. Thus women appear to be able to influence to some extent who is the father of their children, not only by having intercourse with lovers, but also by influencing whether they will become pregnant by their lover. The ways in which reward mechanisms might help this process are described later in this chapter.

Although this research created lively discussion, there was also some scepticism. However, more recent research, including in women (Motta-Mena & Puts 2017), does tend to support the view for cryptic choice by females (Schilthuizen 2015, Yohn, Gergues & Samuels 2017), with some of the evidence described next.

One piece of evidence is that domestic fowls (hens) appear to select which sperm fertilize their eggs, in that when inseminated with sperm of different cocks, the fertilization was non-random (Birkhead, Chaline, Biggins, Burke & Pizzari 2004).

Another piece of evidence is that when a bull mates with a cow, or when a boar (male pig) mates with a sow, there is active contraction of the uterus. The same does not occur with artificial insemination, and that has a much lower success rate in fertilization and pregnancy. There may indeed be active sucking up of liquid into the uterus with movements and reduced pressure in the uterus to achieve this, as shown in mares, rats, and mice (Schilthuizen 2015, Millar 1952). Consistent with these points, something like orgasms, with rhythmic contractions of the uterus, may be more widespread among mammals than was previously thought (Schilthuizen 2015, Troisi & Carosi 1998).

Further evidence is that after the man has ejaculated, and then there is an orgasm in the woman, the pressure in the uterus appears to be lower than in the vagina for several minutes, and this may be part of the mechanism by which an orgasm in the woman facilitates sperm transport from the vagina into the uterus (Fox, Wolff & Baker 1970, Motta-Mena & Puts 2017). It may be that this transport is facilitated by peristaltic movements of the uterus, sucking up the sperm, and directing them upwards through the uterus towards the Fallopian tube and egg (Kunz & Leyendecker 2002).

If female orgasm is involved in influencing who the father is of a baby, then it might be expected that female orgasm might be somewhat variable in whether it occurs, as part of a putative selection process, and female orgasm does appear to be somewhat variable.

In addition, there is evidence from quite different parts of the animal kingdom that females practice cryptic choice to influence who fertilises their eggs (Schilthuizen 2015, Firman et al. 2017). For example, in many insects, the female may have different chambers in which she receives the sperm of different males, and may be able to choose which male will be the father of her offspring by accessing the appropriate chamber. Some animals that do not wish to be fertilised by a particular male can even evert their 'vagina', lick out that male's sperm, and then be ready for another male (Schilthuizen 2015).

Finally, although there are phenomena here that have been described, it is unlikely that they have more than a possible modulatory influence in humans, with other factors being much more important.

7.6 Concealed ovulation and concealed estrus and their consequences for sexual behaviour

Women, and a few non-human primate species, have concealed ovulation. It is not clear to males, or to themselves, when they are fertile. Why do women conceal their ovulation? Diamond (1997) considers evidence that a first process that occurs in evolution is that promiscuity or harems in the mating system give rise to concealed ovulation. This is the 'many fathers' theory. The concealed ovulation (concealed even from the woman, so that she can deceive better – what might be termed 'deceiving conceiving') – makes sure that men do not know who the father is (because they do not know when ovulation has occurred), and thus will not attack the young. (It frequently occurs in the animal kingdom that males kill their female's children if they have been born of other males, a process that enables genes to maximize their own reproductive potential. This occurs because the female will stop lactating and will come back into a reproductive state so that the new male can reproduce. Moreover, it will minimize potential use of his resources in helping to bring up children without his genes.)

A second process can then occur in evolution: monogamy evolves. Monogamy, Diamond (1997) argues, has never evolved in species that have bold advertisement of ovulation. It usually evolved in species with (i.e. that already have) concealed ovulation – the 'daddy-at-home' theory. The concealed ovulation means that fathers stay at home all the time (and help), because they want to be assured of their paternity; and because they think that they are the father, because they have been at home (Simmen-Tulberg & Moller 1993). Thus the consequences of concealed ovulation may be that fathers find it rewarding (and have emotions about) staying at home with their partner to guard a primarily monogamous relationship. Indeed, monogamy can be thought of as a form of mate guarding.

Consistent with these hypotheses, it has been found that free-living Hanuman langur females do have long periods of receptivity during which the time of ovulation is variable, that there is the opportunity for paternity confusion in that ovulation is concealed from the males, that there is a dominant male who tries to monopolize the females, and that nevertheless non-dominant males father a substantial proportion of the offspring (Heistermann, Ziegler, van Schaik, Launhardt, Winkler & Hodges 2001). This is direct evidence that extended periods of sexual receptivity in catarrhine primates may have evolved as a female strategy to confuse paternity.

Concealed ovulation could also play a role in combination with female orgasm to enable female cryptic choice, which would it has been suggested (see Section 7.4) occur if a woman has an orgasm with a man who she wants to be the father of her children. The contribution of the concealed ovulation would be to promote male–male competition.

Thus the interests of females and males may not be consistent, and this leads to the development of measures and countermeasures. Concealed ovulation can be seen as a protection against infanticide. Concealed ovulation promotes polyandry, and this results in multiple matings, and sperm competition and sperm allocation as a response to this. Females may then counter with mechanisms for cryptic choice, such as for example selective orgasms.

Women's estrogen-based sexual ornaments appear to honestly signal reproductive value, and may help her to exercise cryptic choice by making her attractive to men (Thornhill & Gangestad 2015, Motta-Mena & Puts 2017). These ornaments may include young women's breasts, a small waist-to-hip ratio, smooth feminine skin, and the high-pitched voice of women.

Women may also have concealed estrus, it has been argued (Thornhill & Gangestad 2015). Estrus in women is a set of sexual preferences, manifested in the fertile window of the menstrual cycle, for mates with traits that connote male phenotypic and genetic quality. Women's estrus may be an adaptation that functions to obtain genes, including via extra-pair copulation, that enhance offspring reproductive value. Women's estrus is ancient phylogenetically, and has homology and functional similarity with estrus throughout vertebrates. Women's sexuality at infertile cycle points and other infertile times is referred to as 'extended sexuality'. It is common in Old World primates and probably in pair-bonding socially monogamous birds. The kinds of preferences associated with women's extended sexuality are consistent with the hypothesis that its function is to obtain nongenetic material benefits and services from males by exchanging sexual access for them. Concealed estrus is present in women as evidenced by men's limited ability (compared to other male mammals) to detect estrus, women's limited behavioral changes (compared to other female mammals) during estrus, and estrous women's efforts to limit male mate guarding. Concealed estrus may be an adaptation that functions in extra-pair-bond copulation to cuckold the male partner in service of better genes for offspring, while maintaining the material benefits provided by the male partner (Thornhill & Gangestad 2015).

7.7 Sexual selection of sexual and non-sexual behaviour

7.7.1 Sexual selection and natural selection

Darwin (1871) distinguished natural selection from sexual selection, and this distinction has been consolidated and developed (Fisher 1930, Fisher 1958, Hamilton 1996, Dawkins 1986b, Miller 2000, Parker & Pizzari 2015) and applies to humans (Puts 2015). **Natural selection** can be used in a narrow sense to refer to selection processes that lead to the development of characteristics that have a function of providing adaptive or survival value to an individual so that the individual can reproduce, and pass on its genes. In its narrow sense, natural selection can be thought of as 'survival or adaptation selection'. An example might be a gene or genes that specify that the sensory properties of food should be rewarding (and should taste pleasant) when we are in a physiological need state for food. Many of the reward and punishment systems described in this book deal with this type of reward and punishment decoding that has evolved to enable genes to influence behaviour in directions in a high-dimensional space of rewards and punishments that are adaptive for survival and health of the individual, and thus promote reproductive success or fitness of the genes that build such adaptive functionality. We can include kin-related altruistic behaviours (see Chapter 3) because the behaviour is adaptive in promoting the survival of kin, and thus promoting the likelihood that the kin (who contain one's genes) survive and reproduce. Resources and wealth are also understood as making males attractive and being selected by natural selection, in that the wealth and resources may be useful to the female in bringing up her children.

Darwin (1871) also recognized that evolution can occur by **sexual selection**, when what is being selected for has no inherent adaptive or survival value, but is attractive to potential mates (inter-sexual selection, between the sexes), or helps in competing with others of the same sex (intra-sexual selection, within the sexes). The most cited example is the peacock's large tail, which does not have survival value for the peacock (and indeed it is somewhat of a handicap to have a very long tail), but, because it is attractive to the peahen, becomes prevalent in the population. Indeed, part of the reason for the long tail being attractive may be that it is an honest signal of phenotypic fitness (or 'fitness indicator'), in that having a very long tail is a handicap to survival (Zahavi 1975), though the signalling system that reveals this only operates correctly if certain conditions apply[8]. The inherited genes for a long tail may be expressed in the female's sons, and they will accordingly be attractive to females in the next generation. Although the female offspring of the mating will not express the male father's attractive long-tail genes, these genes are likely to be expressed in her sons. The female has to evolve to find the characteristic being selected for in males attractive for this situation to lead to a runaway explosion of the characteristic being selected for by the choosiness of females. Indeed, the fact that the female who chose a long-tailed male has children following her mating with genes for liking long-tailed males, and for generating long tails, is part of what leads to the runaway process that can occur with sexual selection. The fact that the long tail is actually a handicap for the peacock, and so is a signal of general physical fitness in the male, may be one way in which sexual selection can occur stably (Zahavi 1975). The peacock tail example is categorized as sexual selection because the long tail is not adaptive to the individual with the long tail, though of course it is adaptive to have a long tail if females are choosing it because it indicates general physical fitness. However, sexual selection can occur when a revealing or index signal or fitness indicator is not associated with a handicap, but is hard to fake, so that it is necessarily an honest fitness indicator (Maynard Smith & Harper 2003). An example occurs in birds that may show bare skin as part of their courtship, providing a sign that they are parasite resistant (Hamilton & Zuk 1982). Handicaps are costly to produce, and should reduce fitness in contexts other than mating. If the signal is an index signal, it is relatively cost-free, cannot be easily faked, and should correlate with some trait that contributes to fitness in contexts other than mating (Maynard Smith & Harper 2003).

[8] The conditions under which a handicap signalling system can lead to sexual selection are i: the female can correctly infer a male's quality from his advertisement (honesty); ii: signals are costly; and iii: a given signal is more costly for a male of low quality.

Some characteristics of sexual selection that help to separate it from natural or survival selection are as follows:

First, the sexually selected characteristic is sexually dimorphic, with the male typically showing the characteristic. (For example the peacock but not the peahen has the long tail.) This occurs because it is the female who is being choosy, and is selecting males. The female is the choosy one because she has a considerable investment in her offspring, whom she may need to nurture until birth, and then rear until independent, and for this reason has a much more limited reproductive potential than the male, who could in principle father large numbers of offspring to optimize his genetic potential. This is an example of a sexual dimorphism selected by inter-sexual selection. An example of a sexual dimorphism selected by intra-sexual selection is the deer's antlers.

Second, sexually selected characteristics are typically species-specific (consistent with choice by the female of the species of a relatively arbitrary feature in males that may not itself have survival value), whereas naturally selected characteristics may, because they have survival value for individuals, be found in many species within a genus, and even across genera.

Third, and accordingly, the competition is within a species for sexual selection, whereas competition may be across as well as within species for natural (survival) selection.

Fourth, sexual selection operates most efficiently in polygynous species, that is species where some (attractive) males mate with two or more females, and unattractive males are more likely to be childless. Polygyny does seem to have been present to at least some extent in our ancestors, as shown for example by body size differences, with males larger than females. This situation is selected because males compete hard with each other in polygynous species compared to monogamous, where there is less competition. In humans, the male is 10% taller, 20% heavier, 50% stronger in the upper body muscles, and 100% stronger in the hand grip strength than the average female (Miller 2000).

Fifth, the sexually selected characteristics are likely to be apparent after but not before puberty. In humans, one example is the deep male voice.

Sixth, there may be marked differences between individuals, as it is these differences that are being used for mate choice. In contrast, when natural or survival selection is operating efficiently, there may be little variation between individuals.

Seventh, the fitness indicator should be costly or difficult to produce, as in this way it can reflect real fitness, and be kept honest.

Eighth, sexual selection may produce characteristics that wax and then wane. For example, female choice may drive male characteristics to an extreme beyond which little further change is physically possible. There may then be little variation between the male characteristic being selected for. At this point, males who reverse the characteristic may have some advantage, because now they stand out from the crowd, and there is now variation that some females may find attractive (Schilthuizen 2015).

Overall, Darwinian natural or survival selection increases health, strength, and potentially resources, and survival of the individual, and thus ability to mate and reproduce. Inter-sexual sexual selection does not make the individual healthier, but does make the individual more attractive as a mate, as in female choice, an example of intersexual selection. Intra-sexual sexual selection does not necessarily help survival of the individual, but does help in competition for a mate, for example in intimidation of one male by another (Darwin 1871, Kappeler & van Schaik 2004). The behaviours and characteristics involved in sperm competition described in this chapter are produced by intra-sexual sexual selection.

It turns out that many of the best examples of inter-sexual sexual selection are in birds (for example the peacock's tail, and the male lyre bird's tail). Some of the examples in birds may be related to the visual system of birds, which is good at identifying sign stimuli and innate releasing stimuli, and this may facilitate the evolution of elaborate displays. (Is the rhesus macaque's red posterior an exception?) In contrast, mammals have a more general-purpose visual system that can recognize objects invariantly, and does not therefore need to specialize in analysing particular low-level sensory features of stimuli (Rolls 2012e, Rolls 2016c). In mammals, including primates, the selection is often by size, strength, physical prowess, and aggressiveness, which provide for direct physical competition, and are examples of intra-sexual selection (Kappeler & van Schaik 2004).

It has been suggested that sexual selection is important for further types of characteristic in humans. For example, it has been suggested that human mental abilities that may be important in courtship such as kindness, humour, and telling stories, are the type of characteristic that may be sexually selected in humans (Miller 2000). Before assessing this (in Section 7.7.2), and illuminating thus some of what may be sexually selected rewards and punishers that therefore contribute to human affective states, we should note a twist in how sexual selection may operate in humans.

In humans, because babies are born relatively immature and may take years of demanding care before they can look after themselves, there is some advantage to male genes of providing at least some parental care for the children. That is, the father may invest in his offspring. In this situation, where there is a male investment, the male may optimize the chance of his genes faring well by being choosy about his wife. The implication is that in humans, sexual selection may be of female characteristics (by males), as well as of male characteristics (by females). This may mean that the differences between the sexes may not be as large as can often be the case with inter-sexual sexual selection, where the female is the main chooser. One example of how sexual selection may affect female characteristics is in the selection for large breasts. These may be selected to be larger in humans than is really necessary for milk production, by the incorporation of additional fat. This characteristic may be attractive to males (and hence produce affective responses in males) because it is a symbol relating to fertility and child rearing potential, and not because large breasts have any particular adaptive value. It has even been suggested that the large breast size makes them useful to males as a sign of reproductive potential, for their pertness is maximal when a (young) woman's fertility and reproductive potential is at its highest. Although large breasts may be less pert with age, and it might thus be thought to be an advantage for women not to have large breasts, it may be possible that this is offset by the advantageous signal of a pert but large breast when fertility and reproductive potential is at its maximal when young, as this may attract high status males (even though there may be disadvantages later) (Miller 2000). Thus it is possible that inter-sexual selection contributes to the large breast size of some women. The fact that the variation is quite large is consistent with this being a sexually selected, not survival-selected, characteristic. Thus sexual selection of characteristics may occur in women as well as in men (Puts 2015).

Darwin (1871) and Bateman (1948) predicted that the primary sexual difference that generates sexual selection and secondary differentiation of sexual strategies between the sexes is the different size and contributions of the female egg (which is large) and the male sperm which are small, and are produced in much higher numbers. This asymmetry of the gametes is termed anisogamy. The large egg of the female provides nutrients, but also provides cellular organelles that are not produced by the DNA. The male sperm contribute few of these intracellular organelles, it is suggested to minimize the chances of evolutionary competition between the self-reproducing intracellular organelles, which might otherwise by competing do harm to the organism (Schilthuizen 2015). These predictions that anisogamy provides a basis for sex differences in behaviour between females and males have now been supported by major bodies of experimental evidence and theoretical study (Parker & Pizzari 2015).

We may also note that the term 'natural selection' encompasses in its broad sense both 'survival or adaptation selection', and sexual selection. Both are processes now understood to be driven by the selection of genes, and it is gene competition and replication into the next generation that is the driving force of biological evolution (Dawkins 1989, Dawkins 1986b). The distinction can be made that with 'survival or adaptation selection', the genes being selected for make the individual animal stronger, healthier, and more likely to survive and reproduce, whereas sexual selection operates by sexual choice selecting for genes that may have little survival value to the individual, but enable the individual to be selected as a mate in inter-sexual selection, or to compete for a mate in intra-sexual selection, and thus pass on the genes selected by these two types of sexual selection.

Insofar as the states elicited by rewards and punishers are emotional states (see Chapters 2 and 3), this chapter thus extends the understanding of emotion to systems shaped by sexual selection. For example, sexual selection may select symmetric and thus attractive faces which may produce emotional states.

7.7.2 Non-sexual characteristics may be sexually selected for courtship

Miller (2000) has developed the hypothesis that courtship provides an opportunity for sexual selection to select non-sexual mental characteristics such as kindness, humour, the ability to tell stories, creativity, art, and even language. He postulates that these are "courtship tools, evolved to attract and entertain sexual partners". Sexual selection views organisms as advertisers of their phenotypic fitness, and Miller sees these characteristics as such signals. From this perspective, hunting is seen as a costly and inefficient exercise (in comparison with food gathering) undertaken by men to obtain small gifts of meat for women, but at the same time to show how competitive and fit the successful hunter is in relation to other men. Conspicuous waste, and conspicuous consumption, are often signs in nature that sexual selection is at work, with high costs for behaviours that seem maladaptive in terms of survival and natural selection in the narrow sense. The mental characteristics described above are not only costly in terms of time, but may rely on many genes operating efficiently for these characteristics to be expressed well, and so, Miller suggests, may be 'fitness indicators'. Consistent with sexual selection, there is also great individual variability in these characteristics, providing a basis for choice.

One mental characteristic that Miller suggests could have evolved in this way is kindness, which is very highly valued by both sexes (Buss 2015, Buss 2016). In human evolution, being kind to the mother's children may have been seen as an attractive characteristic in men during courtship, especially when relationships may not have lasted for many years, and the children might not be those of the courting male. Kindness may also be used as an indicator of future cooperation. In a sense kindness thus may indicate potential useful benefits, consistent with the fact that across cultures human females tend to prefer males who have high social status, good income, ambition, intelligence, and energy (Buss 2015, Buss 2016). Kindness may also be related to kin altruism (Hamilton 1964) or to reciprocal altruism (Trivers 1971), both of which are genetically adaptive strategies (see Chapter 2)[9]. Although the simple interpretation of all these characteristics is that they indicate a good provider and potential material and genetic benefits (and thus would be subject to natural or survival selection), Miller (2000) argues that at least kindness is being used in addition as a fitness indicator and is being sexually selected. Although morality can be related in part to kin and reciprocal altruism (Ridley 1996) (see Section 11.3), moral behaviour may bring reproductive benefits through the social status that it inspires (Zahavi & Zahavi 1997) or by direct mate choice for moralistic displays during courtship (Tessman 1995, Miller 2000). The suggestion made by Miller (2000) is that the status of moral behaviour helps to attract mates, because it may reflect fitness as the moral behaviour may have costs. He suggests that "*Morality is a system of sexually selected handicaps*".

Miller (2000) (page 258 ff) also suggests that art, language and creativity can be explained by sexual selection, and that they are difficult to account for by survival selection. He suggests that art develops from courtship ornamentation, and uses bowerbirds as an evolutionary example. Male bowerbirds ornament their often enormous and structurally elaborate nests or bowers with mosses, ferns, shells, berries and bark to attract female bowerbirds. The nests are used just to attract females, and after insemination the females go off and build their own cup-shaped nests, lay their eggs, and raise their offspring by themselves with no male support. Darwin himself viewed human ornamentation and clothing as outcomes of sexual selection. Sexual selection for artistic ability does not mean of course that the art itself needs to be about sex. This example helps to show that sexual selection can lead to changes in what is valued and found attractive, in areas that might be precursors to art in humans. Miller (2000) suggests that language evolved as a courtship device in males to attract females. Miller (2000) also suggests that creativity may be related to systems that can explore random new ideas, and also is a courtship device in males to attract females.

One potential problem with this approach is that sexual selection favours fast runaway evolution, because sexual preferences are genetically correlated with the ornaments they favour (as described in section 7.7). Why does mental capacity not develop more rapidly, and with larger sex differences, in humans, if Miller (2000) is right? Why is there not a faster runaway? Miller suggests a number of possible reasons.

1. There is a high genetic correlation between human males and females, with 22/23 chromosomes the same.

2. The female's brain must evolve to be able to appreciate the male's mental adornment – and might even be one step ahead to judge effectively. Further, similar or partly overlapping brain mechanisms may be used to produce (in males) and perceive (in females). In addition, male self-monitoring (and female practice) may help appraisal. Males may even internalize female's appreciation systems, to predict their responses.

[9] Interestingly, the etymology of kindness is Old English cynd, kin, hence looking after kin, relations.

3. There is mutual choice in humans: males choose females because human males do make a parental investment; and females compete for males. Indeed, the selection of a long-term partner is mutual, and this tends to reduce sex differences. Consistent with this, David Buss has shown that, in contrast, human sex differences are more evident in short-term mating (Buss 1989, Buss 2016, Buss 2015). It is likely in fact that sexual selection works mainly through long-term relationships, because of concealed ovulation in women. This means that only in a relatively long-term relationship is it likely that a man will become the father of a woman's child, because only if he mates with her regularly is there a reasonable probability that he will hit her fertile time.

Another criticism of the approach of Miller (2000) is that many of these characteristics may have survival value, and are not purely sexually selected. For example, language has many uses in problem solving, planning ahead, and correcting multiple step plans which are likely to be very important to enable immediate rewards to be deferred, and longer term goals to be achieved (see Chapter 10).

7.8 Brain regions involved in the control of sexual behaviour, and especially in the rewards produced by sexual behaviour

In this section, we consider some of the evidence available at present on the neural mechanisms involved in sexual behaviour. Some of the ways in which the reward systems in the brain may be designed to implement some of the types of behaviour described in this Chapter have been considered by Rolls (2014b).

7.8.1 Olfactory rewards and pheromones

Pheromones, which are typically olfactory stimuli, can trigger a number of different types of sexual behaviour, and thus either affect what is rewarding, or in some cases can act as rewards (Dulac & Torello 2003, Beauchamp & Yamazaki 2003, Dulac & Kimchi 2007).

First, pheromones can produce slow and long-lasting effects by influencing hormones, affecting for example reproductive cycles. They produce the Lee-Boot effect, in which the oestrous cycles of female mice housed together without a male slow down and eventually stop. They act in the Whitten effect, in which the mice start cycling again if they are exposed to the odour of a male or his urine. They act in the Vandenbergh effect, the acceleration in the onset of puberty in a female rodent caused by the odour of a male. They act in the Bruce effect, in which if a recently impregnated female mouse encounters a male mouse other than the one with which she mated, the pregnancy is very likely to fail. The new male can then mate with her. This form of genetic warfare happening after the sperm-warfare stage is clearly to the advantage of the new male's genes, and presumably to the advantage of the female's genes, because it means that her pregnancies will tend to be with males who are not only able to oust other males, but are with males who are with her, so that her offspring will not be harmed by the new male, and may even be protected. The pheromones that produce these effects are produced in males under the influence of testosterone (see Carlson & Birkett (2017)). These effects depend on an accessory olfactory system, the vomeronasal organ and its projections to the accessory olfactory bulb, though this system is not present in humans. The accessory olfactory bulb in turn projects to the medial nucleus of the amygdala, which in turn projects to the preoptic area, anterior hypothalamus, and ventromedial hypothalamus, and these pheromonal effects are produced by influences on hormones such as luteinizing hormone (LH) and prolactin (PRL) (Dulac & Torello 2003). Pheromones can cause groups of women housed together to start cycling together. The evolutionary significance of the synchronized cycling might be to increase male–male competition and selection. In addition, shared care may be facilitated by synchronized breeding, and this could increase the survival of the offspring.

Second, pheromones can act as attracting or rewarding signals, and rapidly influence behaviour. For example, pheromones present in the vaginal secretions of hamsters attract males. In some monkeys, bacteria in the vagina produce more of a pheromone under the influence of an androgen (male sex hormone) produced in small quantities in the adrenal glands, and this pheromone increases the attractiveness of the female to the male (Baum, Everitt, Herbert & Keverne 1977). (In this case, male sexual behaviour is induced by a male hormone produced in females.) Male rats also produce pheromones, which are attractive to females.

The vomeronasal system in rodents utilizes a set of genes that specify approximately 293 types of V1R and 100 types of V2R olfactory pheromone receptor (Dulac & Torello 2003). Pheromones that activate these receptors are involved in behaviours in rodents such as inducing oestrus in females, intermale aggression, and attracting females (Dulac & Torello 2003). This system does appear to be vestigial and disconnected in humans and Old World monkeys (such as macaques) (Stowers & Kuo 2015, Savic 2014). Further, most of the genes in humans that should produce accessory olfactory system pheromone receptors are pseudogenes[10], so that no receptors can be produced, with only 5 of the V1R pheromone genes believed not to be inactivated in humans (Dulac & Torello 2003). If pheromonal effects do operate in humans, they may be produced through the main olfactory system (Savic 2014).

In humans, body odours are not generally described as attractive, but there is a whole industry based on perfume, the odour of a mate may become attractive by conditioning, and there is some evidence that androstenol, a substance found in the underarm sweat of males especially, may increase the number of social interactions that women have with men (Cowley & Brooksbank 1991). It has also been reported that androstadien-3-one, a putative male pheromone, activates the preoptic area in women. Conversely, EST activates the hypothalamus in men. Both activate cortical olfactory areas in both men and women (Savic 2014). In humans, it has also been reported that a putative female pheromone oestra-1,3,5,(10),16-tetraen-3ol-acetate (EST) activates the male anterior medial thalamus and right inferior frontal gyrus at concentrations that cannot be detected consciously (Sobel, Prabhakaran, Hartley, Desmond, Glover, Sullivan & Gabrieli 1999).

In women, there is a significant association between a polymorphism in the gene encoding the human vomeronasal type-1 receptor 1 (VNR1), and a measure of sociosexual behavior driven specifically by a question regarding one-night stands (Henningsson, Hovey, Vass, Walum, Sandnabba, Santtila, Jern & Westberg 2017). This appears to provide reasonable evidence that pheromones do have effects in humans. Hedione, a ligand for the VNR1 receptor, produces activation in the human lateral orbitofrontal cortex, hypothalamus and amygdala (Wallrabenstein, Gerber, Rasche, Croy, Kurtenbach, Hummel & Hatt 2015). (The activation of the lateral orbitofrontal cortex implies that the hedione was not perceived as pleasant, and consistent with this, the activations in the hypothalamus were correlated with the unpleasantness of the hedione. Of course under natural conditions, an odourant would not be presented alone, and activation of the VNR1 receptor by hedione or a natural equivalent might increase the efficacy of some odours.)

[10] A pseudogene is a DNA sequence that is related to a functional gene but cannot be transcribed owing to mutational changes or the lack of regulatory sequences.

In a different line of research, it has been suggested that another way in which animals including humans respond to some pheromones as rewards or as aversive stimuli could be a molecular mechanism for producing genetic diversity by influencing those who are considered attractive as mates. In particular, it was suggested that major histocompatibility complex (MHC)-dependent abortion and mate choice, based on olfaction, was thought to maintain MHC diversity, and functioned both to avoid genome-wide inbreeding and produce MHC-heterozygous offspring with increased immune responsiveness. However, the evidence for this hypothesis is now weak (Overath, Sturm & Rammensee 2014).

7.8.2 Preoptic area and hypothalamus

In males, the preoptic area (see Fig. 7.1) is involved in the control of sexual behaviour (Hull, Meisel & Sachs 2002, Micevych & Meisel 2017, Pfaff & Baum 2018). Lesions of this region permanently abolish male sexual behaviour; electrical stimulation can elicit copulatory activity; metabolic activity is induced (as shown by c-fos) in the preoptic area during copulation; and small implants of testosterone into the preoptic area restore sexual behaviour in castrated rats (Hull et al. 2002). This region appears to have neurons in it that respond to sex-related rewards in primates, in that Aou, Oomura, Lenard, Nishino, Inokuchi, Minami & Misaki (1984) described some preoptic neurons in the male macaque that increased their firing rates when he could see a female macaque seated on a chair that he could pull towards him. The same neurons did not respond to the sight of food (Y. Oomura, personal communication), and so reflected information about the specific type of reward available. They also described neuronal activity changes in the medial preoptic area of the male monkey that were related to the commencement of sexual behaviour, penile erection, and the refractory period following ejaculation. Similarly, neuronal activity changes in the female medial preoptic area were related to the commencement of sexual behaviour and presentation. Increased neuronal activity in the dorsomedial hypothalamic nucleus in the male monkey and in the ventromedial hypothalamic nucleus in the female monkey were synchronized to each mating act. These findings, and studies using local electrical stimulation, suggested the involvement of medial preoptic area neurons in sexual arousal, and of male dorsomedial hypothalamic and female ventromedial hypothalamic neurons in copulation (Aou, Oomura, Lenard, Nishino, Inokuchi, Minami & Misaki 1984).

In females, the medial preoptic area is involved in the control of reproductive cycles. It is probably also involved in controlling sexual behaviour directly (Blaustein & Erskine 2002, Micevych & Meisel 2017). Neurons in it and connected areas respond to vagino-cervical stimulation in a hormone-dependent way (Blaustein & Erskine 2002). The ventromedial nucleus of the hypothalamus (VMH) is involved in some aspects of sexual behaviour, including lordosis (standing still in a receptive position) in rodents, and this behaviour can be reinstated in ovariectomized female rats by injections of oestradiol and progesterone into the ventromedial nucleus (Blaustein & Erskine 2002, Micevych & Meisel 2017). Outputs from the VMH project to the periaqueductal gray of the midbrain, which is also necessary for female sexual behaviour such as lordosis in rodents, via descending influences on spinal cord reflexes implemented via the reticular formation neurons and the reticulospinal tracts (Pfaff, Gagnidze & Hunter 2018). The VMH receives inputs from regions such as the medial amygdala.

The preoptic area receives inputs from the amygdala and orbitofrontal cortex, and thus receives information from the inferior temporal visual cortex (including information about face identity and expression), from the superior temporal auditory association cortex, from the olfactory system, and from the somatosensory system. The operation of these circuits has been described in Chapters 4 and 5. In one example described in Section 4.6.4, Everitt, Cador & Robbins (1989) showed that excitotoxic lesions of the basolateral amygdala dis-

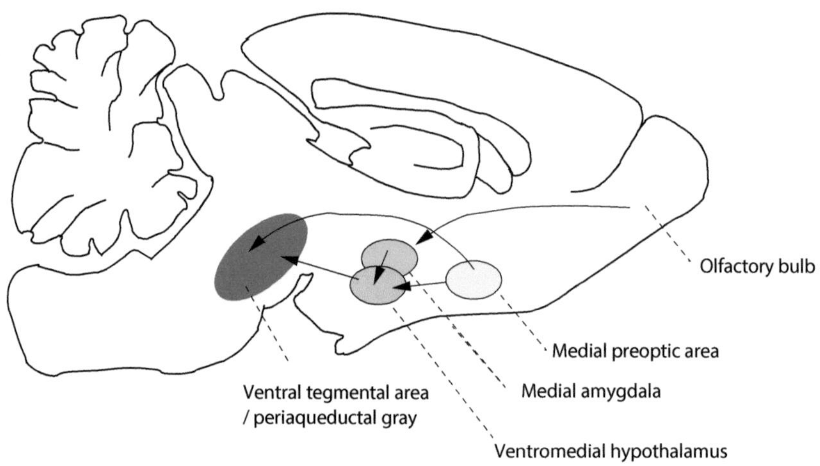

Fig. 7.1 Some of the brain regions implicated in sexual behaviour, shown on a midline view of a rat brain.

rupted appetitive sexual responses maintained by a visual conditioned reinforcer, but not the behaviour to the primary reinforcer for the male rats, copulation with a female rat in heat (see further Everitt (1990) and Everitt & Robbins (1992)). For comparison, medial preoptic area lesions eliminated the copulatory behaviour of mounting, intromission and ejaculation to the primary reinforcer, the female rat, but did not affect the learned appetitive responding for the conditioned or secondary reinforcing stimulus, the light. The conclusion from such studies is that the amygdala is involved in stimulus–reinforcement association learning when the primary reinforcer is a sexual reward. On the other hand, the preoptic area is not involved in such stimulus–reinforcement association learning, but is involved in the rewarding effects of primary sexual rewards. Olfactory inputs reach the medial preoptic area via the medial amygdala and bed nucleus of the stria terminalis, and this pathway provides a route for olfactory stimuli to influence sexual behaviour (Hull et al. 2002). Somatosensory inputs from the genitals also reach the medial preoptic area, via the central tegmental field of the midbrain (Hull et al. 2002). The systems in the hypothalamus and medial preoptic area are influenced by oxytocin in both females and males (Veening et al. 2015). In males, peripheral oxytocin facilitates ejaculation, and brain oxytocin facilitates erection, and overactivity in these systems is implicated in premature ejaculation (Veening et al. 2015). Antidepressant drugs by their influence on the 5-hydroxytryptamine (5-HT) system can influence ejaculation and sexual behaviour (Veening et al. 2015).

The outputs of the preoptic area include connections to the lateral tegmental field in the midbrain, and in this region neurons are found that respond in relation to different aspects of male sexual behaviour (Shimura & Shimokochi 1990). However, it is likely that only some outputs of the orbitofrontal cortex and amygdala that control sexual behaviour act through the preoptic area. The preoptic area route may be necessary for computationally simple aspects of sexual behaviour such as copulation in males, but the attractive effect of sexual stimuli may survive damage to the medial preoptic area (see Carlson & Birkett (2017)), suggesting that, as for feeding, outputs of the amygdala and orbitofrontal cortex can influence behaviour through other pathways (see Chapters 4 and 5).

During early development in males, the steroid hormone testosterone masculinizes the brain, and the effects produced include sexual dimorphism in a part of the preoptic area, which is larger in males than females (Morris, Jordan & Breedlove 2004). Before birth, boys and girls already differ hormonally. At about week 7 of human gestation, the testes begin to produce hormones, resulting in a substantial sex difference in testosterone concentrations (Hines 2010, Hines, Constantinescu & Spencer 2015). This sex difference appears to be maximal between approximately weeks 8 and 24 of gestation. In regard to children's play, evidence from studies of genetic disorders, of maternal treatment with hormones, and of normal variability in hormones all point to the same conclusion: testosterone concentrations prenatally influence children's subsequent sex-typed toy, playmate and activity preferences (Hines 2010). A consistent finding is that girls exposed to unusually high levels of androgens prenatally, owing to congenital adrenal hyperplasia, show increased male-typical play and reduced female-typical play. Similarly, children whose mothers took androgenic progestins during pregnancy show increased male-typical toy and activity preferences, whereas the opposite is the case for children whose mothers took anti-androgenic progestins (Hines 2010, Hines et al. 2015). The effects of the early hormone environment also extend to personality characteristics that show sex differences. Probably the best-established links in this area involve empathy, which is typically higher in females, and physical aggression, which is typically higher in males (Hines 2010).

During puberty there are many changes in sexual behaviour and reward systems, and in other behaviours including impulsivity, and associated with these some changes in brain connectivity and function occur, in for example the medial prefrontal cortex, amygdala, and striatum, but much remains to be understood, including to what extent these changes are steroid-dependent (Walker, Bell, Flores, Gulley, Willing & Paul 2017, Suleiman, Galvan, Harden & Dahl 2017).

7.8.3 Orbitofrontal cortex and related areas

In an example illustrating part of the importance of the orbitofrontal cortex and of somatosensory reinforcers, evidence from fMRI indicates that the pleasantness of touch is represented especially in the orbitofrontal cortex (see Fig. 4.4). Presumably the pleasant effects of sexual touch are also represented in this and connected brain areas (see, e.g., Tiihonen, Kuikka, Kupila, Partanen, Vainio, Airaksinen, Eronen, Hallikainen, Paanila, Kinnunen & Huttunen (1994)). It is presumably by these neural circuits in the orbitofrontal cortex and amygdala that the effects related to the control of sexual behaviour described above are implemented, and much of the decoding of the relevant stimuli, and then their interpretation as primary reinforcers, or learning about their reinforcing properties by stimulus–reinforcement association learning, occurs. A number of the effects that occur in sexual behaviour such as sensory-specific satiety are related to a diminution over time of the reward value produced by the same stimulus or individual, and the enhancement of behaviour produced by novel stimuli or individuals. It is also presumably in regions such as the orbitofrontal cortex and amygdala that such effects, which require a representation of individuals, and systems that can show a form of learning with stimulus repetition to implement sensory-specific satiety and novelty effects, are implemented.

In functional neuroimaging studies in humans (Georgiadis & Kringelbach 2012), a distinction has been suggested between brain areas activated by 'wanting' sexual stimuli, and by 'liking' sexual stimuli, following the distinction suggested by Berridge (1996). First, we can note that 'wanting' corresponds to states related to the expected value of stimuli, and to the conditioned incentive and secondary reinforcing effects of stimuli; and that 'liking' corresponds to the outcome value of stimuli, the more primary rewards. Second, we can note that during the 'anticipatory' or 'wanting' phase, the body is preparing itself physiologically and in terms of actions to obtain the goals of sexual behaviour, and so it is not surprising that the emphasis is on conditioned reinforcers and actions to obtain those conditioned reinforcers, whereas during the consummatory phase, the behavioural responses being made, and the brain regions activated, are different. Third, we can note that although the behaviour required for the anticipatory phase is necessarily different from the behaviour required in the value outcome (or consummatory) phase, the actual goals, the reward value being specified by the genes, may be similar (see Section 4.6.2).

In functional neuroimaging studies, activations are sometimes described as being different for sexual arousing stimuli compared to other stimuli in high order areas of the visual cortex (Georgiadis & Kringelbach 2012). However, this does not mean that individual neurons encode the reward value of these sexual stimuli, as the neuroimaging studies could just reflect greater arousal associated with such stimuli modulating activations. For visual stimuli associated with food reward, it has been shown that visual cortex neurons do not encode reward value, in that their responses do not reverse during visual discrimination reversal (Rolls, Judge & Sanghera 1977). The neuroimaging studies can not address this issue, so must not be over-interpreted. Single neuron studies do show that there are sex anticipation or expected reward value neurons in the primate preoptic area (Aou et al. 1984), which receives from the orbitofrontal cortex and amygdala, and that these neurons do not respond to the sight of food, so in line with other specific reward representations described in Chapter 4, there are also sex reward value specific neurons in primates, and on that basis they are likely to be present in humans too. In the neuroimaging studies, activations to these expected sex reward value or anticipatory stimuli are found in the orbitofrontal cortex (including in men strong activation to women with biologically optimal waist-to-hip ratios), anterior cingulate cortex, and amygdala, and regions to which they project as outputs such as the ventral striatum and hypothalamus (Georgiadis & Kringelbach 2012), but the neuroimaging studies do not address the specificity of the sex-related reward vs other reward-related responses, as the activity of thousands of neurons is imaged in any voxel, and the coding of reward specificity is at the neuronal level (which is the computationally relevant level), as shown in Chapter 4.

In the pregenual cingulate cortex activations are more related to erotic images including images of single nudes (probably reflecting its expected reward value inputs from the orbitofrontal cortex), whereas responses more posteriorly towards the midcingulate cortex tended to be associated with penile responses or long blocks of explicit video-type sexual visual stimuli (reviewed by Georgiadis & Kringelbach (2012)), consistent with it being a more action or motor related area (Section 4.7). Dopamine pathways project into the ventral striatum, and interestingly variations in dopamine-related genes both predict ventral striatum responsivity and sexual motivation, the latter indicated by reports about the number of sexual partners and age of first sexual intercourse (see review by Georgiadis & Kringelbach (2012)).

Face expression and face identity are represented in the primate orbitofrontal cortex (Thorpe et al. 1983, Rolls et al. 2006), and attractive faces produce more activation of the human medial orbitofrontal cortex than unattractive faces (O'Doherty et al. 2003). Interestingly, when women look at male faces this leads to an increase in activity in the medial orbitofrontal cortex/ventromedial prefrontal cortex during the late follicular phase (when women are fertile) relative to the luteal phase. This activity is correlated with the perceived attractiveness as well as the individual's estradiol to progesterone ratio (Rupp & Wallen 2009), suggesting a key role for the orbitofrontal cortex in face attractiveness and mate selection (Hahn & Perrett 2014).

During orgasm (which might be thought of as the reward outcome phase of sexual behaviour), there is in women a strong activation of the orbitofrontal cortex, which correlates with the subjective pleasure (Georgiadis, Kortekaas, Kuipers, Nieuwenburg, Pruim, Reinders & Holstege 2006) (see also Georgiadis & Kringelbach (2012)). This is consistent with the representation of the outcome value of other specific rewards in the orbitofrontal cortex, but by different neurons (Chapter 4).

7.9 Conclusion

We can conclude this chapter by emphasizing that reward systems in the brain are likely to be involved in sexual behaviour and pleasure, and that these have probably been built in the brain by genes as their way of increasing their fitness, with hypotheses about these reward systems described by Rolls (2014b). It will be interesting to know how these different reward systems actually operate in the brain. The issue of the role of reward (and punishment) systems in brain design by genetic variation and natural selection is described in Chapter 3.

Much research remains to be performed to understand the details of the implementation of the rewards underlying sexual behaviour described earlier in this chapter in brain regions such as the orbitofrontal cortex, preoptic area, hypothalamus, and amygdala.

8 Decision-making and attractor networks

8.1 Overview of decision-making

We almost always need to choose between different rewards that may be available, that is between different stimuli that produce different emotional states. How do we compare the reward values, and take a decision for one of the rewards on each occasion? It is very important that we make a real choice on a particular occasion, for the medieval tale told by Duns Scotus was of a donkey situated between two equidistant and equally delicious food rewards that might never make a decision and might starve. The implication is that on each particular occasion, even if the rewards are almost equal, there has to be a mechanism in the brain to make a definite and fast choice on one trial, and then stay with that choice until the reward is obtained. The way in which the brain takes such decisions is described in this Chapter.

One way in which the slight randomness caused by the randomness of the firing times of the neurons is useful is that it breaks symmetries of the type just described, so that a choice is made. It is this that accounts for the fact that if the odds are equal for a pair of choices, we may make each choice on approximately 50% of the occasions.

Decisions between rewards – and therefore about which behaviour to perform next – appear to be implemented in the brain by competition between groups of neurons that represent each reward in attractor networks, which are described in this Chapter.

The attractor networks are formed by the excitatory connections between nearby excitatory neurons in the cerebral cortex.

Each decision is represented by a subset of neurons that have strong excitatory connections between them. There are inhibitory neurons which result is competition between the subsets of neurons. The result is that each subset of neurons tends to increase its activity, but only one subset wins, reaches a high firing rate, and then keeps firing for several seconds due to the internal positive feedback.

Decisions are thus made by competition between subsets of neurons each competing to win, and each biased by the decision variables.

This is described as an attractor network, because the network is attracted into the state based on the learned synaptic excitatory connections between the excitatory neurons, even if the inputs to the network are not exact matches for what has been stored.

This type of decision-making network is implemented for different types of decision in different cortical areas. For emotion-related decisions between rewards, the relevant brain region is anterior to the orbitofrontal cortex, in what is sometimes termed the ventromedial prefrontal cortex. For decisions about what action to take to obtain a reward outcome or goal, the brain region is the anterior cingulate cortex.

The same architecture implements short-term memory, in which the continuing firing of a winning subset of the neurons is maintained because of the internal positive feedback implemented by the excitatory connections between nearby cortical neurons.

In all these attractor systems, the decision-making has an element of randomness introduced by the fact that each neuron in the network has some randomness in the exact times at which its action potentials will occur. This randomness is referred to as noise or stochasticity. It is shown that the slight element of randomness is in fact advantageous in the decision-making and in the operation of short-term and long-term memory implemented with this system, and contributes to processes such as creativity.

The field of neuroeconomics addresses how these decision-making systems operate when we have to choose between different amounts of goods each with a different value, and when we are in a probabilistic and risky world, and is described elsewhere (Glimcher 2011a, Glimcher & Fehr 2013, Rolls 2014b).

We have seen in Chapter 4 how the reward value of stimuli is represented on a continuous scale in the orbitofrontal cortex. For example, the firing rate of orbitofrontal cortex neurons with food-related responses decreases steadily as monkeys are fed to satiety, and similarly, activations in the medial orbitofrontal cortex to food become smaller as humans are fed to satiety, and indeed the activations are linearly related to the subjective pleasure (measured by the pleasantness rating on every trial) produced by the taste or flavour of food. Similarly, activations in the human orbitofrontal cortex are correlated with how much money is won on a trial.

In this Chapter, an introduction to how our decision-making mechanisms operate is provided, with fully quantitative details driven by methods originating in theoretical physics described in *Cerebral Cortex: Principles of Operation* (Rolls 2016c) (with demonstration programs available at www.oxcns.org), and *The Noisy Brain: Stochastic Dynamics as a Principle of Brain Function* (Rolls & Deco 2010).

8.2 Decision-making in an attractor network

8.2.1 An attractor decision-making network

Consider the architecture shown in Fig. 8.1a. A set of cortical neurons has recurrent collateral excitatory synaptic connections w_{ij} from the other neurons. The evidence for decision 1 is applied via the λ_1 inputs, and for decision 2 via the λ_2 inputs. The synaptic weights w_{ij} have been associatively modified during training in the presence of λ_1 and at a different time of λ_2. The Hebbian or associative synaptic modification is such that if the presynaptic terminal and the postsynaptic neuron are simultaneously active, the synaptic connections become stronger. There are inhibitory neurons (not shown in Fig. 8.1a) which keep the total firing in the network within bounds, and in fact implement competition between the neuronal populations. As a result of the associative synaptic modification, there are strong connections within the set of neurons activated by λ_1, and strong connections within the set of neurons activated by λ_2. These strengthened synapses provide positive feedback, so that if the whole or part of λ_1 is applied, that set of neurons becomes active, and maintains its activity for a long period even when the input λ_1 is removed. The neurons activated by λ_1 if firing inhibit the neurons activated by λ_2 through the inhibitory interneurons, so that just one population wins the competition and maintains its activity. This thus provides a model of memory, and its retrieval. This is called an attractor network, because a subset of the neurons within either population is sufficient to attract the system into a state in which all the neurons in that population are active, by using the strengthened recurrent collateral synaptic connections. The properties of attractor

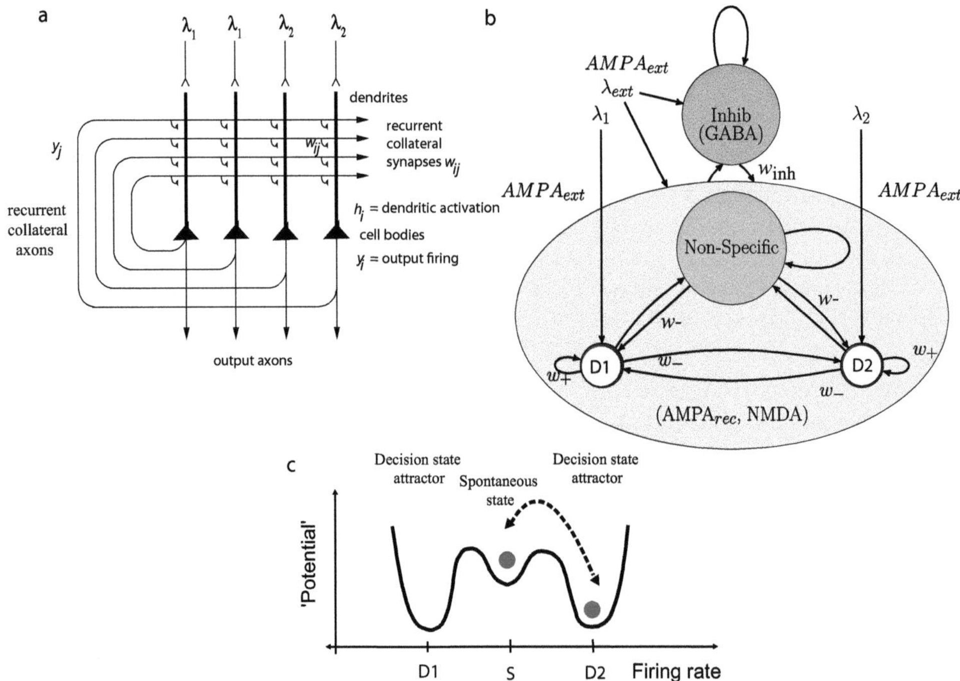

Fig. 8.1 (a) Attractor or autoassociation single network architecture for decision-making. The cell body of each neuron is shown as a triangle (like a cortical pyramidal cell), the dendrite is vertical, and receives recurrent collateral synaptic connections w_{ij} from the other neurons. The evidence for decision 1 is applied via the λ_1 inputs, and for decision 2 via the λ_2 inputs. The synaptic weights w_{ij} have been associatively modified during training in the presence of λ_1 and at a different time of λ_2. When λ_1 and λ_2 are applied, each attractor competes through the inhibitory interneurons (not shown), until one wins the competition, and the network falls into one of the high firing rate attractors that represents the decision. The noise in the network caused by the random spiking times of the neurons (for a given mean rate) means that on some trials, for given inputs, the neurons in the decision 1 (D1) attractor are more likely to win, and on other trials the neurons in the decision 2 (D2) attractor are more likely to win. This makes the decision-making probabilistic, for, as shown in (c), the noise influences when the system will jump out of the spontaneous firing stable (low energy) state S, and whether it jumps into the high firing state for decision 1 (D1) or decision 2 (D2). (b) The architecture of the integrate-and-fire network used to model decision-making (see text). The synaptic weights between the neural populations (decision pools D1 and D2, the non-specific pool, and the inhibitory pool) are 1 except where indicated. In particular, the recurrent weights, indicated by a recurrent arrow, between the neurons within an attractor decision-making pool have strong weights w_+, and between the different excitatory pools have the weak strength w_-. (c) A multistable 'effective energy landscape' for decision-making with stable states shown as low 'potential' basins. Even when the inputs are being applied to the network, the spontaneous firing rate state is stable, and noise provokes transitions from the low firing rate spontaneous state S into the high firing rate decision attractor state D1 or D2. If the noise is greater, the escaping time to a decision state, and thus the decision or reaction time, will be shorter (see Rolls 2016c, Rolls and Deco 2010).

or autoassociation networks are described in detail elsewhere (Rolls 2016c, Deco et al. 2013, Hertz, Krogh & Palmer 1991, Hopfield 1982).

For decision-making, when λ_1 and λ_2 are applied simultaneously, each attractor competes through the inhibitory interneurons (not shown), until one wins the competition, and the network falls into one of the high firing rate attractors that represents the decision. When the network starts from a state of spontaneous firing, the biasing inputs encourage one of the attractors to gradually win the competition, but this process is influenced by the Poisson-like firing (spiking) of the neurons, so that which attractor wins is probabilistic. (Poisson-like indicates that the firing times are random for a given mean firing rate.) If the evidence in favour of the two decisions is equal, the network chooses each decision probabilistically on 50% of the trials. The model shows how probabilistic decision-making could be implemented in the brain. The model also shows how the evidence can be accumulated over long periods of time because of the integrating action of the attractor short-term memory network, with the recurrent collaterals feeding back information to be combined with the continuing inputs λ_1 and λ_2. The model produces shorter reaction or decision times as a function of the magnitude of the difference between the evidence for the two decisions: difficult decisions take longer, partly because the firing rates take longer to reach a decision threshold if the difference between the inputs is small.

8.2.2 The operation of a model of decision-making

To illustrate and analyse the properties of this type of attractor decision-making network, we simulated the decision-making network illustrated in Fig. 8.1 with neurons that were biologically dynamically plausible in that they receive excitatory inputs through dynamically modelled synapses, and integrate the synaptic currents resulting from the input firing received by each synapse to lead to firing of a neuron when the resulting voltage reached a firing threshold (Rolls, Grabenhorst & Deco 2010b). The inputs to the neurons include randomness in the spike times of the inputs to the neurons, to model the noisy operation of the networks in the brain. The 'integrate and fire' simulations were similar to those developed by Brunel & Wang (2001) and Wang (2002), except that we ensured that the spontaneous low firing rate state was stable even when the decision variables were applied, with the aim of more accurately describing for examples the decision times of the network, as described elsewhere (Deco & Rolls 2006, Rolls & Deco 2010, Rolls 2016c).

In the simulations illustrated in Fig. 8.2, there was 2 s of spontaneous activity in which both the decision populations of neurons had a low level of firing of approximately 3 spikes/s. There were 400 excitatory neurons, and the D1 and D2 populations both had 40 neurons. At time = 2 s, the decision variable λ_1 was applied to D1, and λ_2 to D2. On the left are shown difficult decisions in which $\lambda_1 = \lambda_2$, so that the difference ΔI=0. The average firing rate over many trials in which D1 won and entered a high firing rate state is shown in Fig. 8.2a. The firing rates of the different populations including D1, D2, and the inhibitory neurons on a single trial are shown in Fig. 8.2b. Fig. 8.2c shows the rastergrams for the same trial, with each row representing a randomly chosen neuron, and each vertical line the firing of an action potential by the neuron, to illustrating that the firing is similar to that of neurons recorded in the brain. Figure 8.2d shows the firing rates on another difficult trial (ΔI=0) to illustrate the variability shown from trial to trial, with on this trial prolonged competition between the D1 and D2 attractors until the D1 attractor finally won after approximately 1100 ms.

Figure 8.2f shows firing rate plots for the four neuronal populations on an example of a single easy trial (with $\lambda_1 > \lambda_2$ to produce ΔI=160 units), Fig. 8.2g shows the synaptic currents in the four neuronal populations on the same trial, and Fig. 8.2h shows rastergrams for the same trial (Rolls, Grabenhorst & Deco 2010b).

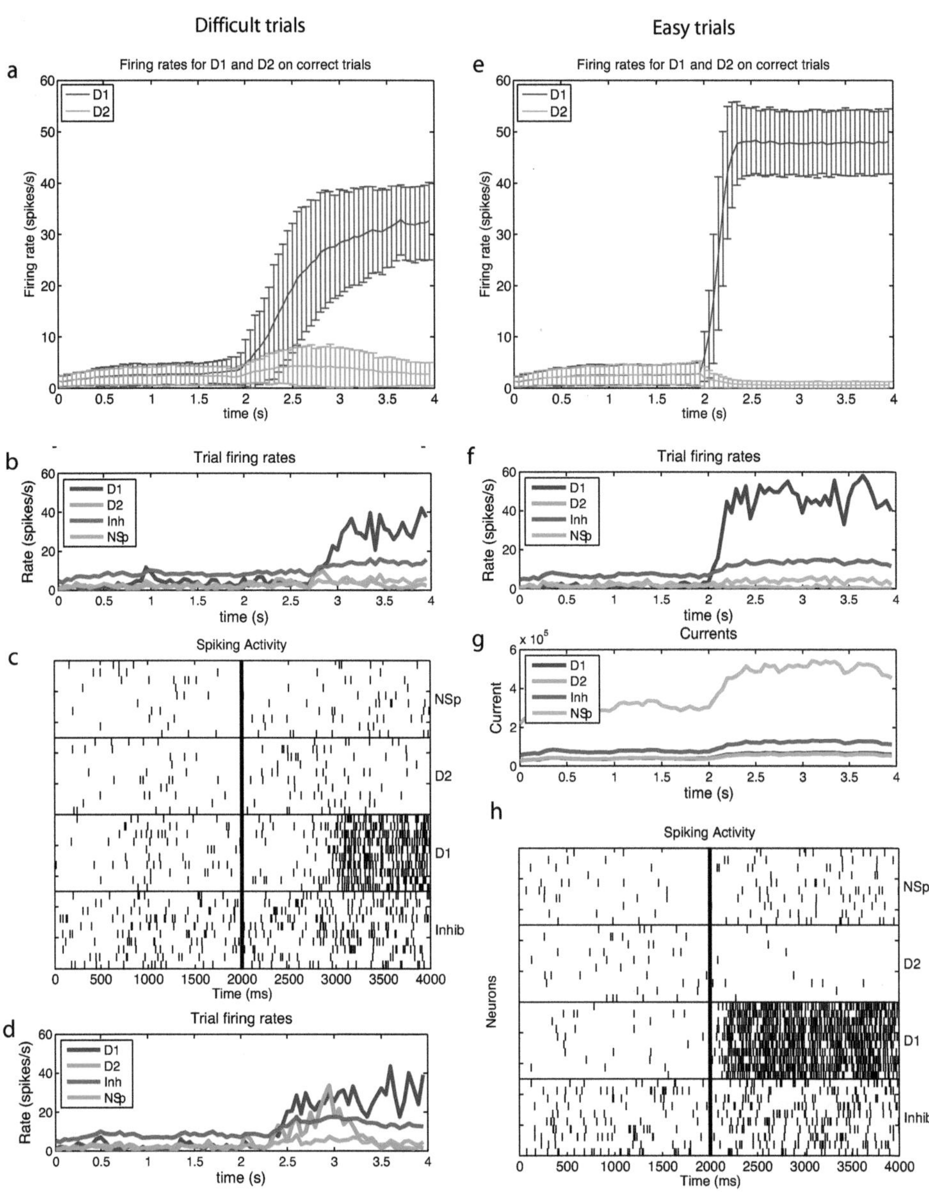

Fig. 8.2 (a) and (e) Firing rates (mean $\pm$ sd) for difficult (ΔI=0) and easy (ΔI=160) trials. The period 0–2 s is the spontaneous firing, and the decision cues were turned on at time = 2 s. D1: firing rate of the D1 population of neurons on correct trials on which the D1 population won. D2: firing rate of the D2 population of neurons on the correct trials on which the D1 population won. A correct trial was one in which in which the mean rate of the D1 attractor averaged > 10 spikes/s for the last 1000 ms of the simulation runs. (b) The mean firing rates of the four populations of neurons on a difficult trial. Inh is the inhibitory population that uses GABA as a transmitter. NSp is the non-specific population of neurons. (c) Rastergrams for the trial shown in b. 10 neurons from each of the four pools of neurons are shown. (d) The firing rates on another difficult trial (ΔI=0) showing prolonged competition between the D1 and D2 attractors until the D1 attractor finally wins after approximately 1100 ms. (f) Firing rate plots for the 4 neuronal populations on a single easy trial (ΔI=160). (g) The synaptic currents in the four neuronal populations on the trial shown in f. (h) Rastergrams for the easy trial shown in f and g. 10 neurons from each of the four pools of neurons are shown. (Reprinted from *Neuroimage*, 33 (2), Edmund T. Rolls, Fabian Grabenhorst, and Gustavo Deco, Choice, difficulty, and confidence in the brain, pp. 694–706, doi.org/10.1016/j.neuroimage.2010.06.073, Copyright © 2010 Elsevier Inc. All rights reserved.)

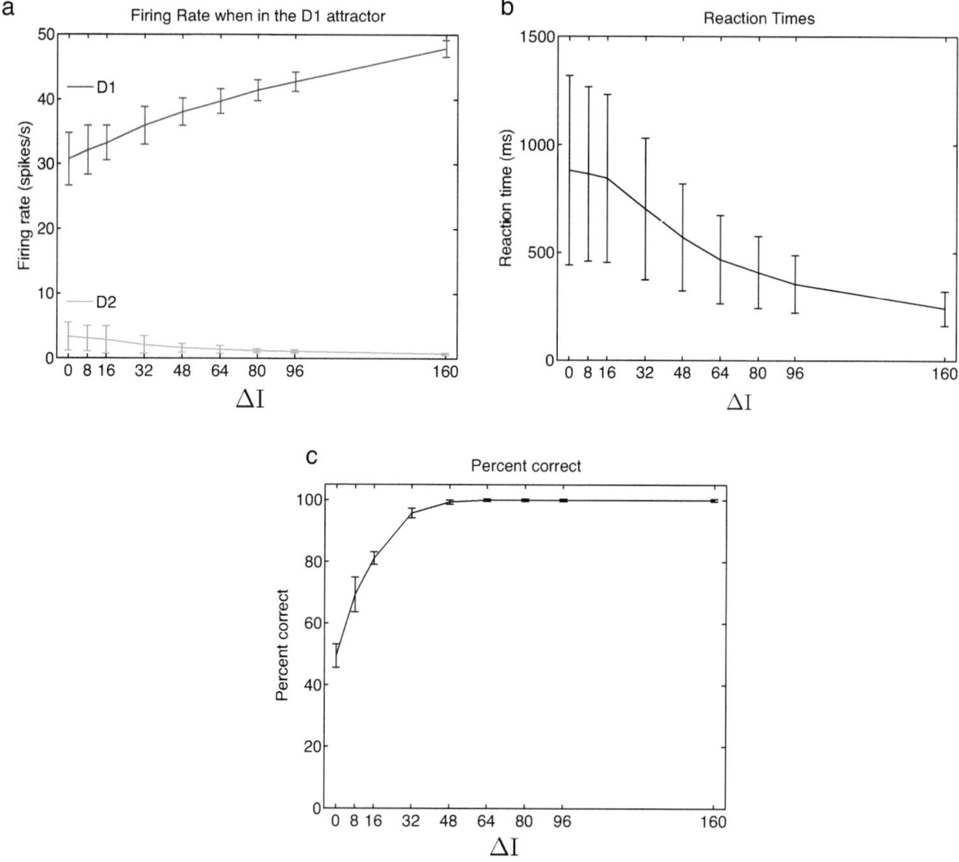

Fig. 8.3 (a) Firing rates (mean $\pm$ sd) on correct trials when in the D1 attractor as a function of ΔI. ΔI=0 corresponds to difficult, and ΔI=160 spikes/s corresponds to easy. The firing rates for both the winning population D1 and for the losing population D2 are shown for correct trials by thick lines. All the results are for 1000 simulation trials for each parameter value, and all the results shown are statistically highly significant. (b) Reaction times (mean $\pm$ sd) for the D1 population to win on correct trials as a function of the difference in inputs ΔI to D1 and D2. (c) Per cent correct performance, i.e. the percentage of trials on which the D1 population won, as a function of the difference in inputs ΔI to D1 and D2. (Reprinted from *Neuroimage*, 33 (2), Edmund T. Rolls, Fabian Grabenhorst, and Gustavo Deco, Choice, difficulty, and confidence in the brain, pp. 694–706, doi.org/10.1016/j.neuroimage.2010.06.073. Copyright 2010, with permission from Elsevier.)

Many important points are illustrated about the operation of integrate-and-fire attractor decision-making networks by what is shown in Fig. 8.2, and in Fig. 8.3 which analyses the decision-making properties across many trials.

First, once one of the populations wins the decision-making and enters a high firing rate state (D1 in the Figure), it inhibits the other decision-making neurons, and the winning population keeps on firing very stably for many seconds. This can happen even if the decision variables λ return to their pre-decision level of firing. The maintenance of the high firing rate winning state shows how short-term memory is implemented in the brain. In the case of emotion, such a high firing rate state might constitute the memory of a decision just taken by the networks, so that other networks in the brain can produce actions to obtain the chosen reward. The ongoing short-term memory state might also reflect the continuing happiness or mood state after an input has triggered the network into its high firing rate attractor state.

Second, the percentage correct is 50% correct when the decision variables are equal (ΔI=0), and gradually increases towards 100% correct as ΔI increases (Fig. 8.3c). This probabilistic decision=making has great adaptive utility, as described later.

Third, the reaction times gradually become faster as ΔI increases (Fig. 8.3b). In fact, there is a long tail of long reaction times with this network under these conditions, which is also found in human experiments (Rolls & Deco 2010).

Fourth, there is only one winning attractor, and both the D1 and D2 neurons do not both end up firing fast. This is a function of the parameters of the network, such as the strength of the recurrent collateral synapses in each set of decision-making neurons; and the amount of inhibition (Rolls 2016c). Graded firing rates, in which a neuron has a set of different firing rates to the set of stimuli, as in the brain, facilitates this (Rolls 2016c). This is fundamental for biologically useful decision-making.

Fifth, the mean firing rate after the network has settled into the correct decision attractor is higher on easy than on difficult trials, if the decision variables are left on as in Fig. 8.2, because then the inputs from the decision variables contribute to the final firing rates. This further makes confidence an emergent property of this type of decision-making network, because when ΔI is high so is the final firing rate of the winning attractor, and the confidence in the decision which can be read from the high firing rates (Rolls et al. 2010b, Rolls, Grabenhorst & Deco 2010c).

8.2.3 Using the model to locate reward-related decision-making attractor networks in the brain

The integrate-and-fire decision-making model just described allows measuring the synaptic currents on easy vs difficult trial types, and from those currents predicting the BOLD signals in fMRI experiments on easy vs difficult trials (Rolls et al. 2010b, Rolls et al. 2010c). The prediction is that in a brain area implementing the decision between two rewards, the BOLD signal should increase approximately linearly with the easiness of the decision.

Two functional neuroimaging investigations were performed to test the predictions of the model just described. Task difficulty was altered parametrically to determine whether there was a close relation between the BOLD signal and task difficulty (Rolls, Grabenhorst & Deco 2010b), and whether this was present especially in brain areas implicated in choice decision-making by other criteria (Grabenhorst, Rolls & Parris 2008b, Rolls, Grabenhorst & Parris 2010d). The decisions were about the pleasantness of olfactory stimuli (Rolls, Grabenhorst & Parris 2010d) or of thermal stimuli applied to the hand (Grabenhorst, Rolls & Parris 2008b).

Figure 8.4 shows experimental data with the fMRI BOLD signal measured on easy and difficult trials of the olfactory affective decision task (left) and the thermal affective decision task (right) (Rolls, Grabenhorst & Deco 2010b). The upper records are for prefrontal cortex medial area 10 in a region identified by the following criterion as being involved in choice decision-making. The criterion was that a brain region for identical stimuli should show more activity when a choice decision was being made than when a rating on a continuous scale of affective value was being made. Figure 8.4 shows for medial prefrontal cortex area 10 that there is a larger BOLD signal on easy than on difficult trials. The top diagram shows the medial prefrontal area activated in this contrast for decisions about which olfactory stimulus was more pleasant (yellow), and for decisions about whether the thermal stimulus would be chosen in future based on whether it was pleasant or unpleasant (red).

Further, there was a clear and approximately linear relation between the BOLD signal and

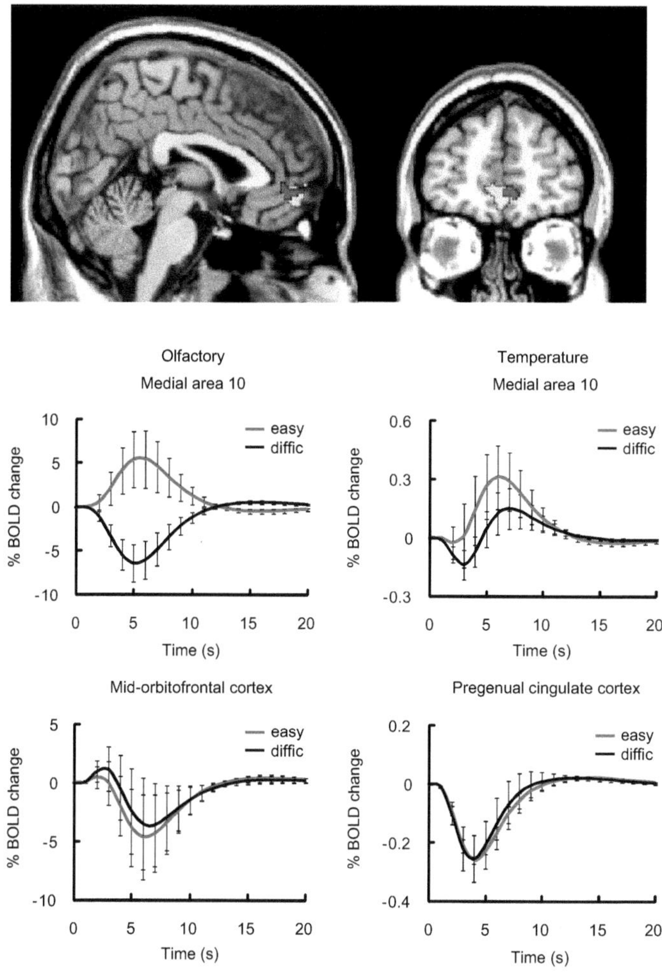

Fig. 8.4 Top: Medial prefrontal cortex area 10 activated on easy vs difficult trials in the olfactory pleasantness decision task (yellow) and the thermal pleasantness decision task (red). Middle: experimental data showing the BOLD signal in medial area 10 on easy and difficult trials of the olfactory affective decision task (left) and the thermal affective decision task (right). This medial area 10 was a region identified by other criteria (see text) as being involved in choice decision-making. Bottom: The BOLD signal for the same easy and difficult trials, but in parts of the pregenual cingulate and mid-orbitofrontal cortex implicated by other criteria (see text) in representing the subjective reward value of the stimuli on a continuous scale, but not in making choice decisions between the stimuli, or about whether to choose the stimulus in future. (Reprinted from *Neuroimage*, 33 (2), Edmund T. Rolls, Fabian Grabenhorst, and Gustavo Deco, Choice, difficulty, and confidence in the brain, pp. 694–706, doi.org/10.1016/j.neuroimage.2010.06.073. Copyright 2010, with permission from Elsevier.)

ΔI for the thermal and for the olfactory pleasantness decision-making task (Rolls et al. 2010b). In addition, the predictions of the model on error trials were also confirmed (Rolls et al. 2010c)

These experimental findings are thus consistent with the predictions made from the model, and provide strong support for the type of model of decision-making described in this book. Moreover, they show that decision confidence, which increases with ΔI, can be read off from fMRI BOLD signals in parts of the brain involved in making choices, as shown in this unifying theory. Further, the findings just described provide evidence that choices between rewards are made in a part of medial prefrontal cortex area 10, sometimes called the ventromedial prefrontal cortex, which is just anterior to the orbitofrontal cortex, where value is represented on a linear scale, and which is the likely source of inputs to the VMPFC decision-making reward network (Rolls et al. 2010b, Rolls et al. 2010c).

8.3 Implications and applications of this approach to decision-making

In this section I describe some implications and applications of this approach to decision-making, with further detail provided elsewhere (Rolls & Deco 2010, Rolls 2012d, Rolls 2014b, Rolls 2016c).

8.3.1 Multiple decision-making systems in the brain

Each cortical area can be conceived as performing a local type of decision-making using attractor dynamics of the type described (Rolls 2016c). Even memory recall is in effect the same local 'decision-making' process. So is short-term memory.

8.3.2 Distributed decision-making

Although the model described here is effectively a single attractor network, I note that the network need not be localized to one brain region. Long-range connections between cortical areas enable networks in different brain areas to interact in the way needed to implement a single attractor network. The requirement is that the synapses between the neurons in any one pool be set up by Hebb-like associative synaptic modification, and this is likely to be a property of connectivity between areas (using forward and backprojections), as well as within areas (Rolls 2016c). In this sense, the decision could be thought of as distributed across different brain areas.

8.3.3 Predicting a decision before the evidence is provided

There is a literature on how early one can predict from neural activity what decision will be taken (Hampton & O'Doherty 2007, Haynes & Rees 2005a, Haynes & Rees 2005b, Haynes & Rees 2006, Haynes, Sakai, Rees, Gilbert, Frith & Passingham 2007, Lau, Rogers & Passingham 2006, Pessoa & Padmala 2005, Rolls, Grabenhorst & Franco 2009). For example, when subjects held in mind in a delay period which of two tasks, addition or subtraction, they intended to perform, then it was possible to decode or predict with fMRI whether addition or subtraction would later be performed from medial prefrontal cortex activations with accuracies in the order of 70%, where chance was 50% (Haynes et al. 2007). A problem with such studies is that it is often not possible to know exactly when the decision was taken at the mental level, or when preparation for the decision actually started, so it is difficult to know whether neural activity that precedes the decision itself in any way predicts the decision that will be taken (Rolls 2011a). In these circumstances, is there anything rigorous that our understanding of the neural mechanisms involved in the decision-making can provide? It turns out that there is (Rolls & Deco 2011b).

While investigating the speed of decision-making using a network of the type described in this chapter, Smerieri, Rolls & Feng (2010) studied the activity that preceded the onset of the decision cues. The results found in simulations in which the firing rate in the spontaneous firing period is measured before a particular attractor population won or lost the competition. The firing rate averaged over approximately 800 winning (correct) vs losing (error) trials for the attractor showed that the firing rate when the attractor will win is on average higher than that for when the attractor will lose at a time that starts in this case approximately 1000 ms before the decision cues are applied. Thus it is possible before the decision cues are applied to predict in this noisy decision-making attractor network something about what decision will be taken for periods in the order of 1 s before the decision cues are applied. (If longer time constants are used for some of the GABA inhibitory neurons in the network, the decision that will be taken can be predicted (probabilistically) for as much as 2 s before the decision cues are applied (Smerieri, Rolls & Feng 2010).)

What could be the mechanism? It appears to be as follows (Rolls & Deco 2011b). There will be noise (randomness, statistical fluctuations) in the neuronal firing that will lead, at different times in the period before the decision cues are applied, to low, but different, firing rates of the two selective populations of neurons that represent the different decisions. If the firing rate of say population D1 (representing decision 1) is higher than that of the D2 population at a time just as the decision-cues are being applied, this firing will add to the effect of the decision cues, and make it more likely that the D1 population will win. These fluctuations in the spontaneous firing rate will have a characteristic time course that will be influenced by the time constants of the synapses etc. in the system, so that if a population has somewhat higher firing at say 500 ms before the cues are applied, it will be a little more likely to also have higher firing a short time later.

8.3.4 The matching law

Another potential application of this model of decision-making is to probabilistic decision tasks. In such tasks, the proportion of choices reflects, and indeed may be proportional to, the expected value of the different choices. This pattern of choices is known as the matching law (Sugrue, Corrado & Newsome 2005). The results illustrated in Fig. 8.3 show comparable behaviour for the decision-making network described here.

This behaviour of the system is quite adaptive, because it means that the less attractive choice is sometimes made, and this can be advantageous in an uncertain world, where the probabilities and amounts of the rewards available for different choice may change over time.

8.3.5 Symmetry-breaking

It is of interest that the noise that contributes to the stochastic dynamics of the brain through the spiking fluctuations may be behaviourally adaptive, and that the noise should not be considered only as a problem in terms of how the brain works. This is the issue raised for example by the donkey in the medieval Duns Scotus paradox, in which a donkey situated between two equidistant food rewards might never make a decision and might starve.

The problem raised is that with a deterministic system, there is nothing to break the symmetry, and the system can become deadlocked. In this situation, the addition of noise can produce probabilistic choice, which is advantageous. We have shown here that stochastic neurodynamics caused for example by the relatively random spiking times of neurons in a finite sized cortical attractor network can lead to probabilistic decision-making, so that in this case the stochastic noise is a positive advantage.

8.3.6 The evolutionary utility of probabilistic choice

Probabilistic decision-making can be evolutionarily advantageous in another sense, in which sometimes taking a decision that is not optimal based on previous history may provide information that is useful, and which may contribute to learning. Consider for example a probabilistic decision task in which choice 1 provides rewards on 80% of the occasions, and choice 2 on 20% of the occasions. A deterministic system with knowledge of the previous reinforcement history would always make choice 1. But this is not how animals including humans behave. Instead (especially when the overall probabilities are low and the situation involves random probabilistic baiting, and there is a penalty for changing the choice), the proportion of choices made approximately matches the outcomes that are available, in what is called the matching law (Sugrue, Corrado & Newsome 2005, Corrado, Sugrue, Seung & Newsome 2005, Rolls, McCabe & Redoute 2008e) (Section 8.3.4). By making the less favoured choice sometimes, the organism can keep obtaining evidence on whether the environment is changing (for example on whether the probability of a reward for choice 2 has increased), and by doing this approximately according to the matching law minimizes the cost of the disadvantageous choices in obtaining information about the environment.

Another example is in food foraging, which probabilistically may reflect the outcomes (Krebs, Davies & West 2012, Kacelnik & Brito e Abreu 1998), and is a way optimally in terms of costs and benefits to keep sampling and exploring the space of possible choices.

Another sense in which probabilistic decision-making may be evolutionarily advantageous is with respect to detecting signals that are close to threshold, in the process of *stochastic resonance* (Rolls & Deco 2010), as follows. If we had a deterministic neuron without noise and a fixed threshold above which spikes were emitted, then if the signal was below the threshold there would be no output, and if the signal was above threshold the neuron would emit a spike, and indeed continuous spike trains if the signal remained above threshold. In particular, if the signal was just below the threshold of the neuron, there would be no evidence that a signal close to threshold was present. However, if noise is present in the system (due for example to the afferent neurons having probabilistic spiking activity similar to that of a Poisson process), then occasionally with a signal close to threshold a spike would occur due to the summation of the signal and the noise. If the signal was a bit weaker, then the neuron might still occasionally spike, but at a lower average rate. If the signal was a bit closer to threshold, then the neuron would emit spikes at a higher average rate. Thus in this way some evidence about the presence of a subthreshold signal can be made evident in the spike trains emitted by a neuron if there is noise in the inputs to the neuron. The noise in this case is useful, and may have an adaptive function (cf. Faisal, Selen & Wolpert (2008)). This process is known as stochastic resonance, and is a well known example of how noise can have beneficial effects in signal detection systems operating close to a threshold (Longtin 1993, Weisenfeld 1993, Stocks 2000, Riani & Simonotto 1994, Shang, Claridge-Chang, Sjulson, Pypaert & Miesenböck 2007, Faisal, Selen & Wolpert 2008, Goldbach, Loh, Deco & Garcia-Ojalvo 2008).

8.3.7 Unpredictable behaviour

An area where the spiking-related noise in the decision-making process may be evolutionarily advantageous is in the generation of unpredictable behaviour, which can be advantageous in a number of situations, for example when a prey is trying to escape from a predator, and perhaps in some social and economic situations in which organisms may not wish to reveal their intentions (Maynard Smith 1982, Maynard Smith 1984, Dawkins 1995). We note that such probabilistic decisions may have long-term consequences. For example, a probabilistic decision in a 'war of attrition' such as staring down a competitor e.g. in dominance hierarchy formation, may fix the relative status of the two individual animals involved, who then tend to maintain that relationship stably for a considerable period of weeks or more (Maynard Smith 1982, Maynard Smith 1984, Dawkins 1995).

Intrinsic indeterminacy may be essential for unpredictable behaviour (Glimcher 2005). For example, in interactive games like matching pennies or rock–paper–scissors, any trend that deviates from random choice by an agent could be exploited to his or her opponent's advantage.

8.3.8 Memory recall

The theory described here of decision-making is effectively a model of the stochastic dynamics of the recall of a memory in response to a recall cue. The memory might be a long-term memory, but the theory applies to the retrieval of any stored representation in the brain. The way in which the attractor is reached depends on the strength of the recall cue, and inherent noise in the attractor network performing the recall because of the spiking activity in a finite size system. The recall will take longer if the recall cue is weak. Spontaneous stochastic effects may suddenly lead to the memory being recalled, and this may be related to the sudden recovery of a memory which one tried to remember some time previously. These processes are considered further by Rolls (2016c).

The theory applies to a situation where the representation may be being 'recalled' by a single input, which is perceptual detection as described in Chapter 7 of Rolls & Deco (2010).

The theory also applies to a situation where the representation may be being 'recalled' by two or more competing inputs λ, which is decision-making as described in this chapter.

The theory also applies to short-term memory, in which the continuation of the recalled state as a persistent attractor is subject to stochastic noise effects, which may knock the system out of the short-term memory attractor, as described in Chapter 3 of Rolls & Deco (2010).

The theory also applies to attention, in which the continuation of the recalled state as a persistent attractor is subject to stochastic noise effects, which may knock the system out of the short-term memory attractor that is normally stable because of the non-linear positive feedback implemented in the attractor network by the recurrent collateral connections, as described by Rolls (2016c) and Rolls & Deco (2010).

8.3.9 Creative thought

Another way in which probabilistic decision-making may be evolutionarily advantageous is in creative thought, which is influenced in part by associations between one memory, representation, or thought, and another. If the system were deterministic, i.e. for the present purposes without noise, then the trajectory through a set of thoughts would be deterministic and would tend to follow the same furrow each time. However, if the recall of one memory or thought from another were influenced by the statistical noise due to the random spiking of neurons, then the trajectory through the state space would be different on different occasions, and we might be led in different directions on different occasions, facilitating creative thought (Rolls 2016c).

Of course, if the basins of attraction of each thought were too shallow, then the statistical noise might lead one to have very unstable thoughts that were too loosely and even bizarrely associated to each other, and to have a short-term memory and attentional system that is unstable and distractible, and indeed this is an account that we have proposed for some of the symptoms of schizophrenia (Rolls 2005, Rolls 2016c, Loh, Rolls & Deco 2007a, Loh, Rolls & Deco 2007b, Rolls, Loh, Deco & Winterer 2008d, Rolls & Deco 2010, Rolls & Deco 2011a, Rolls 2012b) (see Section 8.3.11).

The stochastic noise caused by the probabilistic neuronal spiking plays an important role in these hypotheses, because it is the noise that destabilizes the attractors when the depth of the basins of attraction is reduced. If the basins of attraction were too deep, then the noise might be insufficient to destabilize attractors, and this leads to an approach to understanding obsessive-compulsive disorders (Rolls, Loh & Deco 2008c, Rolls 2012b) (see Section 8.3.11).

8.3.10 Decision-making between the emotional and rational systems

Another application of this type of model is to taking decisions between the implicit and explicit systems in emotional decision-making (see Section 10.1 and Rolls (2014b)), where again the two different systems could provide the biasing inputs λ_1 and λ_2 to the model.

If decision-making in the cortex is largely local and typically specialized, it leaves open the question of how one stream for behavioural output is selected. This type of 'global decision-making' is considered in Sections 10.1 and 6.3.

8.3.11 Dynamical neuropsychiatry: schizophrenia, obsessive-compulsive disorder, and memory changes in normal aging

The stability of the decision-making network described here is influenced by the spiking-related noise in the system, and can be affected by quite small changes in the parameters such as the strength of the excitatory recurrent collaterals and the amount of inhibition. This has led to a new set of computational models aimed at better understanding of disordered mental states such as schizophrenia and obsessive-compulsive disorder, and also the changes in memory than can occur in normal aging, as described elsewhere (Rolls 2016c, Loh et al. 2007a, Rolls et al. 2008d, Rolls & Deco 2011a, Rolls & Deco 2010, Rolls 2012b, Rolls et al. 2008c, Rolls & Deco 2015a).

An application to depression is described in Chapter 9.

9 Depression

9.1 Introduction

Major depressive disorder is ranked by the World Health Organization as the leading cause of years-of-life lived with disability (Drevets 2007, Gotlib & Hammen 2009, Hamilton, Chen & Gotlib 2013). Major depressive episodes, found in both major depressive disorder and bipolar disorder, are pathological mood states characterized by persistently sad or depressed mood. Major depressive disorders are generally accompanied by: (1) altered incentive and reward processing, evidenced by lack of motivation, apathy, and anhedonia (lack of pleasure); (2) impaired modulation of anxiety and worry, manifested by generalized, social and panic anxiety, and oversensitivity to negative feedback; (3) inflexibility of thought and behaviour in association with changing reinforcement contingencies, apparent as ruminative thoughts of self-reproach, pessimism, and guilt, and inertia toward initiating goal-directed behaviour; (4) altered integration of sensory and social information, as evidenced by mood-congruent processing biases; (5) impaired attention and memory, shown as performance deficits on tests of attention set-shifting and maintenance, and autobiographical and short-term memory; and 6) visceral disturbances, including altered weight, appetite, sleep, and endocrine and autonomic function (Drevets 2007, Gotlib & Hammen 2009).

This Chapter describes depression, its brain mechanisms, and a new attractor-based theory of some of the brain mechanisms that are related to depression (Rolls 2016d).

9.1.1 The economic and social cost of depression

The economic cost of depression is enormous. For example, the cost to Europe of work-related depression was estimated to be €617 billion annually in 2013, and is rising (Matrix 2013). The total was made up of costs to employers resulting from absenteeism (€272 billion), loss of productivity (€242 billion), health care costs of €63 billion, and social welfare costs in the form of disability benefit payments (€39 billion).

In addition, there is a major personal burden to sufferers and their families of depression. Moreover, in most countries the number of people who suffer from depression during their lives falls within an 8-12% range, so that if the numbers of people who suffer from depression, and the effects on their families is included, the effects of advances in our understanding of depression will affect the lives of millions of people worldwide.

9.1.2 The triggers and causes of depression: non-reward systems

There are two main types of depression.

One is **reactive**, in which an event triggers depression. This is typically an event in which a reward or rewards are no longer available. An example might be a death in the family, in which a loved one is no longer present. Another might be losing a job, in which all the social and financial benefits of work may be withdrawn.

Some of the triggers of depression have been described in more detail (Rantala, Luoto, Krams & Karlsson 2018). They include:

1. Infection (during which sickness and depression might be adaptive by conserving metabolic resources for the use of the immune system to fight the infection). Although a contribution of activity in the immune system may contribute to depression (Bhattacharya, Derecki, Lovenberg & Drevets 2016), this on its own would not seem to account for all the symptoms of depression, such as low self-esteem, and anhedonia.
2. Long-term stress, in which steroid hormone levels may be increased (Gold 2015, McEwen, Gray & Nasca 2015). These steroid hormones, such as corticosterone, are adaptive in the short-term by preparing the body for action, but in the long term, can contribute to depression, and are associated with many changes in the brain, including a reduction of excitatory synaptic connections in some brain areas such as the hippocampus (McEwen et al. 2015). The stress may be produced in the first instance by non-reward or punishment, and this concept links research on stress to the approach to emotion and depression described in this book. The 'love and trust' hormone oxytocin is low in the periphery in depression, and may perhaps normally (when not depressed) help to counteract some of the effects of stress (McQuaid, McInnis, Abizaid & Anisman 2014).
3. Loneliness, which can be a non-reward and stressor in that humans benefit from social interactions in many ways (Rolls 2012d). Indeed, a solitary individual is more vulnerable to predators, hostile conspecifics and other forces of nature than individuals in social groups (Rantala et al. 2018).
4. Traumatic experience, such as injury, which can lead to stress.
5. Hierarchy conflict, in which successful competition between individuals may be adaptive (Rolls 2014b). Depression may function as a signal that an individual has given up after a hierarchy conflict; and may also lead to a change of behaviour as a response to non-reward.
6. Grief, as in the loss of a loved one. The grief may be the subjective state associated with the loss of the reward. The change produced by a loss of the reward may in evolutionary history be adaptive by stopping behaviour for the previously rewarded stimulus, and leading to new behaviour. Forty-two per cent of individuals whose spouse had passed away fulfilled the diagnostic criteria of clinical depression a month after the spouse's death (Rantala et al. 2018).
7. Romantic rejection, again a major non-reward, where the romantic attachment has the biological utility of leading to pair-bonding and successful reproduction in humans and birds, in which two parents promote gene fitness because the young are immature at birth (Rolls 2014b).
8. Postpartum (or peripartum) depression, which occurs in 10–15% of women in the six months following childbirth (Kuehner 2017). Postpartum depression may be adaptive in functioning as a signal to kin and the spouse that the mother requires more support.
9. The season, as in seasonal affective disorder (SAD), which may occur in the winter when the days are short. SAD is more common in people with evening chronotypes (Sandman, Merikanto, Maattanen, Valli, Kronholm, Laatikainen,

Partonen & Paunio 2016), and light therapy, especially in the morning, is an effective treatment.

10. Chemicals, such as alcohol and cocaine, the repeated use of which can lead to depression (Rantala et al. 2018).
11. Somatic diseases.
12. Starvation, in which depression may conserve energy (Rantala et al. 2018); or obesity, in which inflammation may be associated with depression.
13. The prevalence of depression is twice as high in women as in men, and a number of factors or triggers may contribute to this (Kuehner 2017). In this context, it is of interest that the oxytocin system in the brain (which is separate from the peripheral oxytocin system) is high in depression, and that androgens may inhibit this system (Dai, Li, Zhu, Hu, Balesar, Swaab & Bao 2017).

Although many of these states elicited by these triggers are adaptive in the sense of evolutionary biology (Rantala et al. 2018) (including in reducing risk-taking behaviour and impulsivity as shown below), some may not be adaptive in humans. Part of the reason for this, I suggest, is that many emotions may be stronger in humans than in our ancestors, because of the evolution of the reasoning system in humans, which enables planning and thinking for multiple steps ahead, which can reveal how great a loss has just occurred, as described in Chapter 3. These stronger emotions in humans may take our emotional system out of the range of rewards, non-rewards, and punishers in which our non-language-using ancestors evolved.

A second main type of depression is when there may be no identifiable event or cause in the environment, but the depression just comes on. This is referred to as **endogenous** (internally generated) depression. The brain systems in this case for non-reward may be too sensitive and imbalanced, resulting in the brain entering a depressed state even without an identifiable external trigger. As we have seen in Section 2.5, different individuals may have different sensitivities to different types of reward and reward contingency, and this is part of the way in which evolution works. But the result may be that some people are very sensitive to non-reward, and are for this reason more likely to become depressed. (Although the term 'endogenous depression' is less common now than in the past, the argument just provided does provide an approach to understanding why in some cases it may be difficult to identify the environmental cause of the depression, if the brain system in some individuals is very sensitive to non-reward, or even is triggered into an attractor state by internal noise in the brain as described in Chapter 8.)

The understanding of emotion described in Chapter 2 leads to a clear approach to understanding depression, which relates to most of the triggers described above. Depression is produced when expected rewards are not available as expected, shown on the non-reward axis in Fig. 9.1. With this non-reward contingency, if an action is possible, perhaps to obtain the reward or to prevent the situation re-occurring in future, then emotions such as anger and rage may be felt (the 'active' condition for non-reward in Fig. 9.1). If no action is possible, then sadness, grief, or depression may result (the 'passive' condition for non-reward in Fig. 9.1). Although most of the triggers of depression listed above may be related to the reinforcement contingency of non-reward, some triggers are related to changes in body state such as starvation or obesity, which may trigger the same brain mechanisms that respond to non-reward as part of an evolutionary adaptive strategy to deal with the current environment.

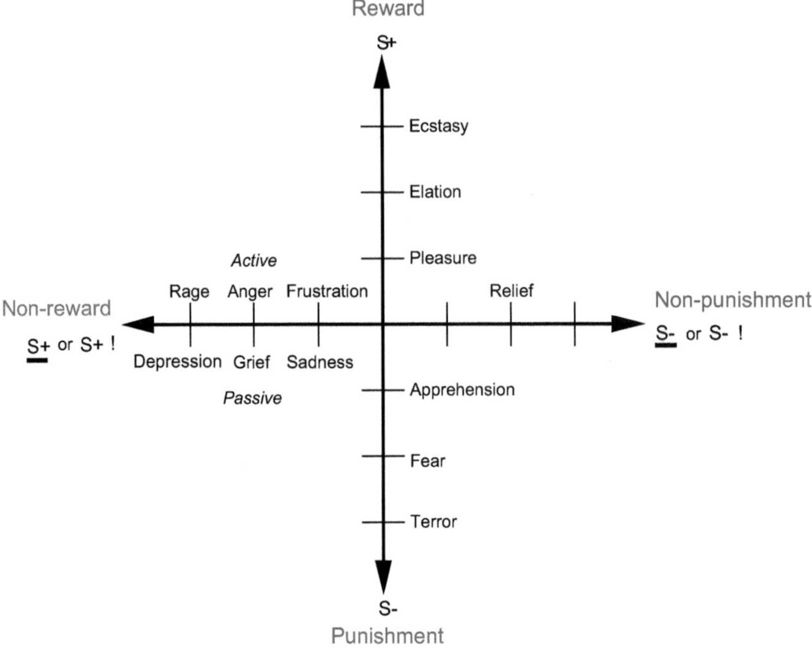

Fig. 9.1 Some of the emotions associated with different reinforcement contingencies are indicated. Intensity increases away from the centre of the diagram, on a continuous scale. The classification scheme created by the different reinforcement contingencies consists with respect to the action of (1) the delivery of a reward (S+), (2) the delivery of a punisher (S–), (3) the omission of a reward (S+) (extinction) or the termination of a reward (S+!) (time out), and (4) the omission of a punisher (S–) (avoidance) or the termination of a punisher (S–!) (escape). Note that the vertical axis describes emotions associated with the delivery of a reward (up) or punisher (down). The horizontal axis describes emotions associated with the non-delivery of an expected reward (left) or the non-delivery of an expected punisher (right). For the contingency of non-reward (horizontal axis, left) different emotions can arise depending on whether an active action is possible to respond to the non-reward, or whether no action is possible, which is labelled as the passive condition. The diagram summarizes emotions that might result for one reinforcer as a result of different contingencies. Every separate reinforcer has the potential to operate according to contingencies such as these. This diagram does not imply a dimensional theory of emotion, but shows the types of emotional state that might be produced by a specific reinforcer. Each different reinforcer will produce different emotional states, but the contingencies will operate as shown to produce different specific emotional states for each different reinforcer.

The brain-related and non-reward contingency approach taken here may be especially useful in the situation that the genetics of depression does not so far suggest a few important genes related to depression that might provide indications about possible treatments, but instead that there may be a large number of genes each of which makes a small contribution (Flint & Kendler 2014).

a. Reversal

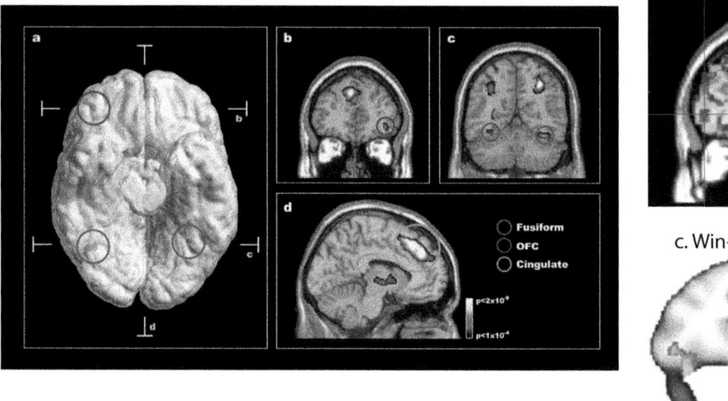

b. Stop-signal task

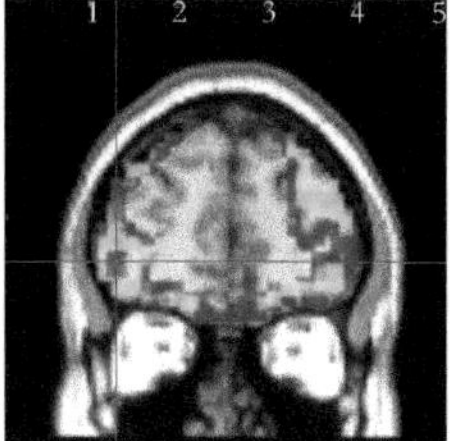

c. Win-stay / lose shift

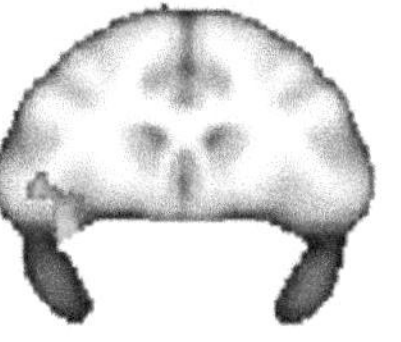

Fig. 9.2 **a. Evidence that the human lateral orbitofrontal cortex is activated by non-reward**. Activation of the lateral orbitofrontal cortex in a visual discrimination reversal task on reversal trials, when a face was selected but the expected reward was not obtained, indicating that the subject should select the other face in future to obtain the reward. a) A ventral view of the human brain with indication of the location of the two coronal slices (b,c) and the transverse slice (d). The activations with the red circle in the lateral orbitofrontal cortex (OFC, peaks at [42 42 -8] and [-46 30 -8]) show the activation on reversal trials compared to the non-reversal trials. For comparison, the activations with the blue circle show the fusiform face area produced just by face expressions, not by reversal, which are also indicated in the coronal slice in (c). b) A coronal slice showing the activation in the right orbitofrontal cortex on reversal trials. Activation is also shown in the supracallosal anterior cingulate region (Cingulate, green circle) that is also known to be activated by many punishing, unpleasant, stimuli (see Grabenhorst and Rolls (2011)). (From *Neuroimage* 20 (2), Morten L. Kringelbach and Edmund T. Rolls, Neural correlates of rapid reversal learning in a simple model of human social interaction, pp. 1371–83, doi.org/10.1016/S1053-8119(03)00393-8, Copyright © 2003 Elsevier Inc. All rights reserved.) **b. Activations in the human lateral orbitofrontal cortex are related to a signal to change behavior in the stop-signal task**. In the task, a left or right arrow on a screen indicates which button to touch. However on some trials, an up-arrow then appears, and the participant must change the behavior, and stop the response. There is a larger response on trials on which the participant successfully changes the behavior and stops the response, as shown by the contrast stop-success - stop-failure, in the ventrolateral prefrontal cortex in a region including the lateral orbitofrontal cortex, with peak at [-42 50 -2] indicated by the cross-hairs, measured in 1709 participants. There were corresponding effects in the right lateral orbitofrontal cortex [42 52 -4]. Some activation in the dorsolateral prefrontal cortex in an area implicated in attention is also shown. (Modified from Deng, Rolls et al, 2017). **c. Bold signal in the macaque lateral orbitofrontal related to win-stay / lose-shift performance, that is, to reward reversal performance**. (Modified from Chau et al, 2015).

9.1.3 Brain systems that underlie depression

We start with the concept that brain systems involved in detecting non-reward are likely to be involved in depression (Fig. 9.1). In the following, I summarize evidence that, on this basis, implicates the lateral orbitofrontal cortex in depression.

The orbitofrontal cortex contains a population of neurons that respond to non-reward and maintain their firing for many seconds after the non-reward, providing evidence that they have entered an attractor state that maintains a memory of the non-reward (Thorpe, Rolls & Maddison 1983, Rolls 2014b) (Section 4.5.3.5). An example of such a neuron is shown in Fig. 4.16 on page 80. These neurons signal that a reward is less than was expected, and are termed negative reward prediction error neurons because they respond to this type of prediction error (Section 4.5.3.5).

The human lateral orbitofrontal cortex is activated by non-reward (not obtaining an expected reward) during reward reversal (Kringelbach & Rolls 2003). This is illustrated in Fig. 9.2a, which shows activations in the lateral orbitofrontal cortex on reversal trials, that is when the human participant chose one person's face, and did not obtain the expected reward.

Activations in the lateral orbitofrontal cortex are also produced by a signal to stop a response that is now incorrect, which is another situation in which behaviour must change in order to be correct (Deng, Rolls et al. (2017), Fig. 9.2b). Orbitofrontal cortex activations in the stop-signal task have further been related to how impulsive the behaviour is (Whelan, Conrod, Poline, Lourdusamy, Banaschewski, Barker, Bellgrove, Büchel, Byrne, Cummins et al. 2012). In this context, it has been suggested that impulsiveness may reflect how sensitive an individual is to non-reward or punishment (Rolls 2014b), with one reason for being impulsive that one may not be very sensitive to non-reward, and the non-rewarding consequences of one's actions. Further, we have shown that people with orbitofrontal cortex damage become more impulsive (Berlin et al. 2004, Berlin et al. 2005).

The lateral orbitofrontal cortex also responds to many punishing, unpleasant, stimuli (Grabenhorst & Rolls 2011, Rolls 2014b) (Fig. 4.14) including bad odour (Rolls, Kringelbach & De Araujo 2003c) and losing money (O'Doherty, Kringelbach, Rolls, Hornak & Andrews 2001a). Consistent with this human neuroimaging evidence and with the macaque neurophysiology (Thorpe, Rolls & Maddison 1983, Rolls 2014b), the macaque lateral orbitofrontal cortex is also activated by non-reward during a reversal task as shown by fMRI (Chau et al. 2015) (Fig. 9.2c).

Further evidence that the orbitofrontal cortex is involved in changing rewarded behaviour when non-reward is detected is that damage to the human orbitofrontal cortex impairs reward reversal learning, in that the previously rewarded stimulus is still chosen during reversal even when no reward is being obtained (Rolls, Hornak, Wade & McGrath 1994a, Hornak, O'Doherty, Bramham, Rolls, Morris, Bullock & Polkey 2004, Fellows & Farah 2003, Fellows 2011).

Now it is well established that not receiving expected reward, or receiving unpleasant stimuli or events, can produce depression (Beck 2008, Drevets 2007, Harmer & Cowen 2013, Price & Drevets 2012, Pryce, Azzinnari, Spinelli, Seifritz, Tegethoff & Meinlschmidt 2011, Eshel & Roiser 2010). A clear example is that if a member of the family dies, then this is the removal of reward (in that we would work to try to avoid this), and the result of the removal of the reward can be depression. More formally, in terms of learning theory, the omission or termination of a reward can give rise to sadness or depression, depending on the magnitude of the reward that is lost, if there is no action that can be taken to restore the reward (the 'passive' condition for non-reward in Fig. 9.1) (Rolls 2014b). If an action can be taken, then frustration and anger may arise to the same reinforcement contingency (Rolls 2014b). This relates the current approach to the learned helplessness approach to depression, in which depression may arise because no actions can be taken to restore rewards (Forgeard, Haigh, Beck, Davidson, Henn, Maier, Mayberg & Seligman 2011, Pryce et al. 2011). A useful therapy for depression may be to help humans to re-appreciate how their actions can lead to rewards, in order to break the cycle of no longer trying to obtain rewards.

9.2 A non-reward attractor theory of depression

The finding that neurons in the lateral orbitofrontal cortex can respond for many seconds following non-reward provides evidence that they have entered an attractor state that maintains a memory of the non-reward (Thorpe, Rolls & Maddison 1983, Rolls 2014b) (Section 4.5.3.5). An example of such a neuron is shown in Fig. 4.16. Attractor networks are described in Chapter 8.

The theory has been proposed that in depression, this lateral orbitofrontal cortex non-reward / punishment attractor network system is more easily triggered, and maintains its attractor-related firing for longer (Rolls 2016d, Rolls 2017b, Rolls 2017d). The greater attractor-related firing of the non-reward / punishment system triggers negative cognitive states held on-line in other cortical systems such as the language system and in the dorsolateral prefrontal cortex which is implicated in attentional control. These other cortical systems then in turn have top-down effects on the orbitofrontal non-reward system that bias it in a negative direction (Rolls 2013a) (see Section 4.5.3.7 and Fig. 4.23), and thus increase the sensitivity of the lateral orbitofrontal cortex to non-reward and maintain its overactivity (Rolls 2016d) (Fig. 9.3). It is proposed that the interaction of non-reward and language / attentional brain systems of these types accounts for the ruminating and continuing depressive thoughts, which occur as a result of a positive feedback cycle between these types of brain system (Rolls 2016d).

Indeed, we have shown that cognitive states can have 'top-down' effects on affective representations in the orbitofrontal cortex (De Araujo, Rolls, Velazco, Margot & Cayeux 2005, Grabenhorst, Rolls & Bilderbeck 2008a, McCabe, Rolls, Bilderbeck & McGlone 2008, Rolls 2013a). Further, top-down selective attention can also influence affective representations in the orbitofrontal cortex (Rolls et al. 2008a, Grabenhorst & Rolls 2008, Ge et al. 2012, Luo et al. 2013, Rolls 2013a), and paying attention to depressive symptoms when depressed may in this way exacerbate the problems in a positive feedback way.

More generally, the presence of the cognitive ability to think ahead and see the implications of recent events that is afforded by language may be a computational development in the brain that exacerbates the vulnerability of the human brain to depression (Rolls 2014b). For example, with language we can think ahead and see that perhaps the loss of an individual in one's life may be long-term, and this thought and its consequences for our future can become fully evident.

The theory is that one way in which depression could result from over-activity in this lateral orbitofrontal cortex system is if there is a major negatively reinforcing life event that produces reactive depression and activates this system, which then becomes self-re-exciting based on the cycle between the lateral orbitofrontal cortex non-reward / punishment attractor system and the cognitive / language system, which together operate as a systems-level attractor (Fig. 9.3). (The generic cortical architecture for such reciprocal feedforward and feedback excitatory effects is illustrated by Rolls (2016c).

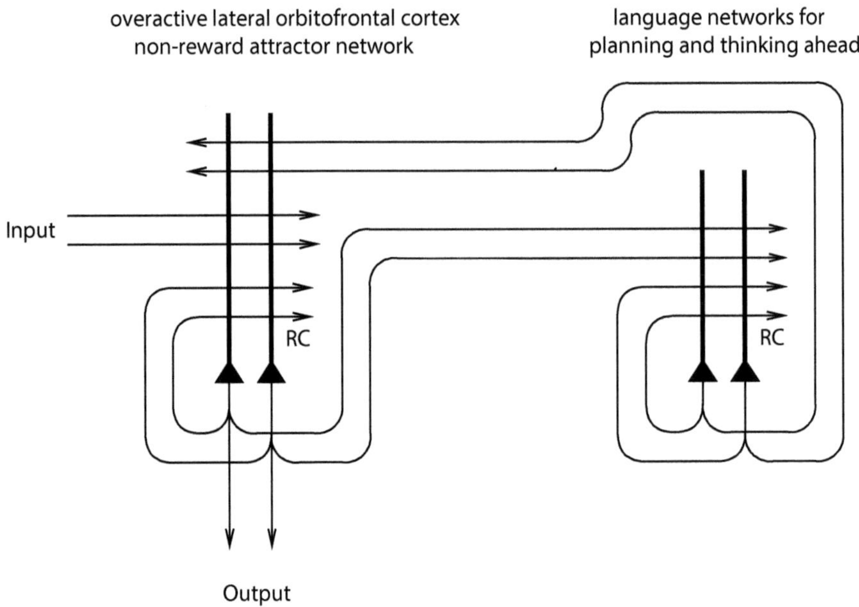

Fig. 9.3 Interaction of orbitofrontal cortex non-reward networks with language networks in depression. Illustration of how an overactive non-reward attractor network in the lateral orbitofrontal cortex could send excitatory information forward to networks for language and planning ahead; which could in turn send excitatory 'top-down' feedback back down to the orbitofrontal non-reward network to maintain its over-activity. It is suggested that such a system with mutual 'long loop' re-excitation contributes to the persistent ruminating thoughts in depression. (After Rolls 2016d.)

The theory is that a second way in which depression might arise is if this lateral orbitofrontal cortex non-reward / punishment system is especially sensitive in some individuals. This might be related for example to genetic predisposition, or to the effects of stress (Gold 2015). In this case, the orbitofrontal system would over-react to normal levels of non-reward or punishment, and start the local attractor circuit in the lateral orbitofrontal cortex (Section 4.5.3.5) (Rolls 2016d, Rolls & Deco 2016), which in turn would activate the cognitive system, which would feed back to the over-reactive lateral orbitofrontal cortex system to maintain now a systems-level attractor with ruminating thoughts. This is described as a 'systems-level' attractor because it includes mutual excitations between different brain areas.

9.3 Evidence consistent with the non-reward attractor theory of depression

There is some evidence for altered structure and function of the lateral orbitofrontal cortex in depression (Drevets 2007, Ma 2015, Price & Drevets 2012). For example, reductions of grey-matter volume and cortex thickness have been demonstrated specifically in the posterolateral OFC (BA 47, caudal BA 11 and the adjoining BA 45), and

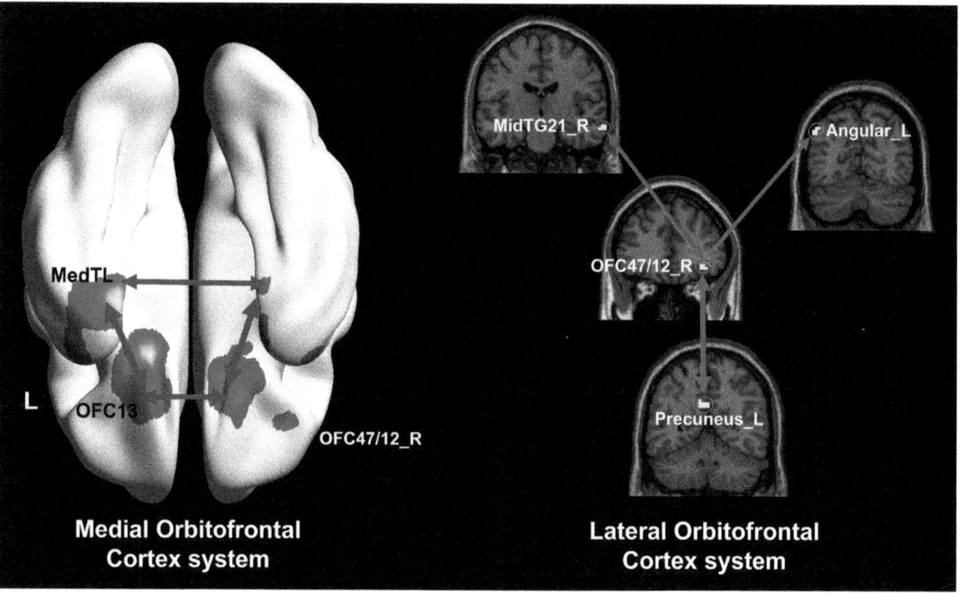

Fig. 9.4 Resting state functional connectivity in depression. The medial and lateral orbitofrontal cortex networks that show different functional connectivity in patients with depression. A decrease in functional connectivity is shown in blue, and an increase in red. MedTL – medial temporal lobe from the parahippocampal gyrus to the temporal pole; MidTG21R – middle temporal gyrus area 21 right; OFC13 – medial orbitofrontal cortex area 13; OFC47/12R – lateral orbitofrontal cortex area 47/12 right. The lateral orbitofrontal cortex cluster in OFC47/12 is visible on the ventral view of the brain anterior and lateral to the OFC13 clusters. (After Cheng, Rolls et al, 2016.)

also in the subgenual cingulate cortex (BA 24, 25) (Drevets 2007, Nugent, Milham, Bain, Mah, Cannon, Marrett, Zarate, Pine, Price & Drevets 2006). In depression, there is increased cerebral blood flow in areas that include the ventrolateral orbitofrontal cortex (which is a prediction of the theory), and also in regions such as the subgenual cingulate cortex and amygdala, and these increases appear to be related to the mood change, in that they become more normal when the mood state remits (Drevets 2007).

In the first brain-wide voxel-level resting state functional connectivity neuroimaging analysis of depression (with 421 patients with major depressive disorder and 488 controls), we have found that one major circuit with altered functional connectivity involved the medial orbitofrontal cortex BA 13, which had reduced functional connectivity in depression with memory systems in the parahippocampal gyrus and medial temporal lobe (Cheng, Rolls, Qiu, Liu, Tang, Huang, Wang, Zhang, Lin, Zheng, Pu, Tsai, Yang, Lin, Wang, Xie & Feng 2016) (Fig. 9.4). (Reduced functional connectivity is measured by a reduced correlation between the activity of two brain areas, and implies that they are communicating less effectively.) The lateral orbitofrontal cortex BA 47/12, involved in non-reward and punishing events, did not have this reduced functional connectivity with memory systems, so that there is an imbalance in depression towards decreased reward-related memory system functionality.

A second major circuit change was that the lateral orbitofrontal cortex area BA 47/12 had increased functional connectivity with the precuneus, the angular gyrus, and the temporal visual cortex BA 21 (Cheng et al. 2016) (Fig. 9.4). This enhanced functional connectivity of the non-reward/punishment system (BA 47/12) with the precuneus (involved in the sense of self and agency), and the angular gyrus (involved in language) is thus related to the explicit affectively negative sense of the self, and of self-esteem, in depression. Further investigations have provided more evidence for increased functional connectivity of the lateral orbitofrontal cortex with the precuneus (Cheng, Rolls, Qiu, Yang, Ruan, Wei, Zhao, Meng, Xie & Feng 2018c), posterior cingulate cortex (providing a route into memory) (Cheng et al. 2018b), and the anterior cingulate cortex (Rolls et al. 2018b), and in a completely different patient population these functional connectivities involving the lateral orbitofrontal cortex were correlated with the Depressive Problems score (Cheng, Rolls, Ruan & Feng 2018d), as described below.

The reduced functional connectivity of the medial orbitofrontal cortex, implicated in reward, with memory systems provides a new way of understanding how memory systems may be biased away from pleasant events in depression. The increased functional connectivity of the lateral orbitofrontal cortex, implicated in non-reward and punishment, with areas of the brain implicated in representing the self, language, and inputs from face and related perceptual systems provides a new way of understanding how unpleasant events and thoughts, and lowered self-esteem, may be exacerbated in depression (Cheng et al. 2016, Rolls, Cheng, Gilson, Qiu, Hu, Li, Huang, Yang, Tsai, Zhang, Zhuang, Lin, Deco, Xie & Feng 2018a).

Because the lateral orbitofrontal cortex responds to many punishing and non-rewarding stimuli (Grabenhorst & Rolls 2011, Rolls 2014b, Rolls 2014c) that are likely to elicit autonomic/visceral responses, as does the supracallosal anterior cingulate cortex, and in view of connections from these areas to the anterior insula which is implicated in autonomic/visceral function (Critchley & Harrison 2013, Rolls 2016b), the anterior insula would also be expected to be overactive in depression, which it is (Drevets 2007, Hamilton et al. 2013, Ma 2015).

Treatments that can reduce depression such as a single dose of ketamine (Zanos & Gould 2018) (see further Section 9.7.2) may act in part by quashing the attractor state in the lateral orbitofrontal cortex at least temporarily. Evidence consistent with this is that the activity of the lateral orbitofrontal cortex is decreased by a single dose of ketamine (Lally, Nugent, Luckenbaugh, Niciu, Roiser & Zarate 2015). This NMDA receptor blocker may act at least in part by decreasing the high firing rate state of attractor networks by reducing transmission in the recurrent collateral excitatory connections between the neurons (Rolls 2016c, Rolls et al. 2008d, Rolls & Deco 2010, Rolls 2012b, Deco et al. 2013, Rolls & Deco 2015a). Given that a ketamine metabolite, hydroxynorketamine, may be related to the antidepressant effects of ketamine and may act via facilitating effects mediated by AMPA receptors (Zanos & Gould 2018), the effects of ketamine might be mediated by increasing the medial orbitofrontal cortex reward-related system (which tends to be reciprocally related to the lateral orbitofrontal non-reward system), or the functional connectivity of the medial orbitofrontal cortex reward system with the hippocampal system which is reduced in depression (Fig. 9.4). Electroconvulsive therapy may have antidepressant effects, may also knock the non-reward system out of its attractor state, and this may contribute to any antidepressant effect.

Electrical stimulation of the brain that may relieve depression (Hamani, Mayberg, Snyder, Giacobbe, Kennedy & Lozano 2009, Hamani, Mayberg, Stone, Laxton, Haber & Lozano 2011, Lujan, Chaturvedi, Choi, Holtzheimer, Gross, Mayberg & McIntyre

2013) may act in part by providing reward that reciprocally inhibits the non-reward system, and/or by interfering with the attractor state. Treatment with antidepressant drugs decreases the activity of this non-reward lateral orbitofrontal cortex system (Ma 2015).

Antidepressant drugs such as Selective Serotonin Reuptake Inhibitors (SSRIs) may treat depression by producing positive biases in the processing of emotional stimuli (Harmer & Cowen 2013), increasing brain responses to positive stimuli and decreasing responses to negative stimuli (Ma 2015). The reward and non-reward systems are likely to operate reciprocally, so that facilitating the reward system, or providing rewards, and thus activating the medial orbitofrontal cortex (O'Doherty, Kringelbach, Rolls, Hornak & Andrews 2001a, Grabenhorst & Rolls 2011, Rolls 2014b) (Fig. 4.14), may operate in part by inhibiting the over-activity in the lateral orbitofrontal cortex non-reward / punishment system (Rolls et al. 2018a).

Further, in research stimulated by the theory and results described here (Rolls 2016d, Cheng et al. 2016), preliminary studies have found that transcranial magnetic stimulation of the lateral orbitofrontal cortex, which may disrupt its activity, may help in the treatment of depression (Feffer, Fettes, Giacobbe, Daskalakis, Blumberger & Downar 2018).

9.4 Advances in understanding the functions of the orbitofrontal cortex and other brain systems in depression

9.4.1 Overview

We have seen evidence that implicates the orbitofrontal cortex in depression in Sections 9.2 and 9.3.

1. Sadness and depression can be caused by not receiving expected rewards, or by receiving punishers.
2. The lateral orbitofrontal cortex is implicated in detecting these reinforcement contingencies and thus in negative emotions, which are produced by these reward contingencies.
3. It has been proposed that this lateral orbitofrontal is overactive in depression, and continues its activity for long periods because of attractor networks implemented within the lateral orbitofrontal cortex, and by long-loop attractor networks between the lateral orbitofrontal cortex and reciprocally connected brain areas.
4. This theory of depression has been supported by functional neuroimaging studies that show increased functional connectivity of the lateral orbitofrontal cortex with other brain areas including the angular gyrus which is involved in language, which may contribute to continuing negative ruminating thoughts; and the precuneus which is involved in the sense of the self, and which may contribute to the low self-esteem that can occur in depression.
5. The medial orbitofrontal cortex is involved in reward processing, pleasure, and happiness, and has decreased connectivity with hippocampal memory systems in depression, which may contribute to the fewer happy memories present in depression.

6. These investigations have been supported by another investigation with participants from the general population in the USA, which showed that similar changes in functional connectivity were found in people who tended to have symptoms of depression (Cheng et al. 2018d).
7. These ideas have been supported by preliminary studies showing that transcranial magnetic stimulation of the lateral orbitofrontal cortex may help in the treatment of depression (Feffer et al. 2018).
8. Thus the investigations described have implications not only for understanding depression better, but also for the treatment of depression.

In this section (9.4), recent advances in understanding the connectivity of brain systems related to depression are described, and many involve links to the orbitofrontal cortex. One of the measures used, functional connectivity, is measured by the correlation of the activity between two brain regions. If the correlation is high, then this implies that if the signal in one brain area increases, this is associated with an increase in the connected brain region. The implication of increased functional connectivity then is that two connected brain areas are 'talking to each other' strongly, and vice versa for decreased functional connectivity. An overview of some of the findings described in this section (9.4) follows.

In sections 9.4.2 and 9.4.8 the evidence on the **orbitofrontal cortex** is extended by showing in a new population of individuals, from the USA, who have not been selected to have depression, that in this general population any tendency to have depressive symptoms is associated with similar changes in functional connectivity of the lateral orbitofrontal cortex found in patients (who were from China) diagnosed with depression. This is important validation of the theory that the orbitofrontal cortex is a key region with altered connectivity related to depression, and is consistent with the theory of depression proposed in Section 9.2.

Another fascinating and new finding on a different group of people is that happiness and subjective well-being are correlated with decreased functional connectivity of the lateral orbitofrontal cortex (Liu, Ma, Rolls, Wei, Zhang, Chen, Meng, Qiu & Feng 2018). This is consistent with the hypothesis that increased non-rewarding processing (which is likely to be related to increased functional connectivity), including that related to sadness and depression, involves *increased* functional connectivity of the lateral orbitofrontal, for happiness is correlated with *decreased* lateral orbitofrontal cortex functional connectivity (Liu et al. 2018). Possible explanations are that people with high well-being are less affected by non-rewarding events; and/or that considerable exposure to non-rewarding events may lead to increased in lateral orbitofrontal cortex connectivity.

In section 9.4.3, the connections from the orbitofrontal cortex to one of the areas to which it projects, the **anterior cingulate cortex**, are considered. It is shown that the medial orbitofrontal, which is involved in processing reward value and pleasure, has high connectivity with the most anterior part of the anterior cingulate cortex (pregenual), which is also activated by rewards. The anterior cingulate cortex is implicated in learning which actions to take to obtain rewards, and the connectivity just described appears to be a way for rewards to reach the anterior cingulate cortex, so that rewards received can influence this type of action to (reward) outcome learning. Correspondingly, it is shown that the lateral orbitofrontal, which is involved in processing non-reward value and unpleasant stimuli, has high connectivity with the supracallosal part of the anterior cingulate cortex (just above the anterior part of the corpus callosum), which is also activated by non-reward and unpleasant stimuli. This provides a route for the costs of actions to be taken into account in learning which actions to take to maximise rewards and minimise the costs of the actions (see further Section 4.7).

It is also shown in Section 9.4.3 that in depression the anterior cingulate cortex has reduced connectivity with the orbitofrontal cortex, and also with temporal lobe areas involved in perception, the parahippocampal gyrus and hippocampus involved in memory, and motor areas. The concept is described that the anterior cingulate cortex, with its representations of rewards and punishers received from the orbitofrontal cortex and which is involved in interfacing these to action systems, appears to contribute to depression by disconnecting rewards and punishers from their action-related and other outputs. This would result is insensitivity to the effects of rewards and punishers, amotivational states, and feelings of helplessness (Rolls et al. 2018b).

Evidence is also described in Section 9.4.3 that a subcallosal part of the anterior cingulate cortex can be activated by negative stimuli, has increased activity in depression, and has been a target for deep brain stimulation to relieve depression (which might act by disrupting activity here), though this has not yet been validated in large-scale studies.

In Section 9.4.4 it is shown that the **posterior cingulate cortex** has significantly increased functional connectivity with the lateral orbitofrontal cortex in depression. The posterior cingulate cortex provides a gateway into the hippocampal memory system for spatial information including information about the self. These findings support the theory that the non-reward system in the lateral orbitofrontal cortex has increased effects on memory systems, which contribute to the rumination about sad memories and events in depression (Cheng et al. 2018b).

In Section 9.4.5, it is shown that in depression the **amygdala**, a brain region implicated in emotion, has reduced functional connectivity with the brain regions with which it is connected, including the orbitofrontal cortex. A possible implication is that because the amygdala is somewhat disconnected in depression, it may be important to focus on other brain regions such as the lateral orbitofrontal cortex that have increased functional connectivity in depression, and may be more closely related to the strong emotional feelings of sadness in depression.

In Section 9.4.6 further evidence is provided that the **precuneus**, a medial parietal cortex region implicated in the sense of self and agency, has increased functional connectivity in depression with the lateral orbitofrontal cortex, a region implicated in non-reward and which is thereby implicated in depression. These findings support the theory that the non-reward system in the lateral orbitofrontal cortex has increased effects on areas in which the self is represented including the precuneus, resulting in the low self-esteem that may be present in depression (Rolls 2016d).

In Section 9.4.7 research is described that goes beyond functional connectivity to **effective connectivity** between different brain areas to measure directed influences of human brain regions on each other (Rolls et al. 2018a). Effective connectivity is conceptually very different, for it measures the effect of one brain region on another in a particular direction, and can in principle therefore provide information more closely related to the causal processes that operate in brain function, that is, how one brain region influences another. In the context of disorders of brain function, the effective connectivity may provide evidence on which brain regions may have altered function, and then influence other brain regions, by comparing effective connectivity in patients and control participants.

The results obtained with the use of effective connectivity are consistent with the hypotheses that some aspects of hippocampal processing, perhaps those related to unpleasant memories, are increased in depression (Rolls 2016d, Cheng et al. 2016); that the temporal cortex has increased effective connectivity to the precuneus which with its connectivity with memory systems and the lateral orbitofrontal cortex may contribute to low self-esteem and negative memories; that the influence of temporal lobe memory systems on specifically the medial orbitofrontal cortex is reduced in depression; and that this in turn may contribute to increased activity in the lateral orbitofrontal cortex non-reward system in depression (Rolls et al. 2018a).

All this new research supports the ideas presented in this Chapter that the orbitofrontal cortex is a key region for understanding how processing is different in depression. Increased connectivity of the lateral orbitofrontal cortex non-reward system in depression may contribute to the increased sadness in depression. The decreased functional connectivity of the medial orbitofrontal cortex reward system may contribute to the reduced happiness in depression. This makes further understanding of these brain areas important for understanding depression better, and potentially for treating depression better.

9.4.2 Orbitofrontal cortex

The human *medial orbitofrontal cortex* has activations related to many rewarding and subjectively pleasant stimuli (Rolls & Grabenhorst 2008, Grabenhorst & Rolls 2011, Rolls 2014b) (Fig. 4.14). In the sense that reward vs non-reward and punishment are reciprocally related in their effects in the medial vs lateral orbitofrontal cortex respectively (O'Doherty, Kringelbach, Rolls, Hornak & Andrews 2001a, Rolls 2014b), the anhedonia of depression can also be related to decreased effects of pleasant rewarding stimuli in the medial orbitofrontal cortex during depression, effects that can be restored by antidepressants (Ma 2015).

The *lateral orbitofrontal cortex / inferior frontal gyrus region* that responds to signals to inhibit a response in the stop-signal task (Deng, Rolls, Ji, Robbins, Banaschewski, Bokde, Bromberg, Buechel, Desrivieres, Conrod, Flor, Frouin, Gallinat, Garavan, Gowland, Heinz, Ittermann, Martinot, Lemaitre, Nees, Papadopoulos Orfanos, Poustka, Smolka, Walter, Whelan, Schumann, Feng & the Imagen consortium 2017) is implicated in impulsive behavior, with damage in this region increasing impulsive behavior (Aron, Robbins & Poldrack 2014). This is of potential importance, for treatment with antidepressants, which would be expected to reduce the over-activity in this ventrolateral prefrontal cortex region, might thereby increase impulsiveness relative to that in the depressed state. Indeed, it is an interesting hypothesis that impulsiveness might reflect under-activity in this ventrolateral prefrontal cortex region, and that depression produced by oversensitivity to non-reward and punishment might reflect over-activity in this lateral orbitofrontal cortex / ventrolateral prefrontal cortex region. In a certain sense, these types of behaviour might reflect opposite ends of a continuum of non-reward/punishment sensitivity. One end of the spectrum of sensitivity to non-reward could be impulsive behaviour (with too little sensitivity to non-reward and punishment); and the other end could be depression (with too much sensitivity to non-reward and punishment). The ventrolateral prefrontal cortex region refers here to a part of the lateral orbitofrontal cortex region BA12/47, and its continuation round the inferior prefrontal convexity to include parts of the inferior frontal gyrus, as found for the stop-signal task (Deng et al. 2017).

It is an interesting thought that these orbitofrontal cortex systems have evolved to have a distribution of efficacy that may serve to produce variation, so important in evolution by natural selection in different environments, in the tendency to initiate behaviour or not. Under-

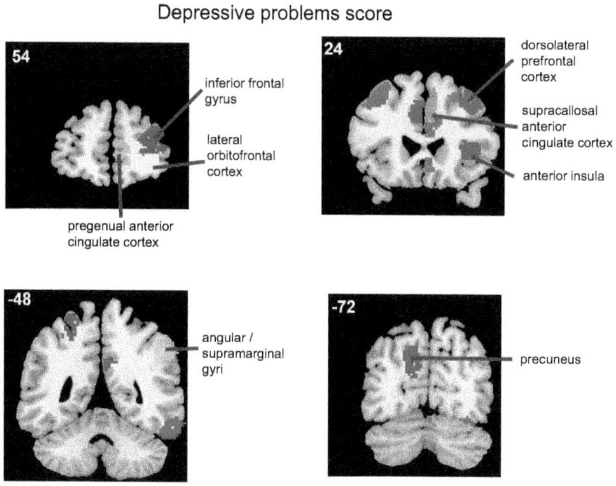

Fig. 9.5 Brain areas with functional connectivities related to the Adult Self-Report Depressive Problems scores from the analysis of Human Connectome Project data in individuals from the normal population. The significance value for the links to be included is $p < 0.005$. The color (red through orange to yellow) reflects the number of correlated links in each of the 250 areas in the atlas by Shen et al (2013). Most of the functional connectivity links are positively correlated with the depression score. The anterior insula region is continuous with and just posterior to the lateral orbitofrontal cortex, and this anteroventral part of the insula is implicated in autonomic function. The number on each slice is the MNY Y coordinate. The right side of the brain is on the right of each image. (Modified from Cheng, Rolls et al, 2018d.)

responsiveness of the lateral orbitofrontal cortex system might lead to individuals with risky, impulsive, behaviour. Over-responsiveness of the lateral orbitofrontal cortex may lead to behaviour very sensitive to non-reward, so that nothing risky is attempted, with at the end of the spectrum depressive behaviour being the outcome. The variation between individuals may reflect the fact that different behavioural strategies can have advantages; and that the genes may maintain this variation, as having variation may be useful for different environments.

Some of the recent findings on the brain functional connectivity differences related to depression have come from patients with depression from large datasets from China and Taiwan. A recent study with a completely different population of people has extended these results, by using participants drawn from the general population in the USA as part of the Human Connectome Project. In this investigation, participants were not selected on the basis of whether they were depressed, but part of the data collected in addition to the resting state fMRI scans consisted of the Adult Self-Report Depressive Problems score, a questionnaire which measures to what extent people may have depressive symptoms. In this general population, we found in a sample of 1017 participants (ages 22–35 years) that the Adult Self-Report Depressive Problems score was positively correlated with functional connectivity involving areas such as the lateral orbitofrontal cortex and the adjacent inferior frontal gyrus, the dorsolateral prefrontal cortex (involved in working memory and attention), the anterior cingulate cortex, the angular gyrus, and the precuneus (implicated in the sense of self) (Fig. 9.5) (Cheng et al. 2018d).

Part of the importance of this investigation (Cheng et al. 2018d) is that it provides strong support for a role of the lateral orbitofrontal cortex in depression. The findings were not on patients selected to have depression, but instead were on a general population in the USA in which a tendency to have depressive symptoms could be assessed, and indeed the correlations arose especially from the presence of 92 people who at some time had been diagnosed with depression. Yet very similar brain regions were identified in this investigation as having increased functional connectivity related to depressive symptoms, as in patients from China with a diagnosis of major depressive disorder. This important cross-validation provides support for the theory that the lateral orbitofrontal cortex is a key brain area that might be targeted in the search for treatments for depression (Rolls 2016d).

It is of interest that in the analysis of correlations of functional connectivities with depressive scores, the hippocampus / parahippocampal gyrus is not prominent in Fig. 9.5; that the angular gyrus is prominent; and that the medial orbitofrontal cortex is not prominent. Part of the importance of these new findings (Cheng et al. 2018d) is that they confirm in a completely different dataset the increased functional connectivity not only of the lateral orbitofrontal cortex, but also of the precuneus and angular gyrus found in patients with major depressive disorder (Cheng et al. 2016).

9.4.3 Anterior cingulate cortex

The supracallosal *anterior cingulate cortex* is activated by many aversive stimuli, and the pregenual cingulate cortex by many pleasant stimuli (Fig. 4.14) (Grabenhorst & Rolls 2011, Rolls 2014b). However, the anterior cingulate cortex appears to be involved in action-outcome learning, where the outcome refers to the reward or punisher for which an action is being learned (Rudebeck et al. 2008, Camille et al. 2011, Grabenhorst & Rolls 2011, Rushworth et al. 2011, Rushworth et al. 2012, Rolls 2014b) (Section 4.7). In contrast, the medial orbitofrontal cortex is implicated in reward-related processing and learning, and the lateral orbitofrontal cortex in non-reward and punishment-related processing and learning (Rolls 2014b). These involve stimulus-stimulus associations, where the second stimulus is a reward (or its omission), or a punisher (Rolls 2014b) (Chapter 2). Now given that emotions can be considered as states elicited by rewarding and punishing stimuli, and that moods such as depression can arise from prolonged non-reward or punishment (Rolls 2014b), the part of the brain that processes these stimulus-stimulus associations, the orbitofrontal cortex, is more likely to be involved in depression than the action-related parts of the cingulate cortex.

The *subgenual (or subcallosal) cingulate cortex* has also been implicated in depression, and electrical stimulation in that region may relieve depression (Mayberg 2003, Hamani et al. 2009, Hamani et al. 2011, Lozano, Giacobbe, Hamani, Rizvi, Kennedy, Kolivakis, Debonnel, Sadikot, Lam, Howard, Ilcewicz-Klimek, Honey & Mayberg 2012, Laxton, Neimat, Davis, Womelsdorf, Hutchison, Dostrovsky, Hamani, Mayberg & Lozano 2013, Lujan et al. 2013) (although it has not been possible to confirm this in a double-blind study (Holtzheimer, Husain, Lisanby, Taylor, Whitworth, McClintock, Slavin, Berman, McKhann, Patil, Rittberg, Abosch, Pandurangi, Holloway, Lam, Honey, Neimat, Henderson, DeBattista, Rothschild, Pilitsis, Espinoza, Petrides, Mogilner, Matthews, Peichel, Gross, Hamani, Lozano & Mayberg 2017)). However, the subgenual cingulate cortex is also implicated in autonomic function (Gabbott et al. 2003), and this could be related to some of the effects found in this area that are related to depression. Whether the subgenual cingulate cortex is activated because of inputs from the orbitofrontal cortex, or performs separate computations is not yet clear. Indeed, the orbitofrontal cortex has the inputs and representations required to compute non-reward, namely representations of expected value, and reward and punishment outcome value (Rolls 2014b) (Section 4.5.3.5), and it is not clear that the subgenual cingulate cortex has the information to perform that computation. Further, the possibility is considered that electrical stimulation of the subcallosal region, which includes parts of the ventromedial prefrontal cortex (Laxton et al. 2013), that may relieve depression, may do so at least in part by activating connections involving the orbitofrontal cortex, other parts of the anterior cingulate cortex, and the striatum (Johansen-Berg, Gutman, Behrens, Matthews, Rushworth, Katz, Lozano & Mayberg 2008, Hamani et al. 2009, Lujan et al. 2013).

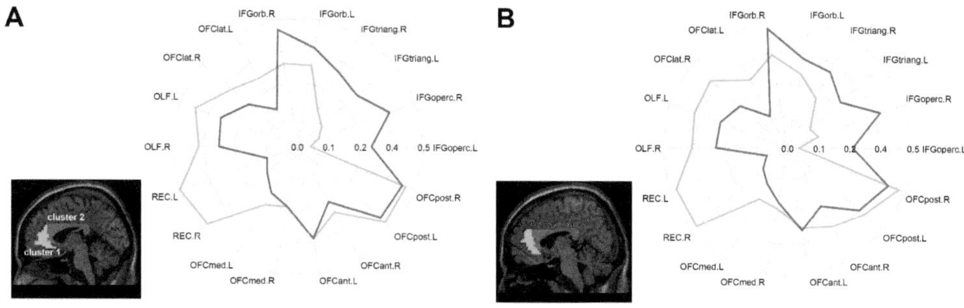

Fig. 9.6 Voxel-level parcellation of the Anterior Cingulate Cortex (ACC) based on its functional connectivity in healthy controls with other brain areas. Cluster 1 (green) is pregenual and subcallosal. Cluster 2 (red) is supracallosal. The circular plot shows the correlations of the voxels in each subdivision of the ACC with the significantly different voxels in orbitofrontal cortex automated anatomical atlas (AAL2, Rolls et al 2015)) areas. The correlations are indicated as the distance from the centre of the circular plot, with the r value for the correlation as shown. The pregenual and subcallosal subdivision (1, green) has strong functional connectivity with the medial orbitofrontal cortex and connected areas (AAL2 areas from OLF to OFCpost). The supracallosal subdivision (2, red) has strong functional connectivity with the lateral orbitofrontal cortex area IFGorb and with adjacent inferior frontal gyrus areas (IFGtriang to IFGoperc). A is left and B is right. (After Rolls, Cheng et al, 2018b.)

In a recent study, the first fully voxel-level resting state functional-connectivity neuroimaging analysis of depression of the anterior cingulate cortex, with 336 patients with major depressive disorder and 350 controls, was performed (Rolls et al. 2018b). Voxels in the anterior cingulate cortex had significantly reduced functional connectivity with the orbitofrontal cortex, temporal lobe areas, the parahippocampal gyrus and hippocampus, and motor areas. The strengths of some of these functional connectivities were correlated with the Beck Depression Inventory and duration of illness measures of the depression, showing that these differences of functional connectivity were related to the depression.

Parcellation was performed based on the functional connectivity of individual anterior cingulate cortex voxels in the controls (Fig. 9.6). A pregenual and subcallosal subdivision (1, green) has strong functional connectivity with the medial orbitofrontal cortex and connected areas (Fig. 9.6), which are implicated in reward (Fig. 4.14). The supracallosal subdivision (2, red), which is activated by unpleasant stimuli and non-reward, has strong functional connectivity with the lateral orbitofrontal cortex and adjacent inferior frontal gyrus areas (Fig. 9.6), also activated by unpleasant stimuli (Fig. 4.14) (Rolls et al. 2018b). These functional connectivities provide support for the hypothesis that the reward-related medial orbitofrontal cortex provides inputs to the pregenual cingulate cortex, also activated by rewards; and that the lateral orbitofrontal cortex, implicated in effects of non-reward and punishers, provides inputs to the supracallosal part of the anterior cingulate cortex, also activated by unpleasant stimuli (Rolls et al. 2018b).

In depression, overall the anterior cingulate cortex had significantly reduced functional connectivity with the orbitofrontal cortex, temporal lobe areas, the parahippocampal gyrus and hippocampus, and motor areas. The anterior cingulate cortex, with its representations of rewards and punishers received from the orbitofrontal cortex and which is involved in interfacing these to action systems, appears to contribute to depression by disconnecting rewards and punishers from their action-related and other outputs. This would result is insensitivity to the effects of rewards and punishers, amotivational states, and feelings of helplessness (Rolls et al. 2018b).

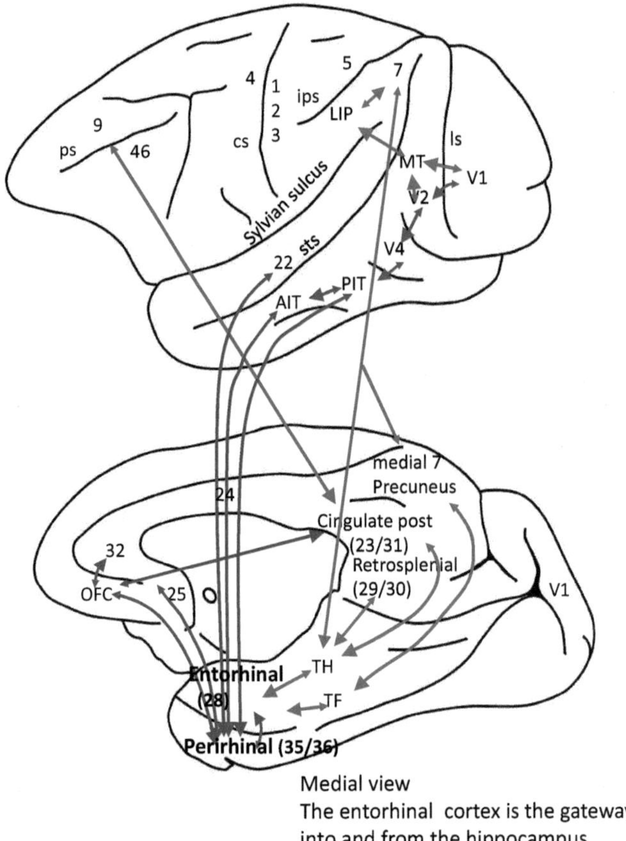

Fig. 9.7 Connections of the primate hippocampus with the neocortex. A medial view of the macaque brain is shown below, and a lateral view is shown above. The hippocampus receives its inputs via the parahippocampal gyrus (areas TF and TH), and the perirhinal cortex (areas 35 and 36), both of which in turn project to the entorhinal cortex (area 28), send inputs to the hippocampus and receive backprojections from the hippocampus as shown in Fig. 2. The forward inputs towards the entorhinal cortex and hippocampus are shown with large arrowheads, and the weaker return backprojections with small arrowheads. The hippocampus receives via the perirhinal cortex areas 35 and 36 which project to the lateral entorhinal cortex areas 28 from the ends of the hierarchically organised ventral visual system pathways (V1, V2, V4, PIT, AIT) that represent 'what' object is present (including also faces, and even scenes), from the anterior inferior temporal visual cortex (AIT, BA21, TE) where objects and faces are represented which receives from the posterior inferior temporal cortex (PIT, BA20, TEO); from the reward system in the orbitofrontal cortex (OFC) and amygdala, and from an area to which the OFC projects, the anterior cingulate cortex BA32 and subgenual cingulate cortex (BA25); from the high order auditory cortex (BA22); and from olfactory, taste, and somatosensory 'what' areas (not shown). These ventral 'what' pathways are shown in blue. The hippocampus also receives via the parahippocampal cortex areas TF and TH inputs (shown in red) from the dorsal visual 'where' or 'action' pathways, which reach parietal cortex area 7 via the dorsal visual stream hierarchy, including V1, V2, MT, MST, LIP, and VIP, and from areas to which they are connected, including the dorsolateral prefrontal cortex BA46 and the posterior cingulate (Cingulate post) and retrosplenial cortex. The hippocampus provides a system for all the high-order cortical regions to converge into a single network in the hippocampal CA3 region (Rolls, 2017e). Other abbreviations: as - arcuate sulcus; cs - central sulcus; ips - intraparietal sulcus; ios - inferior occipital sulcus; ls - lunate sulcus; sts - superior temporal sulcus. (After Rolls and Wirth 2018.)

However, in addition in depression, increased functional connectivity was found between the lateral orbitofrontal cortex and the pregenual and subcallosal parts of the anterior cingulate cortex (Rolls et al. 2018b). This is consistent with the hypothesis that more non-reward information is being transmitted from the orbitofrontal cortex to the anterior cingulate cortex, and that this contributes to the depression (Rolls et al. 2018b).

9.4.4 Posterior cingulate cortex

The posterior cingulate cortex is a region with strong connectivity in primates with the entorhinal cortex and parahippocampal gyrus (areas TF and TH), and thus with the hippocampal memory system (Bubb, Kinnavane & Aggleton 2017, Vogt 2009, Rolls 2018, Rolls & Wirth 2018) (Fig. 9.7). The posterior cingulate cortex is an interesting region of convergence between ventral stream processing involved in the identification of objects, people, face expression, etc using visual, auditory, and tactile multimodal processing, and the dorsal stream processing involved in spatial processing and action in space, providing access for both processing streams to the hippocampal memory system (Vogt 2009, Vogt & Pandya 1987, Vogt & Laureys 2009, Rolls 2018, Rolls & Wirth 2018). The posterior cingulate cortex also has connections with the orbitofrontal cortex (Vogt & Pandya 1987, Vogt & Laureys 2009). The posterior cingulate region (including the retrosplenial cortex) is consistently engaged by a range of tasks that examine episodic memory including autobiographical memory, and imagining the future; and also spatial navigation and scene processing (Leech & Sharp 2014, Auger & Maguire 2013). Self-reflection and self-imagery activate the ventral part of the posterior cingulate cortex (vPCC, the part with which we will be mainly concerned here) (Kircher, Brammer, Bullmore, Simmons, Bartels & David 2002, Kircher, Senior, Phillips, Benson, Bullmore, Brammer, Simmons, Williams, Bartels & David 2000, Johnson, Baxter, Wilder, Pipe, Heiserman & Prigatano 2002, Sugiura, Watanabe, Maeda, Matsue, Fukuda & Kawashima 2005).

To analyze the functioning of the posterior cingulate cortex (PCC) in depression, we performed the first fully voxel-level resting-state functional connectivity neuroimaging analysis of depression of the posterior cingulate cortex, with 336 patients with major depressive disorder and 350 controls (Cheng et al. 2018b). In the 350 controls, it was shown that the posterior cingulate cortex has high functional connectivity with the parahippocampal regions that are involved in memory.

In depression, the posterior cingulate cortex had significantly increased functional connectivity with the lateral orbitofrontal cortex, a region implicated in non-reward and which is thereby implicated in depression (Fig. 9.8). In patients receiving medication, the functional connectivity between the lateral orbitofrontal cortex and the posterior cingulate cortex was decreased back towards that in the controls. These findings support the theory that the non-reward system in the lateral orbitofrontal cortex has increased effects on memory systems, which contribute to the rumination about sad memories and events in depression (Cheng et al. 2018b).

The posterior cingulate cortex also had increased connectivity with BA 45 in the inferior frontal gyrus (Fig. 9.8) (Cheng et al. 2018b), a region involved in speech production which is closely related to the laryngeal motor area (Kumar, Croxson & Simonyan 2016). The increased connectivity between the posterior cingulate cortex system involved in the sense of self and in memory, and the inferior frontal gyrus BA45 speech / language system, may also contribute to the ruminating negative thoughts in depression. (Prefrontal and premotor areas can be active when the thoughts are about actions, even if the actions are not actually being made. In contrast, the primary motor cortex, area 4, is active only if the movements are actually being made (Passingham & Wise 2012).)

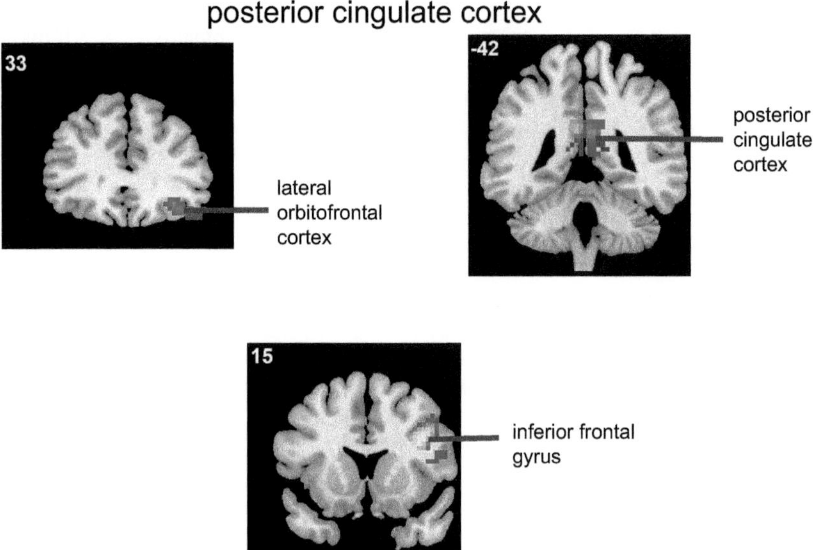

Fig. 9.8 Posterior cingulate cortex. Anatomical location of voxels with significantly different functional connectivity with the posterior cingulate cortex in depression in 125 unmedicated patients vs 254 controls obtained from the voxel-based Association Study (vAS). Red indicates voxels with an increase in functional connectivity in depression, and blue a decrease. Functional connectivity links between pairs of voxels are considered only if they are significantly different with $p < 0.0001$. The right of the brain is on the right of each slice. The Y values are in MNI coordinates. The analysis showed that the main differences in depression for the posterior cingulate cortex are an increase in functional connectivity of the posterior cingulate cortex with the lateral orbitofrontal cortex and a part of the inferior frontal gyrus. (Modified from Cheng, Rolls et al, 2018b.)

9.4.5 Amygdala

In addition to the insula, lateral orbitofrontal cortex, and supracallosal anterior cingulate cortex, which are all activated by unpleasant stimuli (Grabenhorst & Rolls 2011, Rolls 2014b), parts of the *amygdala* are activated by unpleasant stimuli, and parts by pleasant stimuli (Rolls 2014b), and amygdala activation has been related to depression (Harmer & Cowen 2013, Ma 2015, Price & Drevets 2012). However, the amygdala is less involved in non-reward, especially the rule-based reversal of which stimuli are classified as rewarding that is required in a rapid reward reversal task (Rolls 2014b). The orbitofrontal cortex is special in this, because the evidence is that it has attractor states than can be activated by non-reward (Thorpe, Rolls & Maddison 1983, Rolls 2014b), and these attractor states provide a basis for biasing the correct populations of neurons in the orbitofrontal cortex to implement the rapid one-trial reversal (Deco & Rolls 2005a, Rolls 2014b, Rolls & Deco 2016) (Chapter 4). Because the lateral orbitofrontal cortex has recurrent collaterals that can maintain attractor states, it is more likely to be involved in maintaining attractor states elicited by non-reward, including depression, than the amygdala (Rolls 2014b). The amygdala may therefore because of its responsiveness to punishing stimuli be related to depression, but may not be a structure that maintains its activity in an attractor state after non-reward, and during the mood state of depression.

To analyze the functioning of the amygdala in depression, we performed the first voxel-level resting state functional connectivity neuroimaging analysis of depression of voxels in the amygdala with all other voxels in the brain, with 336 patients with major depressive disorder

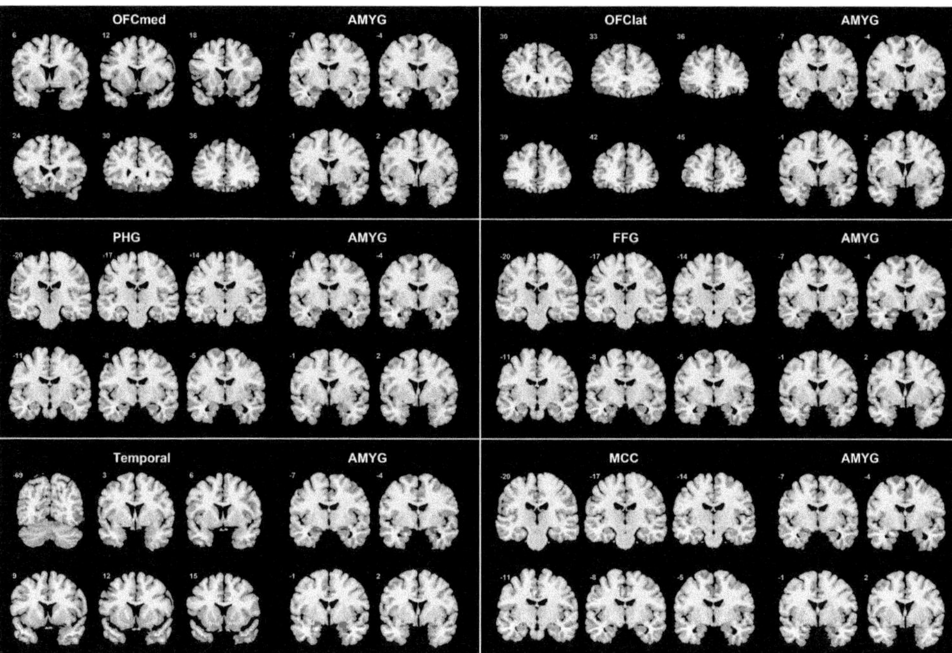

Fig. 9.9 The voxel-level functional connectivity for amygdala voxels that are significantly different in the depressed and the control group, separated by the automated anatomical atlas (AAL2) region in which the significant voxels were located. For each AAL2 area illustrated, the left six slices through that area at the MNI Y level indicated show the locations of the voxels with different functional connectivity with the amygdala. The right four slices at Y=-2, 1, 4, and 7 show the amygdala voxels with different functional connectivity in depressed patients compared to controls for that brain area. Measure of Association (MA) values are shown. Voxels with decreased functional connectivity are shown in blue, and with increased functional connectivity in red/yellow. Voxels are indicated where the functional connectivity with the paired region is $p < 0.05$ (FDR corrected). OFCmed – medial orbitofrontal cortex; OFClat – lateral orbitofrontal cortex; PHG – parahippocampal gyrus; FFG – fusiform gyrus; Temporal – temporal cortical areas; MCC – middle cingulate cortex; FFG – fusiform gyrus. (After Cheng, Rolls et al, 2018a.)

and 350 controls (Cheng, Rolls, Qiu, Xie, Lyu, Li, Huang, Yang, Tsai, Lyu, Zhuang, Lin, Xie & Feng 2018a). Amygdala voxels had decreased functional connectivity with the medial orbitofrontal cortex (involved in reward); the lateral orbitofrontal cortex (involved in non-reward and punishment); temporal lobe areas (involved in visual and auditory perception), including the temporal pole, and inferior temporal gyrus; and the parahippocampal gyrus (involved in memory) (Figs. 9.9 and 9.10). The strengths of the functional connectivity of the amygdala voxels with the medial orbitofrontal cortex and temporal lobe voxels were correlated with the Beck Depression Inventory and duration of illness measures of the depression.

Parcellation analysis in 350 healthy controls based on voxel-level functional connectivity showed that the basal division of the amygdala has high functional connectivity with medial orbitofrontal cortex areas, and the dorsolateral part of the amygdala has especially strong functional connectivity with the lateral orbitofrontal cortex and its related ventral parts of the inferior frontal gyrus. In depression, the basal amygdala division had especially reduced functional connectivity with the medial orbitofrontal cortex which is involved in reward; and the dorsolateral amygdala subdivision had relatively reduced functional connectivity with the lateral orbitofrontal cortex which is involved in non-reward and punishment (Cheng et al. 2018a).

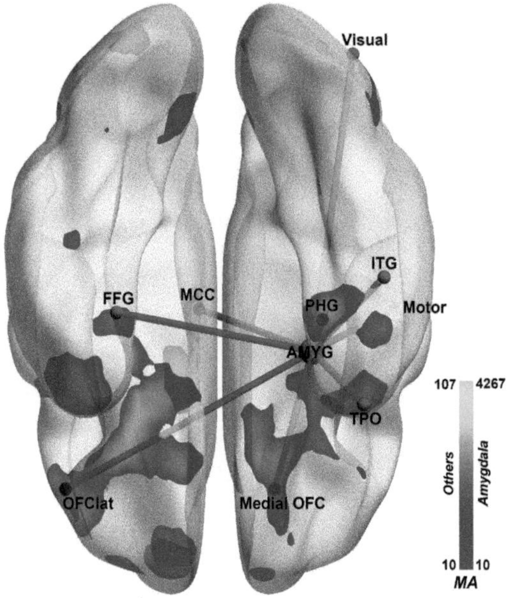

Fig. 9.10 Summary of amygdala functional connectivity differences in depression. The amygdala networks that show different functional connectivity in patients with depression. Ventral view of the brain. A decrease in functional connectivity is shown in blue, and an increase in red, at the voxel level, with the scale shown on the right calibrated using the measure of Association of each voxel (MA, see text). AMYG – amygdala; HIP – hippocampus; ITG – inferior temporal gyrus; MCC – Mid-cingulate cortex; Motor – pre- and post-central gyrus and Rolandic operculum; OFC– orbitofrontal cortex; PHG – parahippocampal area; FFG– fusiform gyrus; TPO– temporal pole; Visual – some occipital areas. Voxels with different functional connectivity from controls are shown by the blue shading, with decreases evident in depression. (After Cheng, Rolls et al, 2018a.)

We can summarize these results (Fig. 9.10) (Cheng et al. 2018a) as follows. First, given that the amygdala has some roles in emotion (Aggleton 2000, Whalen & Phelps 2009, LeDoux 2012, Rolls 2014b), its reduced functional connectivity with the medial orbitofrontal cortex which is involved in reward and positive mood, may contribute to the lowering of mood by being somewhat disconnected from the orbitofrontal cortex in depression.

Second, the functional connectivity reductions of the amygdala with medial temporal lobe areas such as the parahippocampal, perirhinal and entorhinal cortex implicated in memory is similar to that of the medial orbitofrontal cortex, which has greatly reduced functional connectivity with the medial temporal lobe memory system (Cheng et al. 2016), and which with its role in reward may be related to the reduced processing of happy memories, and therefore an imbalance towards unhappy memories, in depression (Cheng et al. 2016, Rolls 2016d).

Third, some voxels in the amygdala had decreased functional connectivity with some temporal cortex areas including the inferior temporal gyrus, temporal pole, and fusiform gyrus, areas known to be involved in visual and multimodal processing (Rolls 2012e, Rolls 2016c). These decreases of these functional connectivities were correlated with the severity of the symptoms and the illness duration, and these functional connectivities were higher in medicated than unmedicated patients. This is thus strong evidence that the reduction of connectivity between temporal cortex areas and the amygdala is important in depression. These temporal cortex areas may introduce inputs relevant to emotion to the amygdala, in that neurons in the primate inferior temporal visual cortex respond to faces (Perrett et al. 1982, Rolls 2011c, Rolls 2012e), and similar neurons are found in the amygdala (Leonard et al. 1985), linking these regions to emotional responses to faces. The hypothesis is that these temporal cortical areas provide important inputs to the amygdala, and that backprojections from the amygdala reach these areas and also earlier cortical including occipital visual areas (Rolls 2014b, Rolls 2016c, Amaral & Price 1984).

Fourth, some amygdala voxels had reduced functional connectivity with the middle cingulate cortex, involved in motor function, in depression (Cheng et al. 2018a). This pathway has been identified in macaques, and it has been suggested is involved in influences of amygdala face processing subsystems on emotional face expressions associated with social communication and emotional constructs such as fear, anger, happiness, and sadness (Morecraft, McNeal, Stilwell-Morecraft, Gedney, Ge, Schroeder & van Hoesen 2007). Interestingly, no effects were found relating the amygdala in depression to a different cingulate area involved in reward and pleasure, the anterior cingulate cortex. This again emphasizes the importance of the orbitofrontal cortex and the regions connected to it in depression (Rolls 2016d).

9.4.6 Precuneus

The precuneus is a medial parietal cortex region implicated in the sense of self and agency, and in autobiographical memory (Cavanna & Trimble 2006, Freton, Lemogne, Bergouignan, Delaveau, Lehericy & Fossati 2014). In our fMRI investigation of functional connectivity in depression, we found that the lateral orbitofrontal cortex had increased functional connectivity in depression with some voxels in the precuneus and posterior cingulate cortex (Cheng et al. 2016). We therefore went on to analyze further the role of the precuneus in depression (Cheng et al. 2018c), as described next.

The precuneus and the adjoining retrosplenial cortex (areas 29 and 30) are key regions related to spatial function, memory, and navigation (Bubb et al. 2017). The retrosplenial cortex provides connections to and receives connections from the hippocampal system, connecting especially with the parahippocampal gyrus areas TF and TH, and with the subiculum (Kobayashi & Amaral 2003, Kobayashi & Amaral 2007, Bubb et al. 2017) (Fig. 9.7). The precuneus can be conceptualized as providing access to the hippocampus for spatial and related information from the parietal cortex (given the rich connections between the precuneus and parietal cortex). Object information from the temporal lobe connects to and from the hippocampus via the perirhinal cortex (Rolls 2015d). This provides a basis for the hippocampus to associate together object and spatial information in the single network in the CA3 region of the hippocampus, to form an episodic memory with object and spatial components (Kesner & Rolls 2015). However, reward-related / emotional information may also be part of an episodic memory, and connections from the orbitofrontal cortex to the hippocampal system via the perirhinal and entorhinal cortex pathway are likely to be one route (Rolls 2014b, Rolls 2015d, Rolls 2016c, Rolls 2017d). Interestingly, the relatively strong functional connectivity between the precuneus and the lateral orbitofrontal cortex described here indicates that reward / punishment-related information also enters this part of the system (Fig. 9.7).

To further analyze the functioning of the precuneus in depression, we performed the first fully voxel-level resting state functional connectivity neuroimaging analysis of depression of the precuneus, with 282 patients with major depressive disorder and 254 controls (Cheng et al. 2018c). In 125 patients not receiving medication, voxels in the precuneus had significantly increased functional connectivity with the lateral orbitofrontal cortex, a region implicated in non-reward and which is thereby implicated in depression (Fig. 9.11). In patients receiving medication, the functional connectivity between the lateral orbitofrontal cortex and precuneus

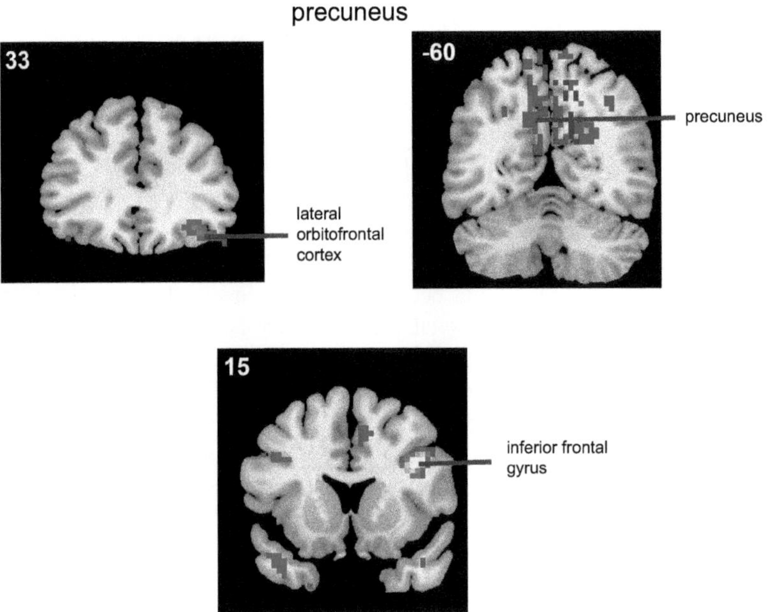

Fig. 9.11 Anatomical location of voxels with significantly different functional connectivity with the precuneus in depression in 125 unmedicated patients vs 254 controls obtained from the voxel-based Association Study (vAS). Red indicates voxels with an increase in functional connectivity in depression, and blue a decrease. Functional connectivity links between pairs of voxels are considered only if they are significantly different with FDR correction $p < 0.05$.) The right of the brain is on the right of each slice. The Y values are in MNI coordinates. This shows that the main differences in depression that is unmedicated are an increase in functional connectivity between the precuneus and the lateral orbitofrontal cortex and an inferior frontal gyrus region. (Modified from Cheng, Rolls et al, 2018c.)

was decreased back towards that in the controls (Cheng et al. 2018c). These findings support the theory that the non-reward system in the lateral orbitofrontal cortex has increased effects on areas in which the self is represented including the precuneus, resulting in low self-esteem (Rolls 2016d).

Functional connectivity was also increased in depression between the precuneus and an inferior frontal gyrus region BA45 that probably is involved in speech production using the larynx and language (Kumar et al. 2016); the angular and supramarginal areas (involved in language); and the temporal cortex including the temporal pole (involved in perception) (Cheng et al. 2018c). The increased connectivity of the precuneus with angular and supramarginal cortical areas involved in language and the inferior frontal gyrus speech / language system may contribute to the negative ruminating thoughts about the self in depression (Cheng et al. 2018c) (Fig. 9.11.

In the 254 controls, it was shown that the precuneus has high functional connectivity with the parahippocampal and dorsolateral prefrontal regions which are involved in memory; and with the parietal cortex. This connectivity, also present in depression, may enable negative memories about the self to be recalled back from memory to influence current thinking (Cheng et al. 2018c).

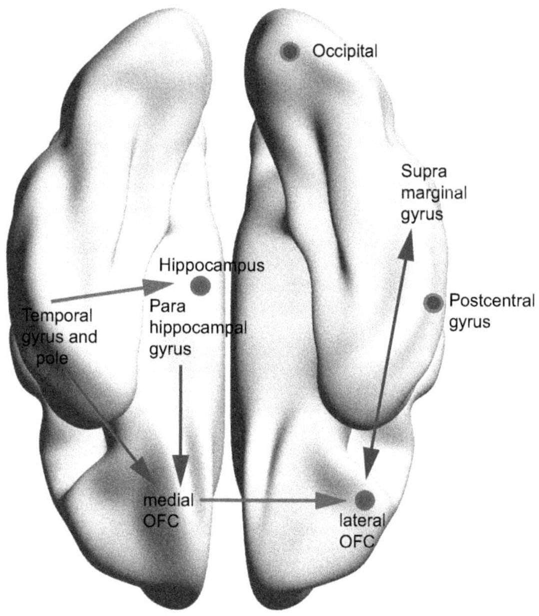

Fig. 9.12 Summary of the networks that show different effective connectivity in patients with depression, shown on a ventral view of the brain. A decrease in effective connectivity in patients with major depressive disorder is shown in blue, and an increase in red. In most cases there was a similar change in the effective connectivity in both directions in depression. The direction of the arrows shows though the direction of the stronger (termed forward) effective connectivity. Regions with an increased value of Σ, reflecting increased activity, are indicated by a red circle; and regions with a decreased value of Σ, are indicated by a blue circle. (After Rolls, Cheng et al, 2018a.)

9.4.7 Effective connectivity in depression

Resting state functional connectivity reflects correlations in the activity between brain areas. The concept is that if the correlations between two brain areas are higher, this may reflect stronger influences between them, including stronger transmission of information from one to the other (Deco & Kringelbach 2014, Cheng et al. 2016). Because the measure of functional connectivity is a correlation, it does not address the direction of the influence between two brain areas.

We have recently gone beyond functional connectivity to effective connectivity between different brain areas to measure directed influences of human brain regions on each other (Rolls et al. 2018a). Effective connectivity is conceptually very different, for it measures the effect of one brain region on another in a particular direction, and can in principle therefore provide information more closely related to the causal processes that operate in brain function, that is, how one brain region influences another. In the context of disorders of brain function, the effective connectivity may provide evidence on which brain regions may have altered function, and then influence other brain regions, by comparing effective connectivity in patients and controls participants. Effective connectivity can also provide a generative model and understanding of brain connectivity.

We utilized a new approach to the measurement of effective connectivity in which each brain area has a simple dynamical model, and known anatomical connectivity is used to provide constraints (Gilson, Moreno-Bote, Ponce-Alvarez, Ritter & Deco 2016). This helps the approach to measure the effective connectivity between the 94 automated anatomical atlas (AAL2) brain areas (Rolls, Joliot & Tzourio-Mazoyer 2015) using resting state functional magnetic resonance imaging. This approach also defines a Σ parameter for each brain area which reflects the variation (variance) of the signal in each brain area.

We found that effective connectivity directed to the medial orbitofrontal cortex from areas including the parahippocampal gyrus, temporal pole, inferior temporal gyrus, and amygdala was decreased in depression (Rolls et al. 2018a) (Fig. 9.12). This is the forward direction for most of these links, i.e. the direction in which the directed connectivity is stronger (Rolls et al. 2018a, Rolls 2016c). This implies less strong positive driving influences of these input regions on the medial and middle orbitofrontal cortex, regions implicated in reward, and thus helps to elucidate part of the decreased feelings of happy states in depression (Rolls 2016d).

The lateral orbitofrontal cortex, an area implicated in non-reward and punishment, had an increased level of activity as reflected in Σ in the depressed group (Fig. 9.12). This was associated with increased effective connectivity from the medial orbitofrontal cortex directed to the lateral orbitofrontal cortex (Fig. 9.12). Given that the medial and lateral orbitofrontal cortex tend to have activations that are related reciprocally to each other, and that there is likely to be less reward-related activity in the medial orbitofrontal cortex in depression, this effective connectivity link may contribute to the increased activity in the lateral orbitofrontal cortex in depression.

The forward links from temporal cortical areas to the precuneus are increased in depression (and are close to significant after FDR correction), and this may relate to representations of the sense of self (Cavanna & Trimble 2006), which become more negative in depression (Rolls 2016d, Cheng et al. 2016, Cheng et al. 2018c).

A notable finding was that Σ was also increased in the right and left hippocampus of patients with depression, reflecting it is suggested some type of heightened memory-related processing. This is in the context that the effective connectivity directed from the temporal pole to the hippocampus is increased in depression (Fig. 9.12).

Together these differences of effective connectivity in depression (Rolls et al. 2018a) are consistent with the hypotheses that some aspects of hippocampal processing, perhaps those related to unpleasant memories, are increased in depression (Rolls 2016d, Cheng et al. 2016); that temporal cortex has increased effective connectivity to the precuneus which with its connectivity with memory systems and the lateral orbitofrontal cortex may contribute to low self-esteem and negative memories; that the influence of temporal lobe memory systems on specifically the medial orbitofrontal cortex is reduced in depression; and that this in turn may contribute to increased activity in the lateral orbitofrontal cortex non-reward system in depression (Rolls et al. 2018a).

The value of effective connectivity in understanding the operation of these systems in depression is that although the functional connectivity (which reflects correlations) between these areas has been shown to be reduced in depression (Cheng et al. 2016), it is only by using effective connectivity that we understand better the direction of the major influence between these brain regions (from the temporal lobe to the medial orbitofrontal cortex), and for example that this directed connectivity is reduced in depression (Rolls et al. 2018a).

9.4.8 Depression and poor sleep quality

Many individuals with depression report poor sleep quality (Becker, Jesus, Joao, Viseu & Martins 2017). What is the relation between depression and sleep? What are the brain systems

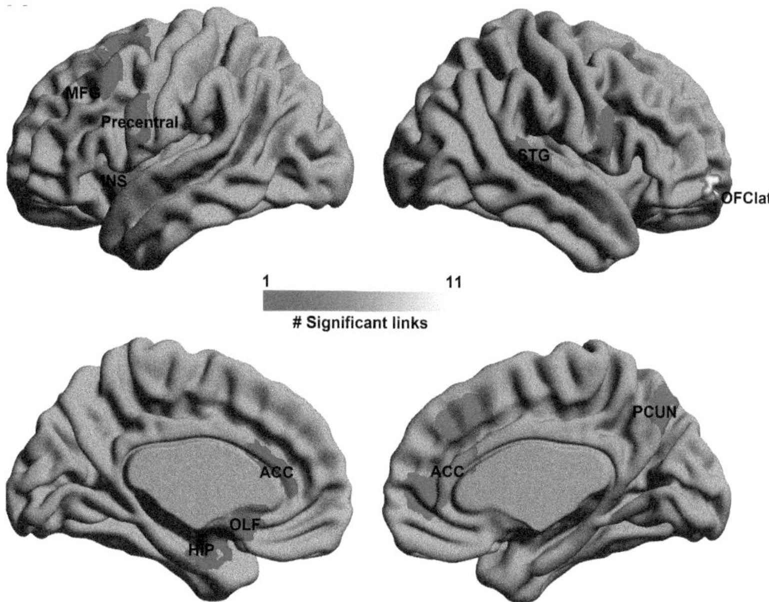

Fig. 9.13 The Shen atlas areas with functional connectivities related to sleep quality, and then selected to be also related to depression. There were 39 such links (significant with NBS correction, $p < 0.05$). ACC – anterior cingulate cortex; HIP- hippocampus; INS – insula; MFG – middle frontal gyrus; OFClat – lateral orbitofrontal cortex; OLF – olfactory tubercle / ventral striatum; PCUN; precuneus; Precentral – precentral gyrus; STG – superior temporal gyrus. (After Cheng, Rolls et al, 2018d.)

that relate to depression and sleep quality? Understanding the answers to these questions may lead to better directed treatments for depression, and may improve sleep quality.

To advance understanding of the brain regions involved in sleep and depression, brain areas that mediate the effect of depression that underlies poor sleep quality were analyzed (Cheng et al. 2018d). The relation between functional connectivity (FC), depressive symptoms (the Adult Self-Report Depressive Problems scores) and poor sleep quality was measured in 1017 participants in the Human Connectome Project (HCP), with cross-validation of the sleep findings in 5342 participants from the UK Biobank.

181 functional connectivity links involving areas such as the precuneus, anterior cingulate cortex and the lateral orbitofrontal cortex related to sleep quality were identified. 39 of these sleep-related links were also related to the depressive scores. The brain areas with increased functional connectivity of these common links related to both sleep and depressive scores included the lateral orbitofrontal cortex; the dorsolateral prefrontal cortex; the anterior and posterior cingulate cortex; the insula; the parahippocampal gyrus and hippocampus; the amygdala; the temporal cortex; and the precuneus (Fig. 9.13). A mediation analysis showed that these functional connectivities in the brain contribute to the relation between depression and poor sleep quality.

The implication is that the increased functional connectivity between these brain regions provides a neural basis for how depression leads to poor sleep quality (Cheng et al. 2018d). This in turn has implications for the treatment of depression, and its effects on poor sleep quality (Cheng et al. 2018d).

Evidence was also found in this general population that the Depressive Problems scores were correlated with functional connectivities between areas that included the lateral orbitofrontal cortex, cingulate cortex; precuneus, angular gyrus, and temporal cortex (Cheng et al. 2018d) (Fig. 9.5). Part of the importance of this is that it provides strong support for a role of the lateral orbitofrontal cortex in depression. Our previous findings on functional and effective connectivity in depression (Cheng et al. 2016, Rolls et al. 2018a, Cheng et al. 2018c, Rolls et al. 2018b, Cheng et al. 2018b, Cheng et al. 2018a) were in hundreds of patients with major depressive disorder and controls in China. The findings in the present study (Cheng et al. 2018d) were not on patients selected to have depression, but instead were on a general population in the U.S.A. in which a tendency to have depressive problems could be assessed. In fact, the correlations arose especially from the presence of 92 people who at some time had been diagnosed with depression. It is important cross-validation that very similar brain regions were identified in the present investigation as having increased functional connectivity related to depressive problems, including the lateral orbitofrontal cortex, precuneus and dorsolateral prefrontal cortex, as in our previous investigations.

This important cross-validation in a completely different population and in people not selected to have depression (Cheng et al. 2018d) provides support for the theory that the lateral orbitofrontal cortex is a key brain area that might be targeted in the search for treatments for depression (Rolls 2016d).

9.5 Possible subtypes of depression

There is growing interest in possible subtypes of depression, for it may be possible to treat different subtypes differently, for example by targeting different brain systems, or by different types of cognitive therapy (Downar, Blumberger, Rizvi, Daskalakis, Kennedy & Giacobbe 2018, Drysdale, Grosenick, Downar, Dunlop, Mansouri, Meng, Fetcho, Zebley, Oathes, Etkin, Schatzberg, Sudheimer, Keller, Mayberg, Gunning, Alexopoulos, Fox, Pascual-Leone, Voss, Casey, Dubin & Liston 2017).

One subtype may be related to anhedonia, a reduction in pleasure and in reward-related learning. This could be related to reduced functioning of the medial orbitofrontal cortex and related brain systems such as the ventral striatum. Pathological distortions of activity in this system (i.e. hypoactivity for conventional positive incentives and hyperactivity for negative incentives) may relate to this symptom of major depressive disorder: anhedonia. Patients with high anhedonia show a poor response to serotonergic antidepressants and to rTMS.

A second possible subtype may be related to prominent (almost compulsive) negative thoughts, and to increased anxiety and neuroticism. This subtype may include a tendency to counterproductive reappraisal of innocuous stimuli as hypothetically harmful or negative. There may also be suicidal ideation. This subtype could be related to increased sensitivity and persistence of networks in the lateral orbitofrontal cortex non-reward / punishment and related networks.

A third possible subtype may have reduced cognitive control and response inhibition, and increased impulsivity. Individuals in this subtype may for example have difficulty in resisting binge eating. The type of impulsivity is that reflected in delay discounting (in which there is impulsive choice of immediate rewards) and clinical measures (e.g. the Barratt impulsivity scale). This may be related to anterior cingulate cortex and related networks.

9.6 Implications for treatments

9.6.1 Brain-based treatments

This non-reward / punishment attractor network sensitivity theory of depression has implications for treatments. These implications can be understood and further explored in the context of investigations of the factors that influence the stability of attractor neuronal networks with integrate-and-fire neurons with noise introduced by the close to Poisson spiking times of the neurons (Chapter 8) (Wang 2002, Rolls 2016c, Deco, Rolls & Romo 2009, Rolls & Deco 2010, Deco et al. 2013, Loh et al. 2007a, Rolls & Deco 2015a).

One implication is that anti-anxiety drugs, by increasing inhibition, might reduce the stability of the high firing rate state of the non-reward attractor, thus acting to quash the depression-related attractor state.

A second implication is that it might be possible to produce agents that decrease the efficacy of NMDA receptors in the lateral orbitofrontal cortex, thereby reducing the stability of the depression-related attractor state. The evidence that there are genes that are selective for NMDA receptors for the neurons in different populations is that there are separate genetic knock-outs for NMDA receptors in the CA3 and CA1 regions of the hippocampus (Nakazawa, Quirk, Chitwood, Watanabe, Yeckel, Sun, Kato, Carr, Johnston, Wilson & Tonegawa 2002, Tonegawa, Nakazawa & Wilson 2003, Nakazawa, Sun, Quirk, Rondi-Reig, Wilson & Tonegawa 2003, Nakazawa, McHugh, Wilson & Tonegawa 2004).

The present theory suggests that searching for ways to influence the attractor networks in the lateral orbitofrontal cortex by decreasing the activity of neurons in this region may be of considerable interest. It should be noted that the present theory is a theory specifically of non-reward and punishment-related attractor networks in the lateral orbitofrontal cortex and related areas in relation to depression, and that alterations of attractor networks in other cortical areas may be related to other psychiatric disorders such as schizophrenia and obsessive-compulsive disorders (Rolls 2012b, Rolls 2016c).

In terms of the implications of the attractor-based aspect of the present theory, an important point is that the attractor dynamics must be kept stable in the face of the randomness or noise introduced into the system by the almost Poisson firing times of neurons for a given mean firing rate. For example, the spontaneous firing rate state of the non-reward attractor must be maintained stable when no non-reward inputs are present (or otherwise the non-reward attractor would jump into a high firing rate non-reward state for no external reason, contributing to depression). The inhibitory transmitter GABA may be important in maintaining this type of stability (Rolls & Deco 2010).

Moreover, the high firing rate state produced by non-reward must not reach too high a firing rate, as this would cause overstability of the non-reward / depression state. In a complementary way, if the high firing rate attractor state is insufficiently high, then that attractor state might be unstable, and the individual might be relatively insensitive to non-reward, not depressed, and impulsive because of not responding sufficiently to non-reward or punishment. The excitatory transmitter glutamate acting at NMDA or AMPA receptors may be important in setting the stability of the high firing rate attractor state. In this respect and in this sense, the tendency to become depressed or to be impulsive may be reciprocally related to each other.

Predictions for treatments follow from understanding these noisy attractor-based dynamics (Rolls & Deco 2010, Rolls 2016c) that are described in Chapter 8, and are considered next.

9.6.2 Behavioural treatments and cognitive therapy

The whole concept of attractor states (Chapter 8) has many implications for the treatment of depression, for rewards and other environmental changes and activities that tend to compete with the non-reward attractor state and quash it may be useful in the treatment of depression. These cognitive approaches might include diverting thought and attention away from the negative stimuli and influences that may contribute to the depression; and directing thought and attention towards rewards, which may help to quash the activity of the non-reward system by the reciprocal interactions between the brain systems involved in reward vs non-reward and punishment.

Particular implications of the attractor-based approach to depression include the following.

First, falling into an attractor state is an inherently non-linear process, and once in the attractor state, the system is stable and is difficult to perturb out of the attractor state, as shown in Chapter 8. An implication is that treatments will need to take this stability of attractor networks into account, and use effective perturbations to make the system move out of its stable attractor. These treatments might be at the purely behavioural or cognitive therapy level. The aim would be to help those with depression to understand some of the factors now thought to lead to depression, and to thereby help them to engage in behavioural changes that would knock the system out of its non-reward attractor. These might include strategies to prevent rumination by the patient deliberately interrupting sad ruminating thoughts, and engaging in activity that might involve performing very different behaviours that would compete with their non-reward attractor. This might involve tasks that require a lot of attention (perhaps activities such as sailing or golf), or that might involve obtaining rewards, which would tend to suppress the non-reward attractor because of the reciprocal relation between the medial orbitofrontal cortex reward system and the lateral orbitofrontal cortex non-reward/punishment system.

This strategy overlaps with the learned helplessness approach to depression, in which placing individuals for a prolonged period in which their actions do not lead to rewards results in the individuals not only obtaining a great deal of non-reward, but also learning to stop trying, as whatever is tried is ineffective (hence the term 'learned helplessness') (Seligman 1978). Setting up situations in which the individuals learn how to obtain rewards again is a beneficial treatment in this situation.

Second, there are multiple attractor loops, each one of which may contribute to the stability of the depressed state, and each one of which may need correction. For example, in Fig. 9.4 we see that in addition to the local attractor network in the lateral orbitofrontal cortex, there is increased functional connectivity between the lateral orbitofrontal cortex and the angular gyrus, which is involved in language (Cheng et al. 2016). This latter is a long loop attractor (implemented by reciprocal backprojections as well as forward connections between cortical areas (Rolls 2016c)), and may have different factors and time-courses that control its activity, such as what one is thinking about with one's syntactic system. In this example, either the short or the long loop might trigger the non-reward system back into its non-reward attractor state, and this needs to be taken account of in behavioural or cognitive treatment. One interesting aspect of this example is that because the syntactic system operates as a single information processing channel (Rolls & Deco 2015b, Rolls 2016c), filling it with positive thoughts would make it difficult to perform multiple step thinking about negative thoughts. This is relevant to the point made above about taking steps to prevent rumination in depression. It may for example be useful to introduce individuals to the idea that constantly returning to stimuli that relate to non-reward, such as the grave of a loved one, while in many ways admirable, may retrigger grief and possibly depression, unless active steps are taken to make something positive out of the situation.

Third, it is important to understand that both depression and non-impulsiveness may be related to non-reward, and that depressed people will, as part of an evolutionarily adaptive strategy, tend not to take risks. This may be important to at least understand when individuals are making financial or economic decisions, so that they can take this into account.

Fourth, noise in the brain caused by the stochastic spiking times of neurons is an important aspect of attractor dynamics, and could contribute to depression, which might occur without an external event causing it (Chapter 8).

Fifth, attractor networks in the brain bias each other and implement top-down attention by this computational process (Rolls 2016c). This again tends to enhance the stability of non-reward networks, because when in the non-reward state, this will tend to bias sensory and memory systems towards sad perceptions and sad memory recall.

Sixth, there are different types of non-reward. Not receiving an expected food reward leaves one adaptively in a state in which trying to obtain the food reward is a goal for action. Not receiving an expected social reward leaves one adaptively in a state in which trying to obtain the social reward is a goal for action. An implication is that understanding what the trigger is for the depression, the type of non-reward or punisher, is likely to be important in treating the depression behaviourally or cognitively.

Seventh, it is argued in this book that different individuals have different sensitivities to different types of reward, non-reward, and punisher, and that this provides a basis for differences in personality. It is argued that this is part of the way in which evolution works, by altering individuals' sensitivities to these goals (Rolls 2012d). This concept in turn should lead us to approach problems such as depression with the understanding that we are dealing with a high-dimensional space of specific rewards, non-rewards, and punishers, different dimensions of which may make different contributions to depression in different individuals.

Now, some of the behavioural and cognitive strategies outlined above have been developed in the context of cognitive therapy for depression, pioneered by Aaron Beck (Beck 1979, Beck 2008, Disner, Beevers, Haigh & Beck 2011). Cognitive behaviour therapy for depression has a great deal of success, and this is helpful information, for it indicates that behavioural and cognitive treatments using the attractor mechanism-based approach described here will lead in turn to well-founded treatments based on this more detailed understanding. In fact, the brain-based attractor approach to depression makes the underlying mechanisms much more explicit, and this it is hoped will lead to better explanations to patients of what may be causing their depression, as well as to better cognitive and behavioural as well as brain-based treatments.

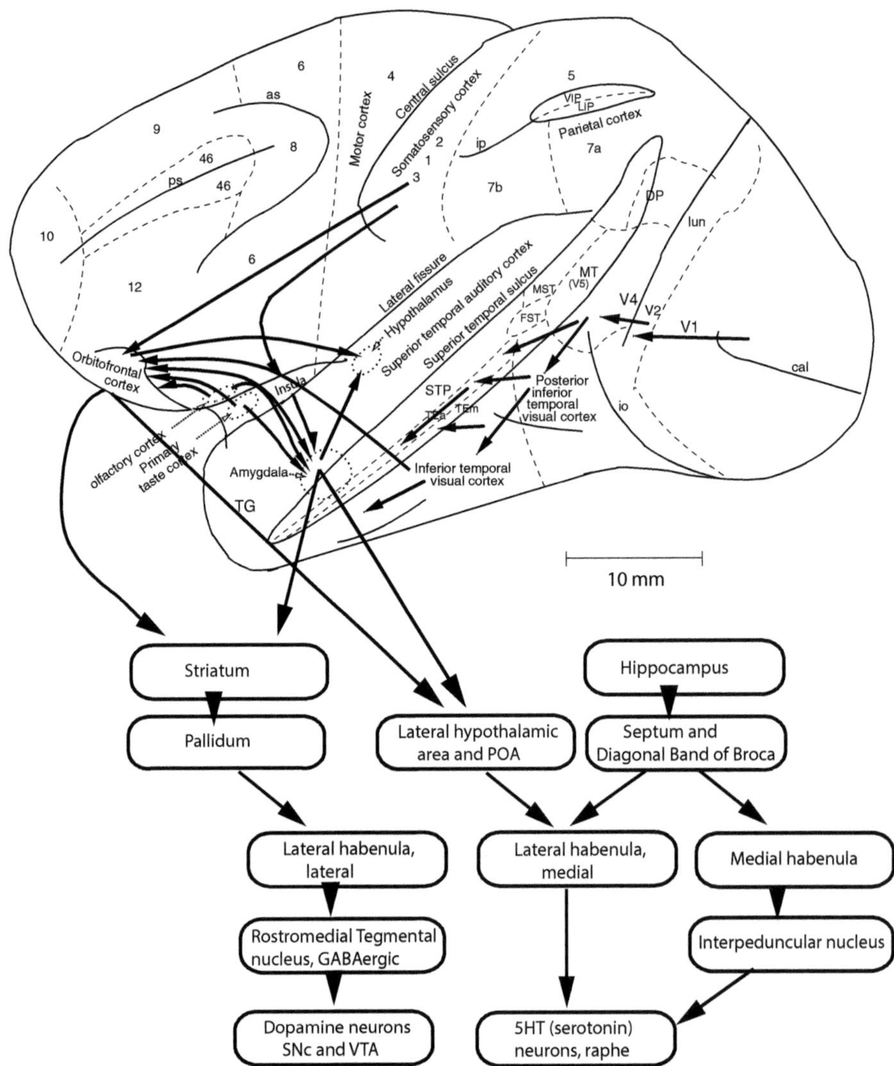

Fig. 9.14 Possible routes for reward and non-reward related information from the orbitofrontal cortex and amygdala to reach the brainstem dopamine and serotonin (5-HT) neurons (see text). as, arcuate sulcus; cal, calcarine sulcus; cs, central sulcus; lf, lateral (or Sylvian) fissure; lun, lunate sulcus; ps, principal sulcus; io, inferior occipital sulcus; ip, intraparietal sulcus (which has been opened to reveal some of the areas it contains); sts, superior temporal sulcus (which has been opened to reveal some of the areas it contains). AIT, anterior inferior temporal cortex; FST, visual motion processing area; LIP, lateral intraparietal area; MST, visual motion processing area; MT, visual motion processing area (also called V5); PIT, posterior inferior temporal cortex; STP, superior temporal plane; TA, architectonic area including auditory association cortex; TE, architectonic area including high order visual association cortex, and some of its subareas TEa and TEm; TG, architectonic area in the temporal pole; V1–V4, visual areas V1–V4; VIP, ventral intraparietal area; TEO, architectonic area including posterior visual association cortex. The numerals refer to architectonic areas, and have the following approximate functional equivalence: 1,2,3, somatosensory cortex (posterior to the central sulcus); 4, motor cortex; 5, superior parietal lobule; 7a, inferior parietal lobule, visual part; 7b, inferior parietal lobule, somatosensory part; 6, lateral premotor cortex; 8, frontal eye field; 12, part of orbitofrontal cortex; 46, dorsolateral prefrontal cortex. (After Rolls 2017b.)

9.7 Pharmacological treatments for depression

9.7.1 Serotonin (5HT)

A number of antidepressant medications increase serotonin (5-hydroxy-tryptamine, 5HT) signalling in the brain by inhibiting serotonin reuptake from the synaptic cleft, thus increasing the efficacy of the 5HT. They include selective serotonin reuptake inhibitors (SSRIs) such as fluoxetine (Prozac), serotonin norepinephrine reuptake inhibitors (SNRIs), and some tricyclic antidepressants such as imipramine which blocks the reuptake of 5-HT (5-hydroxy-tryptamine, serotonin), NA (noradrenaline), and DA (dopamine), in that order of potency. (They inhibit the presynaptic transporters with that order of efficacy (Soares & Young 2016), and blocking the reuptake increases the concentration in the synapse of the 5HT).

The SSRI drugs may take several weeks to reduce the depression, although some effects are faster, such as effects on whether face expressions are sad (Harmer & Cowen 2013). One reason that the rapid increase of concentration of 5-HT produced by most of the antidepressant drugs does not work rapidly appears to be that there are 5-HT_{1A} autoreceptors on the 5-HT cell bodies in the raphe nucleus (and also on the post-synaptic neurons), and when these are activated by the elevated 5-HT, the potassium conductance is increased, producing hyperpolarization of the 5-HT neurons, which decreases their firing, counteracting any influence of the potentially elevated 5-HT concentrations produced by most antidepressant drugs. It may be that this autoreceptor-mediated negative feedback becomes attenuated with a time course of weeks, and then the antidepressant drugs start to influence depression (see e.g. Celada, Puig, Armagos-Bosch, Adell & Artigas (2004)). Indeed, adaptation of these autoreceptors occurred through a desensitization process over the course of 2–3 weeks of SSRIs administration, allowing the recovery of 5-HT neurons to their normal firing rate in the presence of reuptake inhibition of 5-HT, thus overall increasing 5HT-influenced transmission (Ghasemi, Phillips, Fahimi, McNerney & Salehi 2017). Also, the blockade of 5-HT_{2A} receptors by some atypical antipsychotic drugs may improve the clinical effects of SSRIs, perhaps by an action on the prefrontal cortex (Celada et al. 2004).

However, approximately 33% of patients with major depressive disorder do not respond to treatment with commonly used SSRIs, so at least some subtypes or aspects of depression may not be related to serotonin (Yohn et al. 2017).

Serotonin neurons, whose cell bodies are in the raphe nucleus in the brainstem, have widespread projections throughout the brain, and where serotonin effects relate to antidepressant effects is not yet established. In animal models of depression, there is evidence that there is decreased neurogenesis in the dentate gyrus which is part of the hippocampal system, that antidepressants increase neurogenesis in the dentate gyrus, and that antidepressants have some of their behavioral effects in animal models only if this system is intact (Yohn et al. 2017). The significance of this for understanding depression or bipolar disorder is difficult to ascertain, for the hippocampus is mainly involved in memory, and not in emotion and mood (Rolls 2015d, Kesner & Rolls 2015, Rolls 2016c). Perhaps these differences in the hippocampus are related to the altered memory function in at least depression, with increased rumination of memories associated with different functional connectivity of the hippocampus and related systems in depression (Cheng et al. 2016, Cheng et al. 2018b). For example, the posterior cingulate cortex, which provides a route for information to reach the hippocampus, has increased functional connectivity with the lateral orbitofrontal cortex in depression (Cheng et al. 2018b), as described above.

A somewhat unaddressed issue is where the serotonin neurons in the raphe receive inputs from that might produce depression in the first place. In this context, it has now been suggested that reward and non-reward areas of the brain such as the orbitofrontal cortex and amygdala do provide a source of relevant inputs to the 5-HT neurons, via brain regions such as the habenula and ventral striatum (Rolls 2017b) (Fig. 9.14). The suggestion is that the orbitofrontal cortex and amygdala systems involved in reward and non-reward can operate via a lateral hypothalamic area / lateral preoptic area (POA) to influence the Lateral Habenula, medial part, which in turn can influence the 5-HT (serotonin) neurons in the raphe nuclei. Many antidepressant drugs may influence this cortical to brainstem pathway by influencing the effects of the 5-HT neurons, which terminate in many brain areas. The hippocampal influence via the septal nuclei and diagonal band of Broca may enable reward context to access the same Lateral Habenula, medial part, to 5-HT-neuron system (de Araujo, Ferreira, Tellez, Ren & Yeckel 2012, Rolls 2015a). The medial habenula also receives septal inputs, and projects to the interpeduncular nucleus, and thereby to 5-HT neurons (and probably dopamine neurons) (Fig. 9.14) (Proulx, Hikosaka & Malinow 2014, Loonen & Ivanova 2016).

These connections are shown in the context of some of the pathways involved in reward-related processes and emotion shown on the lateral view of the brain of the macaque monkey in the upper part of Fig. 9.14 (Rolls 2017b). Connections from the primary taste and olfactory cortices to the orbitofrontal cortex and amygdala are shown. Connections are also shown in the 'ventral visual system' from the visual cortical areas V1 to V2, V4, the inferior temporal visual cortex, etc., with some connections reaching the amygdala and orbitofrontal cortex. In addition, connections from the somatosensory cortical areas BA 1, 2, and 3 that reach the orbitofrontal cortex directly and via the insular cortex, and that reach the amygdala via the insular cortex, are shown.

Corresponding pathways that provide a route for reward and emotion-related information to reach the dopamine neurons in the midbrain are also shown in Fig. 9.14. The orbitofrontal cortex, amygdala (and probably anterior cingulate cortex and subgenual cingulate cortex) systems involved in reward and non-reward can operate via a basal ganglia route (striatum, ventral pallidum, and globus pallidus / bed nucleus of the stria terminalis) to influence the Lateral Habenula, lateral part, which in turn via the GABAergic Rostromedial Tegmental nucleus can influence dopamine neurons in the Substantia Nigra pars compacta and ventral Tegmental Area (SNc and VTA). This provides a route for reward, non-reward, and reward prediction error signals of largely cortical origin to influence the dopamine neurons. Details of some of these anatomical connections are provided elsewhere (Proulx et al. 2014, Loonen & Ivanova 2016).

Consistent with these points (Rolls 2017b), in the lateral habenula, neurons that respond to signaled low reward value or to punishment have been described (Matsumoto & Hikosaka 2009b), and so have neurons that reflect negative reward prediction error (Bromberg-Martin & Hikosaka 2011). Similar neurons are found in the globus pallidus glutamatergic excitatory habenula-projecting neurons, providing evidence that the necessary computations are not performed in the lateral habenula (Stephenson-Jones, Yu, Ahrens, Tucciarone, van Huijstee, Mejia, Penzo, Tai, Wilbrecht & Li 2016).

9.7.2 Ketamine

A notable recent discovery is that ketamine, a N-methyl-D-aspartate (NMDA) receptor antagonist, in subanaesthetic doses, produces rapid (within hours) antidepressant responses in patients who are resistant to typical antidepressants, and that the effects may last for two weeks or longer (Zanos & Gould 2018, Iadarola, Niciu, Richards, Vande Voort, Ballard, Lundin, Nugent, Machado-Vieira & Zarate 2015, Maltbie, Kaundinya & Howell 2017, Zanos, Moaddel, Morris, Georgiou, Fischell, Elmer, Alkondon, Yuan, Pribut, Singh, Dossou, Fang, Huang, Mayo, Wainer, Albuquerque, Thompson, Thomas, Zarate & Gould 2016). Clinically, ketamine may be useful with a single dose, or doses may be repeated. The short-term effects of ketamine include blocking excitatory NMDA receptors on cortical pyramidal cells which reduces the excitatory effect produced by the excitatory transmitter glutamate; and blocking excitatory receptors on GABA inhibitory neurons, which will tend to decrease GABAergic neuron firing, resulting in a potential increase in pyramidal cell firing. However, ketamine produces further effects, such as inducing synaptogenesis on excitatory neurons, increased glutamate transmission, reversing the synaptic deficits caused by chronic stress, and effects of a ketamine metabolite hydroxynorketamine (Duman & Aghajanian 2012, Ghasemi et al. 2017, Zorumski, Izumi & Mennerick 2016, Abdallah, Adams, Kelmendi, Esterlis, Sanacora & Krystal 2016, Aleksandrova, Phillips & Wang 2017, Zanos & Gould 2018). Another way in which ketamine may be effective in depression is by reducing inflammatory processes, which are sometimes related to depression (Ghasemi et al. 2017).

Stress is a factor that can lead to depression, and some antidepressants including ketamine enhance neurotrophic factors such as BDNF (brain-derived neurotrophic factor), which may help to reduce the damaging effects of prolonged stress (Yohn et al. 2017, Ghasemi et al. 2017).

To understand exactly how antidepressant drugs have their therapeutic effects, it is important to know how they act not just generally in neural tissue, but on particular brain areas and systems. For example, the evidence described above suggests that decreasing the functioning of the lateral orbitofrontal cortex (involved in non-reward), and increasing the functioning of the medial orbitofrontal cortex (involved in reward), may be useful in the treatment of depression, yet these brain regions are just a small distance apart, so measurements that relate to drug effects in particular brain areas may be important in understanding and developing new antidepressant treatments.

Indeed, one potentially fruitful link would be to develop drugs that have potency particularly for some of the brain areas now known to be involved in emotion, such as the lateral vs medial orbitofrontal cortex, amygdala, and cingulate cortex. Another potentially fruitful link is to investigate with neuroimaging the brain changes that occur in depression and in the treatment of depression with antidepressants, to gain further evidence in humans about the brain systems involved in depression, and potentially, with the use of transmitter-specific techniques available with positron emission tomography (PET), to continue to investigate neuropharmacological and neurochemical aspects of depression in humans, as well as the effects of deep brain stimulation (see Section 4.5.4).

9.8 Mania and bipolar disorder

So far in this Chapter (9), we have been considering unipolar depression.

Bipolar disorder includes recurrent periods of mania and depression. The severity of the mania is greatest in bipolar I disorder, moderate in bipolar II disorder, and lower in cyclothymia. During mania, behaviors may include increased energy, grandiosity, less sleep, risk preference / impulsivity, euphoria, aggression, high reward seeking, hypersexuality, and hyperactivity (Anderson, Haddad & Scott 2012, Soares & Young 2016). During depression there may be anhedonia, risk aversion, increased sleep, reduced libido, reduced energy, feeling tired, feeling helpless, and a greater risk of suicide (Anderson et al. 2012, Soares & Young 2016).

The incidence of bipolar disorder is 1–2%. The heritability is fairly high (80–90%), but the disease is polygenic, with many genes each contributing a little (Anderson et al. 2012, Soares & Young 2016).

9.8.1 Mania, increased responsiveness to reward, and decreased responsiveness to non-reward

What is the relation between mania and depression? Could it be that in mania, there is something that in terms of reward/non-reward systems, is almost the opposite of depression? Might there be in mania *increased sensitivity to reward, and decreased sensitivity to non-reward / punishment*? The latter might manifest itself as increased impulsiveness in mania. That is a suggestion that might be considered to be the opposite of what has been described for depression in the previous part of this Chapter.

It turns out that there is support for this hypothesis. It indeed appears that the risk for mania is characterized by a hypersensitivity to goal- and reward-relevant cues (Nusslock, Young & Damme 2014). This hypersensitivity can lead to an excessive increase in approach-related affect and motivation during life events involving rewards or goal striving and attainment. In the extreme, this excessive increase in reward-related affect is reflected in manic symptoms, such as pursuit of rewarding activities without attention to risks, elevated or irritable mood, decreased need for sleep, increased psychomotor activation, and extreme self-confidence. Some evidence consistent with the hypothesis is that patients with bipolar I disorder and their relatives showed greater activation of the medial orbitofrontal cortex in response to reward delivery (Wessa, Kanske & Linke 2014). Also, reduced deactivation of the medial orbitofrontal cortex (where rewards are represented) during reward reversal might reflect a reduced error signal in bipolar disorder patients and their relatives in the lateral orbitofrontal cortex. (The activation of the lateral orbitofrontal cortex by non-reward in healthy individuals is illustrated in Fig. 9.2.) This type of responsiveness has been found to be very different in mania, with apparently decreasing activations in the lateral orbitofrontal cortex during expectation of increasing loss, the opposite of what is found in healthy participants (Bermpohl, Kahnt, Dalanay, Hagele, Sajonz, Wegner, Stoy, Adli, Kruger, Wrase, Strohle, Bauer & Heinz 2010) which we discovered in the orbitofrontal cortex (O'Doherty, Kringelbach, Rolls, Hornak & Andrews 2001a). In this context, of potentially reduced sensitivity or even abnormal function of the lateral orbitofrontal cortex non-reward system in mania, it is relevant that manic bipolar patients continue to pursue immediate rewards despite negative consequences (Wessa et al. 2014). Further, impulsivity in mania is pervasive, encompassing deficits in attention and behavioral inhibition. In addition, impulsivity is greater if the illness is severe (with for example frequent episodes, substance use disorders, and suicide attempts) (Swann 2009). The significance of this is that impulsivity may reflect decreased sensitivity to non-reward, which is represented by activations in the lateral orbitofrontal cortex, where non-reward is represented (see above).

Thus mania may reflect a state in which there is decreased sensitivity of non-reward systems and hence increased impulsiveness due to reduced sensitivity of the lateral orbitofrontal cortex, and at the same time, increased sensitivity to reward reflected in activations in the medial orbitofrontal cortex and pregenual cingulate cortex. Although these medial and lateral orbitofrontal cortex systems may show reciprocally related activations within an individual, with for example increasing activations in the medial orbitofrontal cortex to increasing monetary gains and decreasing activations in the lateral orbitofrontal cortex, and vice versa to increasing monetary loss (O'Doherty et al. 2001a), the reward and non-reward systems could be, and indeed are likely to, have their sensitivity set by independent genes, providing a basis for some patients to be depressed, and others to show both mania and depression. Indeed, Rolls' theory of emotion (Rolls 2014b) (Chapter 2) would go beyond this, and suggest that the sensitivity to many different rewards (e.g. food when hungry, water when thirsty, pleasant touch, sensitivity to reputation), and correspondingly to many different non-rewards, may be set by genes somewhat independently. This provides a relation to personality (Rolls 2014b), with the implication that people with depression may be particularly sensitive to certain non-rewards or punishers, and people with mania may be particularly sensitive to particular rewards. This has important implications for therapy, which might be well-directed towards particular sensitivities to particular non-rewards and particular rewards in different individuals.

9.8.2 Attractor networks, mania, increased responsiveness to reward, and decreased responsiveness to non-reward

The question then arises of the extent to which attractor network operations contribute to mania.

In terms of responses to inputs that increase the expectancy of reward, a short-term attractor system, probably in the orbitofrontal cortex, is likely to be present, to bridge any temporal interval between the expected reward signal and the actual outcome. This could in principle be oversensitive in mania. When the reward, the outcome, is delivered, it might also be useful to have a short-term attractor, to help reset a rule attractor for which stimulus is currently rewarding. However, it would be maladaptive if these reward-expectancy or reward-outcome attractors normally operated for more than perhaps 10 s, for this would tend to break the important contingency between input stimuli and outcomes. In addition to these short-term attractors, there also needs to be a longer term attractor process to reflect mood state, which typically operates on a much longer time scale. This might again be an attractor (with separate competing attractors for different mood states), and this attractor might be re-activated by the longer loop through the language / planning system, which by recalling a recent reward might calculate the long-term benefits, helping to keep the mood state prolonged. This whole 'long-loop' attractor might also be more sensitive in mania.

Given that there is increased impulsiveness in mania, it is also a possibility that the lateral orbitofrontal cortex non-reward attractor network system is less responsive in mania, for lack of responsiveness to non-reward is expected to lead to impulsive behaviour, behaviour that is not restrained by non-reward or punishment. Given that there is some reciprocity between activations in the medial and lateral orbitofrontal cortex (O'Doherty et al. 2001a, Rolls et al. 2018a), it is a possibility that simultaneous low responsiveness of a lateral orbitofrontal cortex non-reward system, and high responsiveness of a medial orbitofrontal cortex reward system, are both contributors to the mania of bipolar disorder.

These are interesting concepts for future empirical exploration.

9.8.3 Other aspects of bipolar disorder

Bipolar disorder involves successive periods of mania and depression. The causes of the cycling between these states is not very clear. However, the circadian rhythm is disrupted in bipolar disorder, with a shortened sleep time, and a more rapid onset of rapid-eye movement (dreaming) sleep. Further, melatonin production, which is high at night, is more suppressed by light in bipolar patients than in controls (Soares & Young 2016). At least some individuals with bipolar disorder have differences in the clock genes that control circadian rhythms (Soares & Young 2016). Whereas light therapy may be used in depression (and is effective especially early in the morning), dark therapy may be used in mania (Soares & Young 2016).

The treatments used for bipolar disorder include those used to treat depression, for in the depressed phase the risk of suicide is increased. Antidepressants such as the SSRIs increase the synaptic efficacy of serotonin, as described in Section 9.7. Treatments such as these may be used in the depressed phase of bipolar disorder (Soares & Young 2016).

In the manic phase, 'mood stabilizers' such as lithium and valproate may be prescribed (Soares & Young 2016). Both may act by enhancing the activity of GABA (inhibitory) neurons and decreasing excitatory neuron activity (Soares & Young 2016).

There are differences in the hippocampal system in bipolar disorder. There is evidence for decreased (GABA) inhibitory neuron efficacy in hippocampal CA3, associated with altered gene expression, and also with a reduced number of GABA neurons (Benes & Subburaj 2016). The significance of this for understanding bipolar disorder is difficult to ascertain, for, as noted above, the hippocampus is mainly involved in memory, and not in emotion and mood (Rolls 2015d, Kesner & Rolls 2015, Rolls 2016c). Perhaps these differences in the hippocampus are related to the altered memory function in at least depression, with increased rumination of memories associated with different functional connectivity of the hippocampus and related systems in depression (Cheng et al. 2016, Cheng et al. 2018b).

10 Rational vs emotional routes to action, and consciousness

10.1 Multiple routes to action; reasoning vs emotion

10.1.1 Some of the different routes to action produced by emotion-related stimuli

Fig. 4.3 on page 54 shows two major routes to behaviour related to emotional stimuli. The first may involve the habit system (in which the basal ganglia are implicated), and a system for goal-directed action-outcome learning, in which the cingulate cortex is implicated. This route is sometimes described as operating implicitly, which implies without consciousness, though the issue of conscious feelings is deferred until Section 10.2.

The second route is described as involving a **reasoning system** that may use some form of language involving syntax (grammar) to plan several steps ahead. It is this second route on which I focus in this Chapter, for it enables actions to be performed for completely different goals than those specified by genes as primary reinforcers which can use the first route just described for output. This reasoning system is very important for understanding human emotion, because its decisions can be made in a completely different way, and do not necessarily lead to decisions that are consistent with those specified by the gene-defined reinforcers that are important in the first 'emotion-related' route to behavioural output. I argue in this Chapter that our reasoning system enables us to go beyond what 'Selfish Genes' might encourage (Dawkins 1976), and that when we use the term 'free will', it is to the rational system that we may wish to refer, together with the non-deterministic, probabilistic, nature of brain computation that is described in Chapter 8 (Rolls 2014b).

I will give a simple example to make the point clear. Our genes may predispose us to like foods that are sweet and fatty (with modern supernormal examples ice cream and chocolate), and these may be rewarding to us because of the processes taking place in brain regions such as the orbitofrontal cortex and amygdala. But our reasoning system may know about discoveries in science and medicine that provide evidence that these foods may tend to promote obesity and poor health if eaten in quantity. So our reasoning system may enable us to override what our gene-based emotional system urges, and instead to eat the healthy foods, for the potential advantage to the individual person of a healthy and long life.

10.1.2 Examples of some complex behaviours that may be performed implicitly

A starting point is that many actions can be performed relatively automatically, without apparent conscious intervention, that is implicitly.

An example sometimes given is driving a car for a short distance while the person may be thinking about something else.

Another example is the identification of a visual stimulus that can occur without conscious awareness if the stimulus is very short (as in backward masking) or weak (Rolls & Tovee 1994, Rolls 2003).

Another example is much of the sensory processing and actions that involve the dorsal stream of visual processing to the parietal cortex, such as a patient posting a letter through a letter box at the correct orientation even when the patient may not be aware of what the object is (Milner & Goodale 1995, Goodale 2004, Milner 2008) because of damage to the ventral visual stream which implements object recognition (Rolls 2016c) .

Another example is blindsight, in which humans with damage to the visual cortex may be able to point to objects even when they are not aware of seeing an object (Weiskrantz 1997, Weiskrantz 1998, Weiskrantz 2009).

Similar evidence applies to emotions, some of the processing for which can occur without conscious awareness (De Gelder, Vroomen, Pourtois & Weiskrantz 1999, Phelps & LeDoux 2005, LeDoux 2008, LeDoux & Pine 2016).

Consistent with the hypothesis of multiple routes to action, only some of which involve conscious awareness, is the evidence that split-brain patients may not be aware of actions being performed by the 'non-dominant' hemisphere (Gazzaniga & LeDoux 1978, Gazzaniga 1988, Gazzaniga 1995).

Also consistent with multiple, including non-verbal, routes to action, patients with focal brain damage, for example to the prefrontal cortex, may emit actions, yet comment verbally that they should not be performing those actions (Rolls et al. 1994a, Hornak et al. 2003). In both these types of patient, confabulation may occur, in that a verbal account of why the action was performed may be given, and this may not be related at all to the environmental event that actually triggered the action (Gazzaniga & LeDoux 1978, Gazzaniga 1988, Gazzaniga 1995, Rolls et al. 1994a).

10.1.3 A reasoning, rational, route to action

The second ('explicit') route in (at least) humans involves a computation with many 'if ... then' statements, to implement a plan to obtain a reward. In this case, the reward may actually be deferred as part of the plan, which might involve working first to obtain one reward, and only then to work for a second more highly valued reward, if this was thought to be overall an optimal strategy in terms of resource usage (e.g. time). In this case, syntax is required, because the many symbols (e.g. names of people) that are part of the plan must be correctly linked or bound. Such linking might be of the form: 'if A does this, then B is likely to do this, and this will cause C to do this ...'. The requirement of syntax for this type of planning implies that involvement of a syntactic system in the brain is required (see Fig. 4.3). **Thus the explicit language system in humans may allow working for deferred rewards by enabling use of a one-off, individual, plan appropriate for each situation.** This explicit system may allow immediate rewards to be deferred, as part of a long-term plan. This ability to defer immediate rewards and plan syntactically in this way for the long term may be an important way in which the explicit system extends the capabilities of the implicit emotion systems that respond more directly to rewards and punishers, or to rewards and punishers with fixed expectancies such as can be learned by reinforcement learning.

Consistent with the point being made about evolutionarily old emotion-based decision systems vs a recent rational system present in humans (and perhaps other animals with syntactic processing) is that humans trade off immediate costs/benefits against cost/benefits that are delayed by as much as decades, whereas non-human primates have not been observed to engage in unpreprogrammed delay of gratification involving more than a few minutes (Rachlin 1989, Kagel, Battalio & Green 1995, McClure, Laibson, Loewenstein & Cohen 2004, Rosati 2017).

Another building block for such planning operations in the brain may be the type of short-term memory in which the prefrontal cortex is involved. This short-term memory may be, for example in non-human primates, of where in space a response has just been made. A development of this type of short-term memory system in humans to enable multiple short-term memories to be held in place correctly, preferably with the temporal order of the different items in the short-term memory coded correctly, may be another building block for the multiple step 'if .... then' type of computation in order to form a multiple step plan. Such short-term memories are implemented in the (dorsolateral and inferior convexity) prefrontal cortex of non-human primates and humans (Goldman-Rakic 1996, Petrides 1996, Deco & Rolls 2003, Rolls 2016c), and may be part of the reason why prefrontal cortex damage impairs planning and executive function (Gilbert & Burgess 2008).

We may examine some of the advantages and behavioural functions that language, present as the most recently added layer to the above system (Fig. 4.3), would confer.

One major advantage would be the ability to plan actions through many potential stages and to evaluate the consequences of those actions without having to perform the actions. For this, the ability to form propositional statements, and to perform syntactic operations on the semantic representations of states in the world, would be important.

Also important in this system would be the ability to have second-order thoughts about the type of thought that I have just described (e.g. I think that she thinks that ..., involving 'theory of mind'), as this would allow much better modelling and prediction of others' behaviour, and therefore of planning, particularly planning when it involves others. Second-order thoughts are thoughts about thoughts. Higher-order thoughts refer to second-order, third-order, etc., thoughts about thoughts... This capability for higher-order thoughts would also enable reflection on past events, which would also be useful in planning [10].

In contrast, non-linguistic behaviour would be driven by learned reinforcement associations, learned rules etc., but not by flexible planning for many steps ahead involving a model of the world including others' behaviour.

It is important to state that the language ability referred to here is not necessarily human verbal language (though this would be an example). What it is suggested is important to multiple step planning is the syntactic manipulation of symbols, and it is this syntactic manipulation of symbols that is the sense in which language is defined and used here. The type of syntactic processing need not be at the natural language level (which implies a universal grammar), but could be at the level of mentalese (Rolls 2014b, Rolls 2004c, Fodor 1994, Rolls & Deco 2015b).

In summary, I understand **reasoning, and rationality**, to involve syntactic manipulations of symbols. Reasoning thus typically may involve multiple steps of 'if .. then' conditional statements, all executed as a one-off or one-time process (see below), and is very different from associatively learned conditional rules typically learned over many trials, such as 'if yellow, a left choice is associated with reward'.

[10] A thought may be defined briefly as an intentional mental state, that is a mental state that is about something. Thoughts include beliefs, and are usually described as being propositional (Rosenthal 2005). An example of a thought is "It is raining". A more detailed definition is as follows. A thought may be defined as an occurrent mental state (or event) that is intentional – that is a mental state that is about something – and also propositional, so that it is evaluable as true or false. Thoughts include occurrent beliefs or judgements. An example of a thought would be an occurrent belief that the earth moves around the sun / that Maurice's boat goes faster with two sails / that it never rains in southern California.)

10.1.4 The Selfish Gene vs The Selfish Phenotype

I have provided evidence in the earlier part of this section (10.1) that there are two main routes to decision-making and action. The first route selects actions by gene-defined goals for action, and is closely associated with emotion. The second route involves multistep planning and reasoning which requires syntactic processing to keep the symbols involved at each step separate from the symbols in different steps. (This second route is used by humans and perhaps by closely related animals.) Now the 'interests' of the first and second routes to decision-making and action are different. As argued convincingly by Richard Dawkins in *The Selfish Gene* (Dawkins 1976, Dawkins 1989), and by others (Hamilton 1964, Ridley 1993a, Hamilton 1996), many behaviours occur in the interests of the survival of the genes, not of the individual (nor of the group), and much behaviour can be understood in this way. I have extended this approach by arguing that an important role for some genes in evolution is to define the goals for actions that will lead to better survival of those genes; that emotions are the states associated with these gene-defined goals; and that the defining of goals for actions rather that actions themselves is an efficient way for genes to operate, as it leaves flexibility of choice of action open until the animal is alive (Rolls 2014b). This provides great simplification of the genotype, as action details do not need to be specified, just rewarding and punishing stimuli, and also provides flexibility of action in the face of changing environments faced by the genes. Thus the interests that are implied when the first route to action is chosen are those of the 'selfish genes', not those of the individual.

However, the second route to action allows, by reasoning, decisions to be taken that might not be in the interests of the genes, might be longer term decisions, and might be in the interests of the individual. An example might be a choice not to have children, but instead to devote oneself to science, medicine, music, or literature. The reasoning, rational, system presumably evolved because taking longer-term decisions involving planning rather than choosing a gene-defined goal might be advantageous at least sometimes for genes. But an unforeseen consequence of the evolution of the rational system might be that the decisions would, sometimes, not be to the advantage of any genes in the organism. After all, evolution by natural selection operates utilizing genetic variation like a Blind Watchmaker (Dawkins 1986a). In this sense, the interests when the second route to decision-making is used are at least sometimes those of the 'selfish phenotype'. (Indeed, we might euphonically say that the interests are those of the '*selfish phene*' (where the etymology is Gk $\phi\alpha\iota\nu\omega$ (phaino), 'appear', referring to appearance, hence the thing that one observes, the individual). Hence the decision-making referred to in this Section (10.1) is between a first system where the goals are gene-defined, and a second rational system in which the decisions may be made in the interests of the genes, or in the interests of the phenotype and not in the interests of the genes. Thus we may speak of the choice as sometimes being between the 'Selfish Genes' and the 'Selfish Phenes'.

Now what keeps the decision-making between the 'Selfish Genes' and the 'Selfish Phenes' more or less under control and in balance? If the second, rational, system chose too often for the interests of the 'Selfish Phene', the genes in that phenotype would not survive over generations. Having these two systems in the same individual will only be stable if their potency is approximately equal, so that sometimes decisions are made with the first route, and sometimes with the second route. If the two types of decision-making, then, compete with approximately equal potency, and sometimes one is chosen, and sometimes the other, then this is exactly the scenario in which stochastic processes in the decision-making mechanism are likely to play an important role in the decision that is taken. The same decision, even with the same evidence, may not be taken each time a decision is made, because of noise in the system.

The system itself may have some properties that help to keep the system operating well. One is that if the second, rational, system tends to dominate the decision-making too much, the first, gene-based emotional system might fight back over generations of selection, and enhance the magnitude of the reward value specified by the genes, so that emotions might actually become stronger as a consequence of them having to compete in the interests of the selfish genes with the rational decision-making process.

Another property of the system may be that sometimes the rational system cannot gain all the evidence that would be needed to make a rational choice. Under these circumstances the rational system might fail to make a clear decision, and under these circumstances, basing a decision on the gene-specified emotions is an alternative. Indeed, Damasio (1994) argued that under circumstances such as this, emotions might take an important role in decision-making. In this respect, I agree with him, basing my reasons on the arguments above. He called the emotional feelings gut feelings, and, in contrast to me, hypothesized that actual feedback from the gut was involved. His argument seemed to be that if the decision was too complicated for the rational system, then send outputs to the viscera, and whatever is sensed by what the periphery sends back could be used in the decision-making, and would account for the conscious feelings of the emotional states. My reading of the evidence is that the feedback from the periphery is not necessary for the emotional decision-making, or for the feelings, nor would it be computationally efficient to put the viscera and more generally the periphery in the loop given that the information starts from the brain (Section 2.4.1 and Rolls (2014b)).

Another property of operation is that the interests of the second, rational, system, although involving a different form of computation, should not be too far from those of the gene-defined emotional system, for the arrangement to be stable in evolution by natural selection. One way that this could be facilitated would be if the gene-based goals felt pleasant or unpleasant in the rational system, and in this way contributed to the operation of the second, rational, system. This is something that I propose is the case. This provides an account of why rewards feel good.

10.1.5 Decision-making between the implicit and explicit systems

The question then arises of how decisions are made in animals such as humans that have both the implicit, direct reward-based, and the explicit, rational, planning systems (see Fig. 4.3). One particular situation in which the first, implicit, system may be especially important is when rapid reactions to stimuli with reward or punishment value must be made, for then the direct connections from structures such as the orbitofrontal cortex to the basal ganglia may allow rapid actions. Another is that when there may be too many factors to be taken into account easily by the explicit, rational, planning, system, then the implicit system may be used to guide action.

In contrast, when the implicit system continually makes errors, it would then be beneficial for the organism to switch from automatic, direct, action based on obtaining what the orbitofrontal cortex system decodes as being the most positively reinforcing choice currently available, to the explicit conscious control system which can evaluate with its long-term planning algorithms what action should be performed next. Indeed, it would be adaptive for the explicit system to be regularly assessing performance by the more automatic system, and to switch itself in to control behaviour quite frequently, as otherwise the adaptive value of having the explicit system would be less than optimal.

Another factor that may influence the balance between control by the implicit and explicit systems is the presence of pharmacological agents such as alcohol, which may alter the balance towards control by the implicit system, may allow the implicit system to influence more the explanations made by the explicit system, and may within the explicit system alter the relative value it places on caution and restraint vs commitment to a risky action or plan.

There may also be a flow of influence from the explicit, verbal system to the implicit system, in that the explicit system may decide on a plan of action or strategy, and exert an influence on the implicit system that will alter the reinforcement evaluations made by and the signals produced by the implicit system. An example of this might be that if a pregnant woman feels that she would like to escape a cruel mate, but is aware that she may not survive in the jungle, then it would be adaptive if the explicit system could suppress some aspects of her implicit behaviour towards her mate, so that she does not give signals that she is displeased with her situation[11]. Another example might be that the explicit system might, because of its long-term plans, influence the implicit system to increase its response to for example a positive reinforcer. One way in which the explicit system might influence the implicit system is by setting up the conditions in which, for example, when a given stimulus (e.g. person) is present, positive reinforcers are given, to facilitate stimulus–reinforcement association learning by the implicit system of the person receiving the positive reinforcers. Conversely, the implicit system may influence the explicit system, for example by highlighting certain stimuli in the environment that are currently associated with reward, to guide the attention of the explicit system to such stimuli.

However, it may be expected that there is often a conflict between these systems, in that the first, implicit, system is able to guide behaviour particularly to obtain the greatest immediate reinforcement, whereas the explicit system can potentially enable immediate rewards to be deferred, and longer-term, multistep, plans to be formed. This type of conflict will occur in animals with a syntactic planning ability, that is in humans and any other animals that have the ability to process a series of 'if ... then' stages of planning. This is a property of the human language system, and the extent to which it is a property of non-human primates is not yet fully clear. In any case, such conflict may be an important aspect of the operation of at least the human mind, because it is so essential for humans to decide correctly, at every moment, whether to invest in a relationship or a group that may offer long-term benefits, or whether to pursue immediate benefits directly (Nesse & Lloyd 1992).

Decision-making as implemented in neural networks in the brain is now becoming understood, and is described in Chapter 8. As shown there, two attractor states, each one corresponding to a decision, compete in an attractor single network with the evidence for

[11] In the literature on self-deception, it has been suggested that unconscious desires may not be made explicit in consciousness (or actually repressed), so as not to compromise the explicit system in what it produces (Alexander 1979, Trivers 1985, Nesse & Lloyd 1992).

each of the decisions acting as biases to each of the attractor states. The non-linear dynamics, and the way in which noise due to the random spiking of neurons makes the decision-making probabilistic, makes this a biologically plausible model of decision-making consistent with much neurophysiological and fMRI data (Wang 2002, Rolls & Deco 2010, Deco, Rolls, Albantakis & Romo 2013, Rolls 2016c).

I propose (Rolls 2005, Rolls 2014b) that this model applies to taking decisions between the implicit (unconscious) and explicit (conscious) systems in emotional decision-making, where the two different systems could provide the biasing inputs λ_1 and λ_2 to the model. An implication is that noise will influence with probabilistic outcomes which system takes a decision, depending on the magnitude of the competing inputs from the emotional and rational systems (see Section 8.2.2).

When decisions are taken, sometimes confabulation may occur, in that a verbal account of why the action was performed may be given, and this may not be related at all to the environmental event that actually triggered the action (Gazzaniga & LeDoux 1978, Gazzaniga 1988, Gazzaniga 1995, Rolls 2014b, LeDoux 2008, Rolls 2012d). It is accordingly possible that sometimes in normal humans when actions are initiated as a result of processing in a specialized brain region such as those involved in some types of rewarded behaviour, the language system may subsequently elaborate a coherent account of why that action was performed (i.e. confabulate). This would be consistent with a general view of brain evolution in which, as areas of the cortex evolve, they are laid on top of existing circuitry connecting inputs to outputs, and in which each level in this hierarchy of separate input–output pathways may control behaviour according to the specialized function it can perform. This hierarchical overlaying is an important concept advanced in this book as being important for understanding emotion, the different brain systems involved in different aspects of emotion and decision-making, and the relation between the implicit and explicit systems. When a new layer is added, previous layers may lose some of their importance, as appears to occur in the taste system in which in primates the subcortical processing from the brainstem nucleus of the solitary tract is lost; when the granular orbitofrontal cortex of primates becomes relatively more important than the amygdala; and when language areas are added on top of existing circuitry (Fig. 4.3) (Rolls 2016c).

10.2 A higher order syntactic thought theory of consciousness

The issue of why we have conscious feelings, that is the phenomenal problem of conscious, and how in terms of brain processing it feels like something to us, is the 'hard' problem of consciousness, to which philosophers and neuroscientists contribute. However, it is not clear what evidence would persuade us to believe one theory vs another. In this situation, nothing that is said here should be taken to have practical implications. However, I will describe one approach to consciousness, and then compare it with some other approaches. When we are interested in analyzing emotional feelings, it is therefore a 'hard' problem. But nevertheless a fascinating problem.

10.2.1 Rolls' higher order syntactic thought (HOST) theory of consciousness

One major approach to consciousness is the higher order thought (HOT) approach (Rosenthal 1986, Rosenthal 1990, Rosenthal 1993, Dennett 1991, Rolls 1995, Carruthers 1996, Rolls 1997a, Rolls 1997b, Rolls 1999a, Gennaro 2004, Rolls 2004c, Rosenthal

2004, Rolls 2005, Rosenthal 2005, Rolls 2007a, Rolls 2008a, Rolls 2007c, Rolls 2011a, Lau & Rosenthal 2011, Rosenthal 2012, Rolls 2013b, Rolls 2014b). In this approach, consciousness may *be* the state that arises in a system that can think about (or reflect on) its own (or other peoples') thoughts, that is in a system capable of second- or higher-order thoughts On this account, a mental state is non-introspectively (i.e. non-reflectively) conscious if one has a roughly simultaneous thought that one is in that mental state. Following from this, introspective consciousness (or reflexive consciousness, or self consciousness) is the attentive, deliberately focused consciousness of one's mental states. It is noted that not all of the higher-order thoughts need themselves be conscious (many mental states are not). However, according to the analysis, having a higher-order thought about a lower-order thought is necessary for the lower-order thought to be conscious.

I have developed this into a higher order syntactic thought (HOST) theory of consciousness, in which the arbitrary symbol-manipulation using important aspects of language processing and used for planning and especially in correcting plans but not in initiating all types of behaviour is close to what consciousness is about (Rolls 1995, Rolls 1997a, Rolls 1997b, Rolls 1999a, Rolls 2004c, Rolls 2005, Rolls 2007a, Rolls 2008a, Rolls 2007c, Rolls 2011a, Rolls 2013b, Rolls 2014b).

The proposal has as its foundation the type of computation that is being performed, and suggests that it is a property of a higher-order syntactic thought (HOST) system used for correcting multistep plans with its representations grounded in the world that it would feel like something for a system to be doing this type of processing. To do this type of processing, the system would have to be able to recall previous multistep plans, and would require syntax to keep the symbols in each step of the plan separate. In a sense, the system would have to be able to recall and take into consideration its earlier multistep plans, and in this sense *report* to itself, on those earlier plans. Some approaches to consciousness take the ability to report on or make a *commentary* on events as being an important marker for consciousness (Weiskrantz 1997), and the computational approach I propose suggests why there should be a close relation between consciousness and the ability to report or provide a commentary, for the ability to report is involved in using higher-order syntactic thoughts to correct a multistep plan.

An implication of the present approach is that the type of linguistic processing or reporting need not be verbal, using natural language, for what is required to correct the plan is the ability to manipulate symbols syntactically, and this could be implemented in a much simpler type of mentalese or syntactic system (Fodor 1994, Jackendoff 2002, Rolls 2004c) than verbal language or natural language which implies a universal grammar.

This approach to consciousness suggests that the information must be being processed in a system capable of implementing HOSTs for the information to be conscious, and in this sense is more specific than global workspace hypotheses (Baars 1988, Dehaene & Naccache 2001, Dehaene, Changeux, Naccache, Sackur & Sergent 2006, Dehaene, Charles, King & Marti 2014). Indeed, the present approach (Rolls 2014b, Rolls 2016c) suggests that a workspace could be sufficiently global to enable even the complex processing involved in driving a car to be performed, and yet the processing might be performed unconsciously, unless HOST (supervisory, monitory, correcting) processing was involved. Others may be moving in this direction (Dehaene, Lau & Kouider 2017).

The approach suggests that it just is a property of HOST computational processing with the representations grounded in the world that it feels like something. There is to some extent an element of mystery about why it feels like something, why it is phenomenal, but the explanatory gap does not seem so large when one holds that the system is recalling, reporting on, reflecting on, and reorganizing information about itself in the world in order to prepare new or revised plans.

An implication of these points is that my theory of consciousness is a computational theory. It argues that it is a property of a certain type of computational processing that it feels like something. In this sense, although the theory spans many levels from the neuronal to the computational, it is unlikely that any particular neuronal phenomena such as oscillations are necessary for consciousness, unless such computational processes happen to rely on some particular neuronal properties not involved in other neural computations but necessary for higher-order syntactic computations. It is these HOST computations and the system that implements them that this computational theory argues are necessary for consciousness.

As a point of clarification, I note that according to this theory, a language processing system (let alone a working memory (LeDoux 2008)) is not sufficient for consciousness. What defines a conscious system according to this analysis is the ability to have higher-order thoughts, and a first order language processor (that might be perfectly competent at language) would not be conscious, in that it could not think about its own or others' thoughts. One can perfectly well conceive of a system that obeyed the rules of language (which is the aim of some connectionist modelling), and implemented a first-order linguistic system, that would not be conscious. [Possible examples of language processing that might be performed non-consciously include computer programs implementing aspects of language, or ritualized human conversations, e.g., about the weather. These might require syntax and correctly grounded semantics, and yet be performed non-consciously. A more complex example, illustrating that syntax could be used, might be "If A does X, then B will probably do Y, and then C would be able to do Z." A first order language system could process this statement. Moreover, the first order language system could apply the rule usefully in the world, provided that the symbols in the language system (A, B, X, Y etc.) are grounded (have meaning) in the world.]

A second clarification is that the plan would have to be a unique string of steps, in much the same way as a sentence can be a unique and one-off (or one-time) string of words. The point here is that it is helpful to be able to think about particular one-off plans, and to correct them; and that this type of operation is very different from the slow learning of fixed rules by trial and error, or the application of fixed rules by a supervisory part of a computer program.

These are my initial thoughts on why we have consciousness, and are conscious of sensory, emotional and motivational qualia, as well as qualia associated with first-order linguistic thoughts. However, as stated above, one does not feel that there are straightforward criteria in this philosophical field of enquiry for knowing whether the suggested theory is correct; so it is likely that theories of consciousness will continue to undergo rapid development; and current theories should not be taken to have practical implications.

10.2.2 Adaptive value of processing in the system that is related to consciousness

It is suggested that part of the evolutionary *adaptive significance* of this type of higher-order syntactic thought system is that it enables correction of errors made in first-order linguistic or in non-linguistic processing.

Indeed, the ability to reflect on previous events is extremely important for learning from them, including setting up new long-term semantic structures. The hippocampus may be a system for 'declarative' recall of recent memories (see also Squire, Stark & Clark (2004)). Its close relation to 'conscious' processing in humans (Squire has classified it as a declarative memory system) may be simply that it enables the recall of recent memories, which can then be reflected upon in conscious, higher-order, processing, and can thereby guide the formation of new semantic representations (Rolls 2016c, Rolls 2018). Another part of the adaptive value of a higher-order thought system may be that by thinking about its own thoughts in a given situation, it may be able to understand better the thoughts of another individual in a similar situation, and therefore predict that individual's behaviour better (Humphrey 1980, Humphrey 1986).

The *computational hypothesis* is that by thinking about lower-order thoughts, the higher-order thoughts can discover what may be weak links in the chain of reasoning at the lower-order level, and having detected the weak link, might alter the plan, to see if this gives better success. In our example above, if it transpired that C could not do Z, how might the plan have failed? Instead of having to go through endless random changes to the plan to see if by trial and error some combination does happen to produce results, what I am suggesting is that by thinking about the previous plan, one might, for example, using knowledge of the situation and the probabilities that operate in it, guess that the step where the plan failed was that B did not in fact do Y. So by thinking about the plan (the first- or lower-order thought), one might correct the original plan in such a way that the weak link in that chain, that 'B will probably do Y', is circumvented.

To draw a parallel with neural networks: there is a **'credit assignment'** problem in such multistep syntactic plans, in that if the whole plan fails, how does the system assign credit or blame to particular steps of the plan? [In multilayer neural networks, the credit assignment problem is that if errors are being specified at the output layer, the problem arises about how to propagate back the error to earlier, hidden, layers of the network to assign credit or blame to individual synaptic connection; see Rumelhart, Hinton & Williams (1986) and Rolls (2016c).] **My suggestion is that this solution to the credit assignment problem for a one-off syntactic plan is the function of higher-order thoughts, and is why systems with higher-order thoughts evolved. The suggestion I then make is that if a system were doing this type of processing (thinking about its own thoughts), it would then be very plausible that it should feel like something to be doing this.** I even suggest to the reader that it is not plausible to suggest that it would not feel like anything to a system if it were doing this.

I note that it is important that the symbols being manipulated in this HOST system may need to be grounded in the world, that in some sense, the symbols 'matter' to the thinker. This issue of symbol grounding is treated elsewhere (Rolls 2014b).

In line with the argument on the adaptive value of higher-order thoughts and thus consciousness given above, that they are useful for correcting lower-order thoughts, I now suggest that correction using higher-order thoughts of lower-order thoughts would have adaptive value primarily if the lower-order thoughts are sufficiently complex to benefit from correction in this way. The nature of the complexity is specific – that it should involve syntactic manipulation of symbols, probably with several steps in the chain, and that the chain of steps should be a one-off (or in American usage, 'one-time', meaning used once) set of steps, as in a sentence or in a particular plan used just once, rather than a set of well learned rules. The first or lower-order thoughts might involve a linked chain of 'if ... then' statements that would be involved in planning, an example of which has been given above, and this type of cognitive processing is thought to be a primary basis for human skilled performance (Anderson 1996). It is partly because complex lower-order thoughts such as these that involve syntax and language would benefit from correction by higher-order thoughts that I suggest that there is a close link between this reflective consciousness and language. However, whenever this HOST system in the brain is engaged in processing, whatever the first order material being processed, then I suggest that we are conscious.

10.3 Comparison with other theories of consciousness

10.3.1 Higher-order thought theories

Some ways in which the current theory may be different from other higher-order thought theories (Rosenthal 2004, Rosenthal 2005, Rosenthal 2012, Gennaro 2004, Carruthers 2000) is that it provides an account of the evolutionary, adaptive, value of a higher-order thought system in helping to solve a credit assignment problem that arises in a multistep syntactic plan, links this type of processing to consciousness, and therefore emphasizes a role for syntactic processing in consciousness. The type of syntactic processing need not be at the natural language level (which implies a universal grammar), but could be at the level of mentalese or simpler, as it involves primarily the syntactic manipulation of symbols (Fodor 1994, Rolls 2014b, Rolls 2016c).

The current theory holds that it is higher-order linguistic thoughts (HOLTs) (or higher-order syntactic thoughts, HOSTs (Rolls 2004c, Rolls 2007a, Rolls 2011a, Rolls 2014b, Rolls 2016c)) that are closely associated with consciousness, and this might differ from Rosenthal's higher-order thoughts (HOTs) theory (Rosenthal 1986, Rosenthal 1990, Rosenthal 1993, Rosenthal 2004, Rosenthal 2005, Rosenthal 2012) in the emphasis in the current theory on language. Language in the current theory is defined by syntactic manipulation of symbols, and does not necessarily imply verbal (or natural) language.

The reason that strong emphasis is placed on language is that it is as a result of having a multistep, flexible, 'one-off', reasoning procedure that errors can be corrected by using 'thoughts about thoughts'. This enables correction of errors that cannot be easily corrected by reward or punishment received at the end of the reasoning, due to the credit assignment problem. That is, there is a need for some type of supervisory and monitoring process, to detect where errors in the reasoning have occurred. It is having such a HOST brain system, and it becoming engaged (even if only a little), that according to the HOST theory is associated with phenomenal consciousness.

This suggestion on the adaptive value in evolution of such a higher-order linguistic thought process for multistep planning ahead, and correcting such plans, may also be different from earlier work. Put another way, this point is that *credit assignment* when reward or punishment is received is straightforward in a one-layer network (in which the reinforcement can be used directly to correct nodes in error, or responses), but is very difficult in a multistep linguistic process executed once.

Some computer programs may have supervisory processes. Should these count as higher-order linguistic thought processes? My current response to this is that they should not, to the extent that they operate with fixed rules to correct the operation of a system that does not itself involve linguistic thoughts about symbols grounded semantically in the external world. If on the other hand it were possible to implement on a computer such a high-order linguistic thought–supervisory correction process to correct first-order one-off linguistic thoughts with symbols grounded in the real world, then prima facie this process would be conscious. If it were possible in a thought experiment to reproduce the neural connectivity and operation of a human brain on a computer, then prima facie it would also have the attributes of consciousness[12]. It might continue to have those attributes for as long as power was applied to the system. [I note here that the ways in which brains and digital computers operate is completely different, and I have elucidated the differences in Section 26.3 of Rolls (2016c). However, it is still in principle possible to simulate the operation of a brain system on a digital computer, by simulating the dynamics of neurons and of populations of neurons (Rolls 2016c).]

Another possible difference from earlier theories is that raw sensory feels are suggested to arise as a consequence of having a system that can think about its own thoughts. Raw sensory feels, and subjective states associated with emotional and motivational states, may not necessarily arise first in evolution.

A property often attributed to consciousness is that it is *unitary*. The current theory would account for this by the limited syntactic capability of neuronal networks in the brain, which render it difficult to implement more than a few syntactic bindings of symbols simultaneously (Rolls & Treves 1998, McLeod, Plunkett & Rolls 1998, Rolls & Deco 2015b, Rolls 2016c). This limitation makes it difficult to run several 'streams of consciousness' simultaneously. In addition, given that a linguistic system can control behavioural output, several parallel streams might produce maladaptive behaviour (apparent as, e.g. indecision), and might be selected against. The close relationship between, and the limited capacity of, both the stream of consciousness, and auditory–verbal short-term working memory, may be that both implement the capacity for syntax in neural networks (Rolls & Deco 2015b).

The hypothesis that syntactic binding is necessary for consciousness is one of the postulates of the theory I am describing (for the system I describe must be capable of correcting its own syntactic thoughts). The fact that the binding must be implemented in neuronal networks may well place limitations on consciousness that lead to some of its properties, such as its unitary nature.

This raises discussion of the *causal role of consciousness*. Does consciousness cause our behaviour? The view that I currently hold is that the information processing that is related to consciousness (activity in a linguistic system capable of higher-order thoughts, and used for planning and correcting the operation of lower-order linguistic systems) can play a causal role in producing our behaviour (see Fig. 4.3), but as part of a 'levels of explanation' account of the relation between mental events and brain events (Rolls 2016c). [My account of the mind-body (or mind-brain) problem is, in brief, that causality operates within levels, but not between levels. Thus we may speak of one neuronal event as causing another neuronal event a little later. At a higher level of explanation, these neuronal events may be expressed as thought processes. (After all, thoughts must be implemented by neuronal activity in the brain, and most neuroscientists would take this position.) And at the level of thoughts, we can speak about one thought as causing another a little later. But to introduce causality as operating between levels would just introduce confusion, as these events at different levels would be simultaneous, and a property of causality is that time is involved. These important issues are considered in more detail elsewhere (Rolls (2016c) Chapter 26).] It is, I postulate, a property of processing in this system (capable of higher-order thoughts) that it feels like something to be performing that type of processing. It is in this sense that I suggest that consciousness can act causally to influence our behaviour – consciousness is the property that occurs when a

[12] This is a functionalist position. Apparently Damasio (2003) does not subscribe to this view, for he suggests that there is something in the 'stuff' (the 'natural medium') that the brain is made of that is also important. It is difficult for a person with this view to make telling points about consciousness from neuroscience, for it may always be the 'stuff' that is actually important.

linguistic system is thinking about its lower-order thoughts, which may be useful in correcting plans.

The hypothesis that it does feel like something when this processing is taking place is at least to some extent testable (cf. Lau & Rosenthal (2011)): humans performing this type of higher-order linguistic processing, for example recalling episodic memories and comparing them with current circumstances, who denied being conscious, would prima facie constitute evidence against the theory. Most humans would find it very implausible though to posit that they could be thinking about their own thoughts, and reflecting on their own thoughts, without being conscious. This type of processing does appear, for most humans, to be necessarily conscious.

It is suggested that qualia, raw sensory, and emotional, 'feels', arise secondarily to having evolved such a higher-order thought system, and that sensory and emotional processing feels like something because once this emotional processing has entered the planning, higher-order thought, system, it would be unparsimonious for it not to feel like something, given that all the other processing in this system I suggest does feel like something.

The adaptive value of having sensory and emotional feelings, or qualia, is thus suggested to be that such inputs are important to the long-term planning, explicit, processing system. Raw sensory feels, and subjective states associated with emotional and motivational states, may not necessarily arise first in evolution.

Reasons why the ventral visual system is more closely related to explicit than implicit processing include the fact that representations of objects and individuals need to enter the planning, hence conscious, system, and are considered in more detail by Rolls (2003) and by Rolls (2016c).

A slightly weaker position than Rosenthal's (and mine) on this is that a conscious state corresponds to a first-order thought that has the capacity to cause a second-order thought or judgement about it (Carruthers 1996). Another position that is close in some respects to that of Carruthers and the present position is that of Chalmers (1996), that awareness is something that has direct availability for behavioural control, which amounts effectively for him in humans to saying that consciousness is what we can report (verbally) about (see (Rolls 2014b).

10.3.2 Oscillations and temporal binding

The postulate of Crick & Koch (1990) that oscillations and synchronization are necessary bases of consciousness might possibly be related to the present theory if it turns out that oscillations or neuronal synchronization are the way the brain implements syntactic binding. However, the fact that oscillations and neuronal synchronization are especially evident in anaesthetized cats does not impress as strong evidence that oscillations and synchronization are critical features of consciousness, for most people would hold that anaesthetized cats are not conscious. The fact that oscillations and stimulus-dependent neuronal synchronization are much more difficult to demonstrate in the temporal cortical visual areas of awake behaving monkeys (Tovee & Rolls 1992, Franco, Rolls, Aggelopoulos & Treves 2004, Aggelopoulos, Franco & Rolls 2005, Rolls 2016c, Rolls & Treves 2011) might just mean that during the evolution of primates the cortex has become better able to avoid parasitic oscillations, as a result of developing better feedforward and feedback inhibitory circuits (Rolls 2016c).

The suggestion that syntax in real neuronal networks is implemented by temporal binding (Malsburg 1990, Singer 1999) seems unlikely (Rolls 2016c, Rolls & Treves 2011). For example, the code about which visual stimulus has been shown can be read off from the end of the visual system without taking the temporal aspects of the neuronal firing into account; much of the information about which stimulus is shown is available in short times of 30–50 ms, and cortical neurons need fire for only this long during the identification of objects

(Tovee, Rolls, Treves & Bellis 1993, Rolls & Tovee 1994, Tovee & Rolls 1995, Rolls & Treves 1998, Rolls 2003, Rolls 2006a, Rolls 2016c, Rolls & Treves 2011) (these are rather short time-windows for the expression of multiple separate populations of synchronized neurons); and stimulus-dependent synchronization of firing between neurons is not a quantitatively important way of encoding information in the primate temporal cortical visual areas involved in the representation of objects and faces (Tovee & Rolls 1992, Rolls & Treves 1998, Rolls, Franco, Aggelopoulos & Reece 2003b, Rolls, Aggelopoulos, Franco & Treves 2004, Franco, Rolls, Aggelopoulos & Treves 2004, Aggelopoulos, Franco & Rolls 2005, Rolls 2016c, Rolls & Treves 2011, Rolls 2012e).

Further, even the hypothesis that information transmission is facilitated by coherent (phase locked) oscillations (communication through coherence (Fries 2005, Fries 2009)) has considerable difficulties (Rolls, Webb & Deco 2012), in that although there is much emphasis on finding coherence in the brain, there is much less causal evidence that coherence affects the transmission of information. In a test of this, it was found in an integrate-and-fire model of two connected networks in which causal effects of gamma oscillations (approximately 50 Hz) could be analysed, that information transmission between coupled networks occurs at very much lower strengths of the connecting synapses than are required to make the oscillations coherent (Rolls et al. 2012). The finding was thus that information transmission does not require, and is little influenced by, gamma oscillations. The implication is that great care is needed to test whether coherence in the brain has causal effects in influencing information transmission, at least in the gamma band (Rolls et al. 2012, Rolls & Treves 2011).

10.3.3 A high neural threshold for information to reach consciousness

Part in fact of Rolls' theory of consciousness is that it provides a computational reason why the threshold for information to reach consciousness is higher than the threshold for information to influence behaviour in what is referred to as subliminal processing (Dehaene, Changeux, Naccache, Sackur & Sergent 2006).

Evidence that explicit, conscious, processing may have a higher threshold in sensory processing than implicit processing is considered by Rolls (2003, 2006a, 2011a) based on neurophysiological and psychophysical investigations of backward masking (Rolls & Tovee 1994, Rolls, Tovee, Purcell, Stewart & Azzopardi 1994b, Rolls, Tovee & Panzeri 1999b, Rolls 2003, Rolls 2006a, Rolls 2016c, Rolls 2012e). It is suggested there that part of the adaptive value of this is that if linguistic processing is inherently serial and slow, it may be maladaptive to interrupt it unless there is a high probability that the interrupting signal does not arise from noise in the system. In the psychophysical and neurophysiological studies, it was found that face stimuli presented for 16 ms and followed immediately by a masking stimulus were not consciously perceived by humans, yet produced above chance identification, and firing of inferior temporal cortex neurons in macaques for approximately 30 ms. If the mask was delayed for 20 ms, the neurons fired for approximately 50 ms, and the test face stimuli were more likely to be perceived consciously. In a similar backward masking paradigm, it was found that happy vs angry face expressions could influence how much beverage was wanted and consumed even when the faces were not consciously perceived (Winkielman & Berridge 2005, Winkielman & Berridge 2003). This is further evidence that unconscious emotional stimuli can influence behaviour.

10.3.4 James–Lange theory and Damasio's somatic marker hypothesis about feelings

The theory described here is also different from other theories of consciousness and affect. James and Lange (James 1884, Lange 1885) held that emotional feelings arise when feedback from the periphery (about for example heart rate) reach the brain, but had no theory of why some stimuli and not others produced the peripheral changes, and thus of why some but not other events produce emotional feelings.

Moreover, the evidence that feedback from peripheral autonomic and proprioceptive systems is essential for emotions is very weak, in that for example blocking peripheral feedback does not eliminate emotions, and producing peripheral, e.g. autonomic, changes does not elicit emotion (Reisenzein 1983, Schachter & Singer 1962, Rolls 1999a) (see Section 2.4.1).

Damasio's theory of emotion (Damasio 1994, Damasio 2003) is a similar theory to the James–Lange theory (and is therefore subject to some of the same objections), but holds that the peripheral feedback is used in decision-making rather than in consciousness. He does not formally define emotions, but holds that body maps and representations are the basis of emotions. When considering consciousness, he assumes that all consciousness is self-consciousness (Damasio 2003) (p. 184), and that 'the foundational images in the stream of the mind are images of some kind of body event, whether the event happens in the depth of the body or in some specialized sensory device near its periphery' (Damasio 2003) (p. 197). His theory does not appear to be a fully testable theory, in that he suspects that "the ultimate quality of feelings, a part of why feelings feel the way they feel, is conferred by the neural medium" (Damasio 2003) (p. 131). Thus presumably if the processes he discusses (Damasio 1994, Damasio 2003) were implemented in a computer, then the computer would not have all the same properties with respect to consciousness as the real brain. In this sense he appears to be arguing for a non-functionalist position, and something crucial about consciousness being related to the particular biological machinery from which the system is made. In this respect the theory seems somewhat intangible.

10.3.5 LeDoux's approach to emotion and consciousness

LeDoux's approach to emotion (LeDoux 1992, LeDoux 1995, LeDoux 1996, LeDoux 2008, LeDoux 2012) has been largely (to quote him) one of automaticity, with emphasis on brain mechanisms involved in the rapid, subcortical, mechanisms involved in fear. LeDoux (1996), in line with Johnson-Laird (1988) and Baars (1988), emphasizes the role of working memory in consciousness, where he views working memory as a limited-capacity serial processor that creates and manipulates symbolic representations (p. 280). He thus holds that much emotional processing is unconscious, and that when it becomes conscious it is because emotional information is entered into a working memory system. However, LeDoux (1996) concedes that consciousness, especially its phenomenal or subjective nature, is not completely explained by the computational processes that underlie working memory (p. 281). More recently, LeDoux has moved towards a higher order theory of consciousness, and argues that 'general networks of cognition' are involved (LeDoux & Brown 2017). This is a much less well defined processing system than the higher order syntactic thought processing system that I suggest is related to consciousness.

10.3.6 Global workspace theories of consciousness

Rolls' approach to consciousness suggests that the information must be being processed in a system capable of implementing HOSTs for the information to be conscious, and in this sense is more specific than global workspace hypotheses (Baars 1988, Dehaene & Naccache 2001, Dehaene et al. 2006, Dehaene et al. 2014). Indeed, the present approach suggests that a workspace could be sufficiently global to enable even the complex processing involved in driving a car to be performed, and yet the processing might be performed unconsciously, unless HOST (supervisory, monitory, correcting) processing was involved.

10.3.7 Monitoring and consciousness

An attractor network in the brain with positive feedback implemented by excitatory recurrent collateral connections between the neurons can implement decision-making (Wang 2002, Deco & Rolls 2006, Wang 2008, Rolls & Deco 2010) (see Chapter 8). As explained in detail elsewhere (Rolls & Deco 2010), if the external evidence for the decision is consistent with the decision taken (which has been influenced by the noisy neuronal firing times), then the firing rates in the winning attractor are supported by the external evidence, and become especially high. If the external evidence is contrary to the noise-influenced decision, then the firing rates of the neurons in the winning attractor are not supported by the external evidence, and are lower than expected (Fig. 8.3). In this way the confidence in a decision is reflected in, and encoded by, the firing rates of the neurons in the winning attractor population of neurons (Rolls & Deco 2010).

If we now add a second attractor network to read the firing rates from the first decision-making network, the second attractor network can take a decision based on the confidence expressed in the firing rates in the first network (Insabato, Pannunzi, Rolls & Deco 2010). The second attractor network allows decisions to be made about whether to change the decision made by the first network, and for example abort the trial or strategy. The second network, the confidence decision network, is in effect monitoring the decisions taken by the first network, and can cause a change of strategy or behaviour if the assessment of the decision taken by the first network does not seem a confident decision. This is described in detail elsewhere (Insabato, Pannunzi, Rolls & Deco 2010, Rolls & Deco 2010, Rolls 2014b), and shows that a simple system of two attractor networks can enable confidence-based (second-level) decisions to be made, by monitoring the output of the first, decision-making, network.

Now this is the type of description, and language used, to describe 'monitoring' functions, taken to be a high-level cognitive process, possibly related to consciousness (Block 1995, Lycan 1997). For example, in an experiment performed by Hampton (2001) (experiment 3), a monkey had to remember a picture over a delay. He was then given a choice of a 'test flag', in which case he would be allowed to choose from one of four pictures the one seen before the delay, and if correct earn a large reward (a peanut). If he was not sure that he remembered the first picture, he could choose an 'escape flag', to start another trial. With longer delays, when memory strength might be lower partly due to noise in the system, and confidence therefore in the memory on some trials might be lower, the monkey was more likely to choose the escape flag. The experiment is described as showing that the monkey is thinking about his own memory, that is, is a case of meta-memory, which may be related to consciousness (Heyes 2008). However, the decision about whether to escape from a trial can be taken just by adding a second decision network to the first decision network. Thus we can account for what seem like complex cognitive phenomena with a simple system of two attractor decision-making networks (Rolls & Deco 2010, Rolls 2012d).

The implication is that some types of 'self-monitoring' can be accounted for by simple, two-attractor network, computational processes. But what of more complex 'self-monitoring', such as is described as occurring in a commentary that might be based on reflection on previous events, and appears to be closely related to consciousness (Weiskrantz 1997). This approach has been developed into my higher-order syntactic theory (HOST) of consciousness (Section

10 (Rolls 1997b, Rolls 2004c, Rolls 2005, Rolls 2007a, Rolls 2008a, Rolls 2007c, Rolls 2010a, Rolls 2011a, Rolls 2012d, Rolls 2014b, Rolls 2016c)), in which there is a credit assignment problem if a multi-step reasoned plan fails, and it may be unclear which step failed. Now this type of 'self-monitoring' is much more complex, as it requires syntax. The thrust of the argument is that some types of 'self-monitoring' are computationally simple, for example in decisions made based on confidence in a first decision (Insabato et al. 2010, Rolls & Deco 2010), and may have little to do with consciousness; whereas higher-order thought processes are very different in terms of the type of syntactic computation required, and may be more closely related to consciousness (Rolls 1997b, Rolls 2003, Rolls 2004c, Rolls 2005, Rolls 2007a, Rolls 2008a, Rolls 2007c, Rolls 2010a, Rolls 2011a, Rolls 2012d, Rolls 2014b, Rolls 2016c).

Thus the theory of consciousness described in this chapter is different from some other theories of consciousness.

11 Conclusions, and broader issues

11.1 Conclusions

Let us evaluate where we have reached in this book, before we consider some broader issues, including the background that this biological approach to emotion provides for understanding some issues that arise in aesthetics, ethics, and economics, which are developed further in *Neuroculture: On the Implications of Brain Science* (Rolls 2012d).

1. We have a scientific approach to emotion, its nature, and its functions (Chapters 2 and 3). It has been shown that this approach can help with classifying different emotions (Chapter 2), and in understanding what information processing systems in the brain are involved in emotion, and how they are involved (Chapters 4–6).

2. We have reached a quite specific view about how brains are designed around reward and punishment value systems, because this is the way that genes can build a complex system that will produce appropriate but flexible behaviour to increase their fitness, as described in Chapter 3. The way that evolution by natural selection does this is to build us with reward and punishment systems that will direct our behaviour towards goals in such a way that survival and in particular reproductive fitness are achieved. By specifying goals, rather than particular responses, genes leave much more open the possible behavioural strategies that might be required to increase their fitness. Specifying particular responses would be inefficient in terms of behavioural flexibility as environments change during evolution, and also would be more genetically costly to specify (in terms of the information to be encoded and the possibility of error). This view of the evolutionarily adaptive value for genes to build organisms using reward- and punishment-decoding and action systems in the brain places one squarely in line as a scientist from Darwin, and is a key part of my theory of emotion that will I envisage stand the test of time.

The theory helps us to understand much of sensory information processing in the brain, followed by reward and punishment value encoding, followed by action selection to obtain the goals identified by the sensory/reinforcer decoding systems. Value coding systems must be separate from purely sensory or motor systems, and while a goal is being sought, or if a goal is not obtained, the value-related representation must remain to direct further goal-directed behaviour, and it is these continuing goal-related states to which emotion is related.

3. The importance of reward and punishment systems in brain design helps us to understand not only the significance and importance of emotion, but also of motivational behaviour, which frequently involves working to obtain goals that are specified by the current state of internal signals to achieve homeostasis (see Chapter 5 on hunger and Rolls (2005) on thirst) or are influenced by internal hormonal signals (Chapter

7 on sexual behaviour). Indeed, motivation may be seen as a state in which one is working for a goal, and emotion as a state that occurs when the goal, a reinforcer, is obtained or is not obtained, and that may persist afterwards. The concept of gene-defined reinforcers providing the goals for action helps to understand the relation between motivational states (or desires) and emotion, as the organism must be built to be motivated to obtain the goals, and to be placed in a different state (emotion) when the goal is or is not achieved by the action. Emotional states may be motivating, as in frustrative non-reward. The close but clear relation between motivation and emotion is that both involve what humans describe as affective states (e.g. feeling hungry, liking the taste of a food, feeling happy because of a social reinforcer), and both are about goals.

4. We have outlined in Chapters 4–6 what may be the fundamental architectural and design principles of the brain for sensory, reward value, and punishment value information processing in primates *including humans*. These architectural principles include the following:

(a) For potential secondary reinforcers, analysis is to the stage of invariant object identification before reward and punisher associations are learned. The reason for this is to enable correct generalization to other instances of the same or similar objects, even when a reward or punisher has been associated with one instance previously.

(b) The representation of the object is (appropriately) in a form that is ideal as an input to pattern associators that allow the reinforcement associations to be learned. The representations are appropriately encoded in that they can be decoded by dot product decoding of the type that is very neuronally plausible; are distributed so allowing excellent generalization and graceful degradation; have relatively independent information conveyed by different neurons in the ensemble thus allowing very high capacity; and allow much of the information to be read off very quickly, in periods of 20–50 ms (see Chapter 4, Rolls (2016c), and Rolls & Treves (2011)).

(c) An aim of processing in the ventral visual system (which projects to the inferior temporal visual cortex) is to help select the goals, or objects with reward or punisher associations, for actions. Action is concerned with the identification and selection of goals, for action, in the environment. The ventral visual system is crucially involved in this. I thus disagree with Milner & Goodale (1995) that the dorsal visual system is for the control of action, and the ventral visual system for 'perception', e.g. perceptual and cognitive representations. The ventral visual system is concerned with selecting the goals for action. It does this by providing invariant representations of objects, with a representation that is appropriate for interfacing to systems [such as the amygdala and orbitofrontal cortex, see Chapter 4, and Figs. 4.2 and 4.3 in which association cortex would correspond in vision to the inferior temporal visual cortex] which determine using pattern association the reward or punishment value of the object, as part of the process of selecting which goal is appropriate for action. Some of the evidence for this described in Chapter 4 is that large lesions of the temporal lobes (which damage the ventral visual system and some of its outputs such as the amygdala) produce the Kluver-Bucy syndrome, in which monkeys select objects indiscriminately, independently of their reward value, and place them in their mouths. The dorsal visual system helps with executing those actions, for example with shaping the hand appropriately to pick up a selected object. (Often this type of sensorimotor operation is performed implicitly, i.e. without conscious awareness.) In so far as explicit planning about future goals and actions requires knowledge of objects and their reward or punisher associations, it is the ventral visual system that provides the appropriate input for planning future actions. Further, for the same reason, I propose that when explicit, or conscious, planning is required, activity in the ventral visual system will be closely related to consciousness, because it is to objects, represented in the ventral visual system, that we normally apply multi-step planning processes.

(d) For primary reinforcers, the reward decoding may occur after several stages of processing, as in the primate taste system in which reward is decoded only after the primary taste cortex. The architectural principle here is that in primates there is one main taste information-processing stream in the brain, via the thalamus to the primary taste cortex, and the information about the identity of the taste is not biased by modulation of how good the taste is before this, so that the taste representation in the primary cortex can be used for purposes that are not reward-dependent. One example might be learning where a particular taste can be found in the environment, even when the primate is not hungry and therefore the taste is not currently rewarding. In the case of other sensory systems, the reinforcement value may be made explicit early on in sensory processing. This occurs, for example, in the pain system. The architectural basis of this is that there are different channels (nerve fibres) for pain and touch, so that the affective value and the identity of a tactile stimulus can be carried by separate parallel information channels, allowing separate representation and processing of each.

(e) In non-primates including, for example, rodents, the design principles may involve less sophisticated design features, partly because the stimuli being processed are simpler. For example, view-invariant object recognition is probably much less developed in non-primates, with the recognition that is possible being based more on physical similarity in terms of texture, colour, simple features, etc. (Rolls 2016c). It may be because there is less sophisticated cortical processing of visual stimuli in this way that other sensory systems are also organized more simply in rodents, with, for example, some (but not total, only perhaps 30%) modulation of taste processing by hunger early in sensory processing in rodents (Scott, Yan & Rolls 1995, Rolls & Scott 2003) (Section 1.3). Further, while it is appropriate usually to have emotional responses to well-processed objects (e.g. the sight of a particular person), there are instances, such as a loud noise or a pure tone associated with punishment, where it may be possible to tap off a sensory representation early in sensory information processing that can be used to produce emotional responses, and this may occur, for example, in rodents, where the subcortical auditory system provides afferents to the amygdala (see Chapter 4).

(f) Another design principle is that the outputs of the reward and punishment value systems must be treated by the action system as being the goals for action. The action systems must be built to try to maximize the activation of the representations produced by rewarding events, and to minimize the activation of the representations produced by punishers or stimuli associated with punishers. Drug addiction produced by the psychomotor stimulants such as amphetamine and cocaine can be seen as activating the brain at the stage where the outputs of the amygdala and orbitofrontal cortex, which provide representations of whether stimuli are associated with rewards or punishers, are fed into the ventral striatum to influence approach behaviour. The fact that addiction is persistent may be related to the fact that because the outputs of the amygdala and orbitofrontal cortex are after the stage of stimulus–reinforcer learning, and after sensory-specific satiety has been computed, the action system has to be built to interpret the representations they provide as meaning reward value, and a goal for action.

5. Especially in primates, the visual processing in emotional and social behaviour requires sophisticated representation of individuals, and for this there are many neurons devoted to face processing (Rolls 2011c). In addition, there is a separate system that encodes face gesture, movement, and view, as all are important in social behaviour, for interpreting whether a particular individual, with his or her own reinforcement associations, is producing threats or appeasements (Rolls 2011c, Rolls 2012e, Rolls 2014b, Rolls 2016c).

6. After mainly unimodal processing to the object level, sensory systems then project into convergence zones. Those especially important for reward and punishment, emotion and motivation, are the orbitofrontal cortex and amygdala, where primary reinforcers are represented to encode **outcome value**. These parts of the brain appear to be especially important in emotion and motivation not only because they are the parts of the brain where in primates the primary (unlearned) reinforcing value of stimuli is represented, but also because they are the parts of the brain that perform pattern-association learning between potential secondary reinforcers and primary reinforcers to compute **expected value**. They are thus the parts of the brain involved in learning the emotional and motivational **reward value** of stimuli.

The orbitofrontal cortex is involved in the rapid, one-trial, reversal of emotional behaviour when the reinforcement contingencies change, and this may be implemented by switching a rule, as described in Section 4.5.5. These orbitofrontal cortex neurons may be described as *expected value* neurons. This rapid, rule-based, reversal and re-valuation of stimuli to encode their current reward value in one trial and using rules may be a computation made possible by the development of the granular orbitofrontal cortex and connected areas that are not present in rodents (Section 1.3).

7. The different reward valuation systems are specified to have values scaled appropriately by genes to lead to their selection in such a way that reproductive success is maximized. In addition, the reward systems are specific, encode the value of specific rewards and punishers, and have tendencies to self-regulate, so that they operate on a common value scale that leads to the selection of different rewards with appropriately balanced probabilities, and often depending on modulation by internal motivational signals. The presence of many different reward value systems operating with a **common scale of value** helps each reward to be selected to maximize reproductive success. There is no conversion to a common currency, as this would no longer encode the specific reward to which the action system should direct action. The value of a reward or punisher specified by genes may be rescaled by learning, as in taste aversion learning (Scott 2011) and conditioned appetite and satiety (Booth 1985).

8. A principle that assists the selection of different behaviours is sensory-specific satiety, which builds up when a reward is repeated for a number of minutes. A principle that helps behaviour to lock on to one goal for at least a useful period is incentive motivation, the process by which early on in the presentation of a reward there is reward potentiation. There are probably simple neurophysiological bases for these time-dependent processes in the reward (as opposed to the early sensory) systems that involve synaptic habituation and (non-associative) facilitation respectively.

9. With the advances made in the last 30 years in understanding the brain mechanisms involved in reward and punishment, and emotion and motivation, the basis for addiction to drugs is becoming clearer, with dopamine playing an important role, particularly in the conditioned reinforcing effects of stimuli associated with drug usage, which influence 'wanting' for the addictive substance. Further, now that we are starting to understand how different brain systems contribute to emotion, this provides a better foundation for developing pharmacological treatments for depression and anxiety that may target particular brain areas (Chapter 6).

10. The representation in the orbitofrontal cortex appears indeed to represent economic value, in that neuronal responses and neural activations appear to be related closely to what is chosen, and also to the conscious subjective value or pleasantness rating placed on a 'good'. The orbitofrontal cortex activity reflects by these measures of **economic value** the effects of risk (the probability that a reward will be available), of ambiguity (whether the outcome probability is known), of temporal discounting, and of the tradeoff between the amount of the good that is available and the value of the good. Value is represented on a continuous scale in the orbitofrontal cortex, and indeed orbitofrontal cortex activations are linearly related to the subjective pleasantness (medially) or unpleasantness (laterally) of stimuli or events.

11. The reward value placed on different rewards and the punishment value placed on different non-rewards or punishers will be different between different individuals, as a result of genetic variation for natural selection. Also, most humans cannot perform economic calculations of the expected value of different choices, as the human brain operates primarily by similarity comparisons and not by logical calculations of the type implemented in computers (Rolls 2016c). For these reasons, classical microeconomics with its approach of a few axioms and a rational actor can no longer be considered as what really may account for the behaviour of humans and other animals. Instead, classical (micro)economics may be replaced by an understanding in neuroeconomics of how heuristics guided by evolution make different rewards and costs become differently scaled in different individuals, and further how choices may be selected by a decision-making process based on in-built and probabilistic heuristics rather than by correctly computed calculations in a rational, reasoning, decision-making actor.

12. The orbitofrontal cortex represents the value of stimuli. Its neurons respond to stimulus value, and not to behavioural responses. The orbitofrontal cortex provides outputs to:

(a) the anterior cingulate cortex for goal-directed actions taking into account the costs of the actions (Section 4.7), and for which positive value is represented in the pregenual anterior cingulate cortex and negative value more dorsally in the supracallosal anterior cingulate cortex, for interfacing to motor / action representations in the midcingulate cortex;

(b) the basal ganglia for stimulus-response habits (Section 6.3);

(c) the amygdala, which implements Pavlovian learning processes which enable stimuli to elicit approach or withdrawal as well as affective states which may become the goals for instrumental actions;

(d) and with the amygdala, implements Pavlovian learning processes which enable autonomic and endocrine responses to be elicited by conditioned stimuli (Section 4.6).

13. Decision-making is now understood as a non-linear competition between different attractor states in an attractor neuronal network that results in a single winner. The decision variables bias the neurons in the different possible attractor states. The mechanism is understood at the level of integrate-and-fire neurons with biophysically realistic parameters. The decision-making is probabilistic because of statistical fluctuations introduced by the approximately Poisson nature of the timing of the spikes of the neurons for a given mean firing rate.

This understanding is replacing the artificial drift-diffusion mathematical models of decision-making with fitted parameters, not only because the attractor model is more realistic, but also because it allows the exploration of how biological parameters such as ion channel conductances and the effects of different transmitters expressed through different ion channels influence the operation and stability of the decision-making system. This is enabling medically relevant implications to be investigated, for example to neuropsychiatric disorders including schizophrenia and obsessive-compulsive disorder (Rolls 2016c).

14. The attractor approach to decision-making is a unifying approach, for the same mechanism applies not only to decision-making, but also to the operation of short-term memory systems, to the recall of information from long-term memory systems, and to top-down attention (Rolls 2016c). Part of the basis for this is that attractor states are a natural property of cortical systems, which are characterized by excitatory local recurrent collaterals which implement positive feedback; associative synaptic plasticity of these connections; and inhibition between the neurons implemented by GABA neurons (Rolls 2016c).

15. The probabilistic operation of the decision-making process caused by the spiking-related statistical fluctuations in finite-sized neuronal networks has many advantages, including different decisions and memory recall on different occasions even with similar inputs, giving rise to non-deterministic behaviour of the system. This probabilistic behaviour has a useful impact in many situations, including sometimes choosing less favourable options to update knowledge, predator avoidance, social interactions, and creativity (Rolls & Deco 2010, Rolls 2016c). The probabilistic behaviour of the mechanism also makes the brain non-deterministic, and there are implications for free-will.

16. These non-linear decision-making attractor networks that result not only in 'decisions' but also in categorization are found in many parts of the cortex, typically after earlier stages of more linear processing performing analysis of the stimulus. There is not therefore just one decision-maker in the brain, but multiple decision processes for different types of decision. One type of decision for example is the direction of global optic flow made in the dorsal visual system (Rolls 2016c, Rolls & Deco 2010). In the context of value and hence emotion systems, there is evidence that the more anterior, ventromedial parts of the prefrontal cortex (vmPFC), including medial prefrontal cortex area 10, are involved in the decision-making between stimuli of different value, and follow in the hierarchy the more linear representation of reward value in the orbitofrontal cortex.

17. With respect to the dopamine system, it appears that the activity of the dopamine neurons does not represent reward, and is not correlated with hedonic or emotional states (see Chapter 6). Part of the evidence for this is that the dopamine neurons may fire in relation to a reward prediction error, rather than in relation to reward itself, and that damage to the dopaminergic system does not impair hedonic responses or 'liking'. Dopamine pathways do influence systems involved in Pavlovian (classically conditioned) incentive salience effects mediated by the ventral striatum, and may thereby influence 'wanting'. However, there are inconsistencies with the dopamine reward prediction error hypothesis, with respect for example to whether the dopamine system is implicated in salience (as many dopamine neurons respond to aversive, novel, and alerting stimuli) vs reward error prediction, and whether a reward prediction error signal could facilitate the learning of stimuli associated with punishment (see Chapter 6).

18. In addition to the implicit system for action selection, in humans and perhaps related animals there is also an explicit system that can use language to compute actions to obtain deferred rewards using a one-off plan. The language system enables one-off multistep plans that require the syntactic organization of symbols to be formulated in order to obtain rewards and avoid punishers. There are thus two separate systems for producing actions to rewarding and punishing stimuli in humans and potentially in related animals. These systems may weight different courses of action differently, and produce conflict in decision-making, in that each can produce behaviour for different goals (immediate vs long-term goals involving multiple step planning). Understanding our evolutionary history is useful in enabling us to understand our emotional decision-making processes, and the conflicts that may be inherent in how they operate.

19. It is argued that the decisions taken by the emotional system are in the interests of selfish genes, in which the value systems have their foundations. The reasoning, rational, system enables longer-term decisions to be taken by planning ahead, and for the decisions to be in the interests of the individual, the phenotype, instead of the genes. This is another important sense (additional to the sense that genes and environment usually make joint contributions) in which the behaviour of humans and other animals with reasoning systems can be said to be not determined by our genes.

This rational, reasoning, 'explicit' decision-making system provides a basis for the operation of societies in which social contracts underpinned by reasoned understanding provide a basis for stability, and for gene-specified emotional value systems not to provide the only goal (Rolls 2012d). Understanding the emotional system is very important, for it has major influences on behaviour, and helps us to understand not only individual differences and personality, but also influences on behaviour that may have their origins partly in the different interests of males and females (Chapter 7). Understanding the emotional and the rational systems, and their very different types of computation, has many implications for understanding processes as far ranging as aesthetics, economics, politics, and religion (Rolls 2012d).

20. Pleasure is a subjective state reported in humans that is associated with a reward. Just as reward is specific, with many different types of reward, so is pleasure. It is possible that emotional feelings (including pleasure), part of the much larger problem of consciousness, arise as part of a process that involves thoughts about thoughts, which have the adaptive value of helping to correct one-off multistep plans. This is the approach described in Chapter 10, but there seems to be no clear way to choose which theory of consciousness is moving in the right direction, and caution must be exercised here, and current theories should not be taken to have implications.

21. Functional neuroimaging and neuropsychological data in humans (see Chapters 4 and 6) are consistent with many of the conclusions based on primate data including neurophysiology which provide the fundamental evidence needed to make computational models of how the brain functions as an information processing system exchanging information between its computing elements, the neurons (see Rolls (2016c)). In addition, the human findings provide interesting new evidence on how top-down cognitive and attentional effects can influence emotions in areas such as the orbitofrontal and anterior cingulate cortex (Section 4.5.3.6). The mechanisms by which cognitive states have top-down effects on emotion are probably similar to the biased competition mechanisms that subserve top-down attentional effects (Rolls & Deco 2002, Deco & Rolls 2003, Deco & Rolls 2005b, Rolls 2016c), though whole linked processing streams of cortical processing may be influenced in a top-down biased activation process (Rolls 2013a) (see also Section 4.9).

22. In relation to animal welfare, the suggestion arises that in addition to being guided by health, it may be useful to be guided by how the animals set their priorities for different rewards and punishers. This follows from the hypothesis that the brain is designed round reward/punisher evaluation systems, and behaviour optimizes obtaining the goals defined by the genes. The degree to which different genes make different reinforcers important, and how they depend on for example motivational state, then directly influence the value the animal places on a provision. The value or choice of the reinforcer thus provides a useful measure of its 'importance to the animal'. When making these measures of the value of different instrumental reinforcers, it is important to be aware of the many factors that can influence the selection of a reinforcer. Examples are the fact that the choice of a reinforcer is very sensitive to incentive motivational effects, priming, delay of reinforcement, and shows rapid extinction if the reinforcer is of low value, as shown by the behaviour when tested under zero drive conditions (Rolls 2005). We may also note that the reinforcer value systems in the brain are generally different to the systems involved in autonomic and endocrine responses (see Chapter 4). The implication is that the systems (for reinforcer value vs autonomic/endocrine responses) have evolved separately, and that the autonomic/endocrine responses elicited in emotion-provoking situations may not necessarily be a good guide to the instrumental reinforcing value (as measured by choice) or 'importance' of the resource to the animal.

23. The processes and systems involved in emotion have evolved considerably. Some of the principles described in this book include the following:
1. There may be no cortical area in rodents that is homologous to most of the primate including human orbitofrontal cortex (Wise 2008).
2. The primate including human orbitofrontal cortex (OFC) implements reward value, as shown by devaluation experiments such as feeding to satiety.
3. Value is not represented at earlier stages of processing in primates including humans. Invariant visual object recognition is used for many functions including memory formation, so perception is kept separate from emotion.

4. In contrast, in rodents, value is represented even in the first taste relay in the brain, the nucleus of the solitary tract: there is no clear separation between perception and emotion. In rodents, even the taste pathways are connected differently, with subcortical connections bypassing the cortex (including orbitofrontal cortex) and making connections via a pontine taste area directly to the hypothalamus and amygdala.
5. In primates and humans, the orbitofrontal cortex implements one-trial rule-based reversal learning, and this is important in rapidly updating social behaviour. This is rapid updating of value-based representations. Maintaining the current rule in short-term memory and using this to bias neurons in the orbitofrontal cortex (Deco & Rolls 2005a) may be one computation that granular prefrontal cortex facilitates. Rodents may not be able to perform this.
6. The value representation in the primate and human orbitofrontal cortex is domain general, in that the amount and value of goods, and temporal discounting, operate transitively (as shown by trade-offs), providing a basis for economic decision-making. There is evidence that this is not the case in rodents.
7. Goal value-directed choice is usual in primates and humans, whereas fixed action patterns such as pecking in birds are more common elsewhere.
8. Goal-directed choice may be the best measure of value and emotion, for there are many partly separate neural circuits for different emotion-related responses, e.g. autonomic output, freezing, fixed action patterns, and unconditioned approach or withdrawal.
9. In humans, and perhaps some primates, syntactic reasoning and thereby planning allows selfish gene-specified (emotion-related) rewards to be rejected in favour of the long-term interests of the individual, the phenotype.

11.2 Selection of optimal actions by explicit rational thought

As scientists we can see that our behaviour is not ‘determined’ by our genes, for the rational system can make choices that are not subject to the goals that our genes promote.

This scientific understanding of behaviour should lead to societies that, with this understanding, can support the goals, desires, and pleasures that are influenced by genes and by the reasoning system, without producing harm to others. I emphasize that rationality, reasoning, enables humans to go beyond gene-specified or gene-influenced goals. These and related concepts have many implications, including for ethics, religion, aesthetics, politics, and economics (see further *Neuroculture: On the Implications of Brain Science* (Rolls 2012d)).

11.3 Emotion and ethics

I have argued in this book that much of the foundation of our emotional behaviour arises from specification by genes of primary reinforcers that provide goals for our actions. We have emotional reactions in certain circumstances, such as when we see that we are about to suffer pain, when we fall in love, or if someone does not return a favour in a reciprocal interaction. What is the relation between our emotions, and what we think is right, that is our ethical principles? If we think something is right, such as returning something that has been on loan, is this a fundamental and absolute ethical principle, or might it have arisen from deep-seated biologically-based systems shaped to be adaptive by natural selection operating in evolution to select genes that tend to promote the survival of those genes?

Many principles that we regard as ethical principles *might* arise in this biological way (see Rolls (2012d)). For example, as noted in Chapter 2, guilt might arise when there is a conflict between an available reward and a rule or law of society. Jealousy is an emotion that might be aroused in a male if the faithfulness of his partner seems to be threatened by her liaison (e.g. flirting) with another male. In this case the reinforcement contingency that is operating is produced by a punisher, and it may be that males are specified genetically to find this punishing because it indicates a potential threat to their paternity and parental investment, as described in Chapters 7 and 3. Similarly, a female may become jealous if her partner has a liaison with another female, because the resources available to the 'wife' useful to bring up her children are threatened. Again, the punisher here may be gene-specified, as described in Chapter 3. Such emotional responses might influence what we build into some of the ethical principles that surround marriage and partnerships for raising children.

Many other similar examples can be surmised from the area of evolutionary psychology (see e.g. Ridley (1993a, 1996) and Buss (2015)). For example, there may be a set of reinforcers that are genetically specified to help promote social cooperation and even reciprocal altruism, and that might thus influence what we regard as ethical, or at least what we are willing to accept as ethical principles. Such genes might specify that emotion should be elicited, and behavioural changes should occur, if a cooperating partner defects or 'cheats' (Cosmides & Tooby 1999). Moreover, the genes may build brains with genetically specified rules that are useful heuristics for social cooperation, such as acting with a strategy of 'generous tit-for tat', which can be more adaptive than strict 'tit-for-tat', in that being generous occasionally is a good strategy to help promote further cooperation that has failed when both partners defect in a strict 'tit-for-tat' scenario (Ridley 1996). Genes that specify good heuristics to promote social cooperation may thus underlie such complex emotional states as feeling forgiving.

It is suggested that many apparently complex emotional states have their origins in designing animals to perform well in such sociobiological and socioeconomic situations (Ridley 1996, Glimcher & Fehr 2013). In this way, many principles that humans accept as ethical may be closely related to strategies that are useful heuristics for promoting social cooperation, and emotional feelings associated with ethical behaviour may be at least partly related to the adaptive value of such gene-specified strategies.

The situation is clarified by the ideas I have advanced in Chapter 10 and in this chapter about a rational syntactically based reasoning system and how this interacts with an evolutionarily older emotional system with gene-specified rewards. The rational system enables us for example to defer immediate gene-specified rewards, and make longer-term plans for actions that in the long term may have more useful outcomes. This rational system enables us to make reasoned choices, and to reason about what is right. Indeed, it is because of the linguistic system that the naturalistic fallacy becomes an issue. In particular, we should not believe that what is right is what is natural (*the naturalistic fallacy*), because we have a rational system that can go beyond simpler gene-specified rewards and punishers that may influence our actions through brain systems that operate at least partly implicitly, i.e. unconsciously. I now consider further the relation between the biological underpinnings to emotion, and ethics, morals, and morality.

There are many reasons why people have particular moral beliefs, and believe that it is good to act in particular ways. It is possible that biology can help to explain why certain types of behaviour are adopted perhaps implicitly by humans, and become incorporated for consistency into explicit rules for conduct. This approach does not, of course, replace other approaches to what is moral, but it may help in implementing moral beliefs held for other reasons to have some insight into some of the directions that the biological underpinnings of human behaviour might lead. Humans may be better able to decide explicitly what to do when they have knowledge and insight into the biological underpinnings. It is in this framework that the following points are made, with no attempt made to lead towards any suggestions about what is 'right' or 'wrong'. The arguments that follow are based on the hypothesis that there are biological underpinnings based on the types of reward and punishment systems that have been built into our genes during evolution for at least some of the types of behaviour held to be moral.

One type of such biological underpinning is kin selection. This would tend to produce supportive behaviour towards individuals likely to be related, especially towards children, grandchildren, siblings etc., depending on how closely they are genetically related. This does tend to occur in human societies, and is part of what is regarded as 'right', and indeed it is a valued 'right' to be able to pass on goods, possessions, wealth, etc., to children. The underlying basis here would be genes for kin altruism[13]. Although genes may via kin selection tend to favour children and grandchildren, many people feel it is unfair that people get an advantage in life by what they inherit from their parents. There may be some conflicts here, between good for an individual's family vs others, and the good of society which might advance with less friction and more rapidly with anti-nepotism laws.

Another such underpinning might be the fact that many animals, and especially primates, co-operate with others in order to achieve ends which turn out to be on average to their advantage, including genetic advantage. One example includes the coalitions formed by a group of males in order to obtain a female for one of the group, followed by reciprocation of the good turn later (see Ridley (1996)). This is an example of altruism, in this case by groups of primates, which is to the advantage of both groups or individuals provided that neither individual or group cheats, in which case the rules for social interaction must change to keep the strategy stable. Another such underpinning, in this case for property 'rights', might be the territory guarding behaviour that is so common from fish to primates. Another such underpinning might be the jealousy and guarding of a partner shown by males who invest parental care in their partner's offspring. This occurs in many species of birds, and also in humans, with both exemplars showing male parental investment because of the immaturity of the children. This might be a biological underpinning to the 'right' to fidelity in a female partner.

The suggestion I make is that in all these cases, and in many others, there are biological underpinnings that determine what we find rewarding or punishing, designed into genes by evolution to lead to appropriate behaviour that helps to increase the fitness of the genes. When these implicit systems for rewards and punishers start to be expressed explicitly (in language) in humans, the explicit rules, rights, and laws that are formalized are those that set out in language what the biological underpinnings 'want' to occur[14]. Clearly in formulating the explicit rights and laws, some compromise is necessary in order to keep the society stable. When the rights and laws are formulated in small societies, it is likely that individuals in that society will have many of the same genes, and rules such as 'help your neighbour' (but 'make war with "foreigners" ') will probably be to the advantage of one's genes. However, when the society increases in size beyond a small village (in the order of 1000), then the explicitly formalized rules, rights, and laws may no longer produce behaviour that turns out

[13] Kin selection genes spread because of kin altruism. Such genes direct their bodies to aid relatives because those relatives have a high chance of having the same relative-helping gene. This is a specific mechanism, and it happens to be incorrect to think that genes direct their bodies to aid relatives because those bodies 'share genes' in general (see Hamilton (1964); and the chapter on inclusive fitness in Dawkins (1995)).

[14] Before the rules are explicitly formalized, conventions may be developed and spread using language, for example in the form of verbal traditions handed down from generation to generation that may provide possible models for behaviour, such as Homer's *Odyssey*.

to be to the advantage of an individual's genes. In addition, it may no longer be possible to keep track of individuals in order to maintain the stability of 'tit-for-tat' co-operative social strategies (Dunbar 1996, Ridley 1996)[15]. In such cases, other factors doubtless come into play to additionally influence what groups hold to be right. For example, a group of subjects in a society might demand the 'right' to free speech because it is to their economic advantage.

Thus overall it is suggested that many aspects of what a society holds as right and moral, and of what becomes enshrined in explicit 'rights' and laws, are related to biological underpinnings, which have usually evolved because of the advantage to the individual's genes, but that as societies develop other factors also start to influence what is believed to be 'right' by groups of individuals, related to socioeconomic factors. In both cases, the laws and rules of the society develop so that these 'rights' are protected, but often involve compromise in such a way that a large proportion of the society will agree to, or can be made subject to, what is held as right.

To conclude this discussion, we note that what is natural does not necessarily imply what is 'right' (the naturalistic fallacy, pointed out by G. E. Moore) (see, e.g., Singer (1981)). However, our notions of what we think of as right may be related to biological underpinnings, and the point of this discussion is that it can only give helpful insight into human behaviour to realize this. Other ways in which a biological approach, based on what our brains have evolved to treat as rewarding or punishing, can illuminate moral issues, and rights, follow.

'Pain is a worse state than no pain'. This is a statement held as true by some moral philosophers, and is said to hold with no reference to biological underpinnings. It is a self-evident truth, and certain implications for behaviour may follow from the proposition. A biological approach to pain is that the elicitation of pain has to be punishing (in the sense that animals will work to escape or avoid it), as pain is the state elicited by stimuli signalling a dimension of environmental conditions that reduces survival and therefore gene fitness.

'Incest is morally wrong. One should not marry a brother or sister. One should not have intercourse with any close relation.' The biological underpinning is that children of close relations have an increased chance of having double-recessive genes, which are sometimes harmful to the individual and reduce fitness. In addition, breeding out may produce hybrid vigour. It is presumably for this reason that many animals as well as humans have behavioural strategies (influenced by the properties of reward systems) that reduce inbreeding (e.g. philopatry, that is only one sex remaining in the natal unit at the time of puberty; and mate selection influenced by the olfactory receptor/major histocompatibility genes as described in Section 7.8). At the same time, it may be adaptive (for genes) to pair with another animal that has many of the same genes, for this may help complex gene sequences to be passed intact into the next generation. This may underlie the fact that quails have mechanisms that enable them to recognize their cousins, and make them appear attractive, an example of kin selection (Bateson 1983). In humans, if one were part of a strong society (in which one's genes would have a good chance not to be eliminated by other societies), then it could be advantageous (whether male or female) to invest resources with someone else who would provide maximum genetic and resource potential for one's children, which on average across a society of relatively small size and not too mobile would be a person with relatively similar genes and resources (wealth, status etc.) to oneself. In an exception to this, in certain societies there has been a tradition of marrying close relations (e.g. the Pharaohs of Egypt), and part of the reason for this could be maintaining financial and other resources within the (genetic) family.

[15] A limit on the size of the group for reciprocal altruism might be set by the ability both to have direct evidence for and remember person–reinforcer associations for large numbers of different individual people. In this situation, reputation passed on verbally from others who have the direct experience of whether an individual can be trusted to reciprocate might be a factor in the adaptive value of language and gossip (Dunbar 1996, Dunbar 1993).

There may be several reasons why particular behavioural conduct may be selected. A first is that the conduct may be good for the individual and for the genes of the individual, at least on average. An example might be a prohibition on killing others in the same society (while at the same time defending that kin group in times of war). The advantage here could be for one's own genes, which would be less at risk in a society without large numbers of killings. A second reason is that particular codes of conduct might effectively help one's genes by making society stable. An example here might be a prohibition on theft, which would serve to protect property. A third reason is that the code of conduct might actually be to other, powerful, individuals' advantage, and might have been made for that reason into a rule that others in society are persuaded to follow. A general rule in society might be that honesty is a virtue, but the rule might be given a special interpretation or ignored by members of society too powerful to challenge. As discussed in Chapter 7, different aspects of behaviour could have different importance for males and females (Goetz & Shackelford 2009). This could lead men and women to put different stress on different rules of society, because they have different importance for men and women. One example might be being unfaithful. Because this could be advantageous to men's genes, this may be treated by men as a less serious error of conduct than by women. However, within men there could be differential condemnation, with men predisposed to being faithful being more concerned about infidelity in other men, because it is a potential threat to them. In the same way, powerful men who can afford to have liaisons with many women may be less concerned about infidelity than less powerful men, whose main genetic investment may be with one woman.

Society may set down certain propositions of what is 'right'. One reason for this is that it may be too difficult on every occasion, and for everyone, to work out explicitly what all the payoffs of each rule of conduct are. A second reason is that what is promulgated as 'right' could actually be to someone else's advantage, and it would not be wise to expose this fully. One way to convince members of society not to do what is apparently in their immediate interest is to promise a reward later. Such deferred rewards are often offered by religions (Rolls 2012d). The ability to work for a deferred reward using a one-off plan in this way becomes possible, it was suggested earlier in this chapter, with the evolution of the explicit, propositional, system.

The overall view that one is led to is that some of our moral beliefs may be explicit, verbal, formulations of what may reflect factors built genetically by kin selection into behaviour, namely a tendency to favour kin, because they are likely to share some of an individual's genes. In a small society this explicit formulation may be 'appropriate' (from the point of view of the genes), in that many members of that society will be related to that individual. When the society becomes larger, the relatedness may decrease, yet the explicit formulation of the rules or laws of society may not change. In such a situation, it is presumably appropriate for society to make it clear to its members that its rules for what is acceptable and 'right' behaviour are set in place so that individuals can live in safety, and with some expectation of help from society in general.

Other factors that can influence what is held to be right might reflect socioeconomic advantage to groups or alliances of individuals. It would be then in a sense up to individuals to decide whether they wished to accept the rules, with the costs and benefits provided by the rules of that society, in a form of Social Contract. Individuals who did not agree to the social contract might wish to transfer to another society with a different place on the continuum of costs and potential benefits to the individuals, or to influence the laws and policies of their own society. Individuals who attempt to cheat the system would be expected to pay a cost in terms of punishment meted out by the society in accordance with its rules. This approach is developed further in *Neuroculture* (Rolls 2012d).

11.4 Emotion and aesthetics

Those interested in literature are sometimes puzzled by the following situation, which can perhaps be clarified by the theory of emotion developed here. The puzzle is that emotions often seem very intense in humans, indeed sometimes so intense that they produce behaviour that does not seem to be adaptive, such as fainting instead of producing an active escape response, or freezing instead of avoiding, or vacillating endlessly about emotional situations and decisions, or falling hopelessly in love even when it can be predicted to be without hope or to bring ruin. The puzzle is not only that the emotion is so intense, but also that even with our rational, reasoning, capacities, humans still find themselves in these situations, and may find it difficult to produce reasonable and effective decisions and behaviour for resolving the situation. The reasons for this include, I suggest, the following.

In humans, the reward and punishment systems may operate implicitly in comparable ways to those in other animals. But in addition to this, humans have the explicit system, which enables us consciously to look and predict many steps ahead (using language and syntax) the consequences of environmental events, and also to reflect on previous events (see Chapter 10). The consequence of this explicit processing is that we can see the full impact of rewarding and punishing events, both looking ahead to see how this will impact us, and reflecting back to previous situations that we can see may never be repeated. For example, in humans grief occurs with the loss of a loved one, and this may be much more intense than might occur simply because of failure to receive a positively reinforcing stimulus, because we can look ahead to see that the person will never be present again, can process all the possible consequences of that, and can remember all the previous occasions with that person. In another example, someone may faint at the sight of blood, and this is more likely to occur in humans because we appreciate the full consequences of major loss of blood, which we all know is life-threatening.

Thus what happens is that reinforcing events can have a very much greater reinforcing value in humans than in other animals, because we have so much cognitive, especially linguistic, processing that leads us to evaluate and appreciate many reinforcing events far more fully than can other animals. Thus humans may decode reinforcers to have supernormal intensity relative to what is usual in other animals, and the supernormal appreciated intensity of the decoded reinforcers leads to super-strong emotions. The emotional states can then be so strong that they are not necessarily adaptive, and indeed language has brought humans out of the environmental conditions under which our emotional systems evolved. For example, the autonomic responses to the sight of blood may be so strong, given that we know the consequences of loss of blood, that we faint rather than helping. Another example is that panic and anxiety states can be exacerbated by feeling the heart pounding, because we are able to use our explicit processing system to think and worry about all the possible causes. One can think of countless other examples from life, and indeed make up other examples, which of course is part of what novelists do.

A second reason for such strong emotions in humans is that the stimuli that produce emotions may be much stronger than those in which our emotional systems evolved. For example, with man-made artefacts (such as cars and guns which may injure many people simultaneously, or a large bus speeding towards one, both of which produce super-normal stimuli), the sights and related stimuli that can be produced in terms of damage to humans are much more intense that those present when our emotional systems evolved. In this way, the things we see can in some cases produce super-strong emotions. Indeed, the strength and sometimes maladaptive consequences of human emotions have preoccupied literature and literary theorists for the last 2,400 years, since Aristotle.

A third reason for the intensely mobilizing, and sometimes immobilizing, effects of emotions in humans is that we can evaluate linguistically, with reasoning, the possible courses of action open to us in emotional situations. Because we can evaluate the possible effects of reinforcers many steps ahead in our plans, and because language enables us to produce flexible one-off plans for actions, and enables us to work for deferred rewards based on one-off plans (see Chapter 10), the ways in which reinforcers are used in decision-making becomes much more complex than in those animals that cannot produce similar one-off plans using language. The consequence of this is that decision-making can become very difficult, with so many potential but uncertain reinforcement outcomes, that humans may vacillate. They are trying to compute by this explicit method the most favourable outcome of each plan in terms of the net reinforcements received, rather than using reinforcement implicitly to select the highest currently available reinforcer.

A fourth reason for complexity in the human emotional system is that there are, it is suggested, two routes to action for emotions in humans, an implicit (unconscious) and an explicit route (see Chapter 10). These systems may not always agree. The implicit system may tend to produce one type of behaviour, typically for immediately available rewards. The explicit system may tend to produce another planned course of action to produce better deferred rewards. Conflict between these systems can lead to many difficult situations, will involve conscience (what is right as conceived by the explicit system) and the requirement to abide by laws (which assume a rational explicit system responsible for our actions). It appears that the implicit system does often control our behaviour, as shown by the effects of frontal lobe damage in humans, which may produce deficits in reward-reversal tasks, even when the human can explicitly state the correct behaviour in the situation (see Chapters 4 and 10). The conflicts that arise between these implicit and explicit systems are again some of the very stuff on which literature often capitalizes.

A fifth reason for complexity in the human emotional system is that we, as social animals, with major investments in our children who benefit from long-term parental co-operation, and with advantages to be gained from social alliances if the partners can be trusted, may be built to try to estimate the goals and reliability of those we know. For example, it may matter to a woman with children whether her partner has been attracted by / is in love with / a different woman, as this could indicate a reduction of help and provision. Humans may thus be very interested in the emotional lives of each other, as this may impact on their own lives. Indeed, humans will, for this sort of reason, be very interested in who is co-operating with whom, and gossip about this may even have acted as a selective pressure for the evolution of language (Dunbar 1996, Dunbar 1993). In these circumstances, fascination with unravelling the thoughts and emotions of others (using the capacity described as theory of mind (Frith & Frith 2003, Gallagher & Frith 2003)), and empathy which may facilitate this (Singer, Seymour, O'Doherty, Kaube, Dolan & Frith 2004), would have adaptive value, though it is difficult computationally to model the minds and interactions of groups of other people, and to keep track of who knows what about whom, as this requires many levels of nested syntactical reference. Our resulting fascination with this, and perhaps the value of experience of as wide a range of situations as possible, may then be another reason why human emotions, and guessing others' emotions in complex social situations, may also be part of the stuff of novelists, playwrights, and poets. Indeed, it may be important for us to find it attractive to engage in this type of processing because of its potential adaptive value, and this may be part of the reason why we find drama, novels, and poetry so fascinating.

A sixth reason for complexity in the human emotional system is that high level cognitive processing can reach down in to the emotional systems and influence how they respond. This was demonstrated in the experiment by DeAraujo, Rolls et al. (2005) in which it was shown that processing at the linguistic level, in the form of a word label, can influence processing as far down in sensory processing as the secondary olfactory cortex in the orbitofrontal cortex, the first stage in cortical processing at which the reward- or punishment-related (hence affective) significance of stimuli is made explicit in the neuronal representations of stimuli. An implication of this is that cognitive factors such as the current cultural, cognitive, interpretation of literature or music may influence how the literature or music is perceived emotionally (Reddy 2001). Correspondingly, when in the 18th and 19th centuries sentiment developed as a cultural aspect of emotion in literature, the great cognitive emphasis on sentiment can be predicted to have influenced how people responded emotionally to novels written at that time. Thus the current cognitive and cultural context may have an effect not just on the high-level cognitive processing involved in emotion, but may also reach down into the systems (such as the orbitofrontal cortex) where emotion is first made explicit in brain processing, and influence at that level the emotional feelings that occur.

When at the performance of a drama or when reading a novel, the emotional feelings that occur may be partly related to the empathetic states that are being elicited as part of the way in which we are built to try to understand the feelings of others, so as better to predict their behaviour. Of course at the drama or when reading a novel, we know with our explicit system that these are not real events that have direct consequences for us, and top-down cognitive attentional processes (see Section 4.5.3.6) may influence to what extent we allow the incoming events to elicit emotional responses in us, using probably a biased competition attentional mechanism (Rolls & Deco 2002, Deco & Rolls 2003, Deco & Rolls 2005b, Rolls 2013a, Rolls 2016c).

This approach is developed further, and applied to aesthetics more widely, in *Neuroculture* (Rolls 2012d) and elsewhere (Rolls 2011d, Rolls 2014a, Rolls 2015e, Rolls 2017a).

11.5 Close

This book started by raising the following questions. What are emotions? Why do we have emotions? What is their adaptive value? What are the brain mechanisms of emotion, and how can disorders of emotion be understood? Why does it feel like something to have an emotion? Why do emotions sometimes feel so intense? How do we take decisions? When we know what emotions are, why we have them, how they are produced by our brains, and why it feels like something to have an emotion, and how decisions are taken, we will have a broad-ranging explanation of emotion and decision-making. How close have we come to this?

This book provides answers to these questions. The 'why' question is answered by a Darwinian, evolutionary, theory of the adaptive value of emotion in terms of the design of animals and the brain, for the book shows that if genes specify a range of rewards and punishers (primary reinforcers) as the goals for action, then this is an efficient way for genes to influence adaptively the behaviour of the organism to promote fitness (of the genes). Part of the adaptive value, simplicity, and efficiency of this design is that the behaviour itself is not determined or specified by the genes, which need to specify just the goals for actions. This means that during the lifetime of the organism, appropriate actions to obtain the goals can be learned, allowing great flexibility of the behaviour. Another part of the adaptive value of the design is that arbitrary, previously neutral, stimuli can become associated with a primary reinforcer by stimulus–reinforcer association learning, so that there is great flexibility in learning in the lifetime of the organism about which stimuli are associated with primary reinforcers, and should also act as emotional stimuli, and lead towards attainment of the goals specified by the primary reinforcers. This is I believe a fundamental approach to understanding why we have emotions.

This Darwinian account of the 'why' question fits naturally with the operational definition of emotions as states (with particular functions) elicited by instrumental reinforcers (Chapter

2), for the reinforcers define the goals for action, that is rewards and punishers, and it is the rewards and punishers that are operationally related to emotional states. The definition thus should not be thought of as a behaviourist definition of emotion, but as a definition linked to the deep biological adaptive value of designing animals around reward and punishment systems. In addition, the definition is not behaviourist in the sense that cognitive states can elicit emotions, and that emotions can influence cognitive states (see for example Sections 2.6 and 4.9). Further, the definition is not limited to an account of a narrow range of emotions, but can encompass a very wide range of emotions, as outlined in Chapter 2. An advantage of the approach is that it clearly specifies what emotions are, and what their adaptive value is.

The 'how' question about the implementation of emotion in the brain is addressed not only by a wealth of data from neuroscience, but also by a set of principles of the brain organization for emotion set out at the start of this chapter. An advantage of the approach to emotion described here is that it leads to well formulated questions about how to investigate the brain mechanisms that underlie emotion, for the approach indicates that it is important to understand where primary reinforcers are decoded and represented in the brain, how and where stimulus–reinforcer association learning occurs in the brain, how action–outcome (i.e. action–reinforcer) learning occurs, and the ways in which rewards and punishers influence decision-making as outlined in Chapter 8.

In relation to decision-making, it is shown that there are multiple routes via which rewards and punishers, that is emotion-provoking stimuli and the states they elicit, can influence behaviour (see Section 10.1). An important division is into the implicit ways in which rewards directly influence choice via processes such as Pavlovian approach and action–outcome learning, and an explicit route via which immediate rewards can be deferred using a long-term one-off explicit plan which may enable alternative rewards to be obtained in the long term. This is the 'dual routes to action' account developed in Chapter 10 and Section 10.1.

In relation to emotional feelings, it is emphasized that this is part of the much larger problem of consciousness. My own approach to this is described in Chapter 10, but it is pointed out that this is just one approach, that there do not seem to be clear criteria by which any particular theory can be confirmed, and that in the circumstances such theories should not be taken to have practical implications. Nevertheless, these are interesting issues.

It is also shown how a scientific approach to emotion can illuminate some of the biological underpinnings on top of which ethical and moral principles are developed (Section 11.3). A scientific approach to emotion also provides comments about the role of emotion in literature and aesthetics (Section 11.4 and Rolls (2012d)).

This approach to emotion also fits well with the development of a precise and quantitative understanding of how emotion and decision-making are implemented, using the computational approaches described by Rolls (2016c).

In this book, I show how it is now possible to follow processing in the brain from the sensory representation and perception of objects including visual and taste objects that are independent of reward value; to brain regions where reward value (both outcome value and expected value) are represented, which are crucial components of decision-making; to brain mechanisms that actually implement the choice part of the decision-making, with a mechanism that is common to categorization and decision-making in other brain systems and cortical areas. I believe that this represents a major advance in neuroscience that we are able to understand at the level of mechanisms all of these processes, and to see how they are linked together in the brain to implement much of our behaviour. Moreover, all of this neural understanding is linked to an understanding of the adaptive value of this organization of behaviour, how emotion is a key component, and even how the subjective feeling of pleasure may arise and be related to these processes.

Thus we may suggest that we are getting closer to a scientific understanding and explanation of emotion and of decision-making; and that we have some useful principles and guidelines for investigations that will further enhance our understanding.

Appendix 1 Glossary

A.1 General

An **affective state** is a term used to describe an emotional state (Chapter 2). It may have a connotation of subjective experience.

An **Attractor network** is formed by a set of neurons with positive connections between the neurons. Different subsets of neurons have especially strong connections between themselves, with each subset representing one memory or decision. Negative feedback inhibitory neurons implement competition between the neurons so that typically only one subset wins the competition. If an input is received that is close to one of the stored memories or decisions, then the network is attracted towards and recalls one of the stored memories. These networks, and how they are involved in **decision-making** are described in Chapter 8. An attractor network in the brain may store as many as 10,000 memories, if there are 10,000 connections to a neuron from the other neurons in the network. The operation of these networks with equations and quantitative analyses is described by Rolls (2016c).

Effective connectivity measures the effect of one brain area on another, that is a directed effect. The measure of activity is typically the BOLD signal, and the measurement involves comparing the signals in successive time-steps, with the underlying idea that if a first brain area has activity just before a second brain area, then the first brain area may be having a directed effect on a second brain area. In the cortex, there are typically connections in both directions between two cortical areas, and we sometimes refer to the direction as forward for the stronger connectivity, because in cortical hierarchies, the forward connectivity is generally stronger, as described by Rolls (2016c).

An **emotion** can be described operationally as a state elicited by an instrumental reinforcer (Chapter 2).

Fitness is the reproductive potential of genes. Through the process of natural selection and reproduction, fit genes are selected for the next generation.

Functional connectivity measures the correlation between the measure of activity (typically the BOLD signal) in two brain regions. A high functional connectivity implies that two brain areas are relatively strongly connected functionally. The relation might be produced by one area influencing the other, by the two areas influencing each other, or by a common input from another brain area. Functional connectivity does not imply that there is necessarily a direct anatomical connection, for the effects could be mediated through other brain areas.

Functional magnetic resonance imaging (fMRI) measures a blood oxygenation level dependent **(BOLD) signal**. When neural activity in a brain area increases, the blood flow increases, and this change of blood flow can be measured by the change in the amount of deoxyhaemoglobin (which is paramagnetic) in a brain region. The spatial resolution is in the order of 3 mm and so reflects the activity of hundreds of thousands of neurons, and the temporal resolution is in the order of several seconds.

Functional neuroimaging measures the activity of the brain either while the participant is resting, or during a task. The methods commonly used include functional magnetic resonance imaging of the brain (fMRI), positron emission tomography (PET), and magnetoencephalography (MEG).

A **pattern association network** learns the association between an input pattern (such as the sight of food) and the stimulus to be recalled (such as the taste of food). It can be used to compute **expected value**. This type of network is illustrated in Fig. 4.24, and is described quantitatively by Rolls (2016c).

A reward **prediction error** is positive if the **reward outcome** (e.g. the taste of food) is greater than the **expected value** (e.g. what is expected from the sight of food). Dopamine neurons appear to encode this error, useful in **reinforcement learning** (see Chapter 6). A reward **prediction error** is negative if the reward outcome (e.g. the taste of food) is less than the expected value (e.g. what is expected from the sight of food). This is sometimes referred to as **non-reward**. Some neurons in the orbitofrontal cortex encode negative reward prediction error, as described in Section 4.5.3.5, and may be related to depression, as described in Chapter 9.

Reward value refers to the value of a good, and is a term used in neuroeconomics and decision-making (Glimcher & Fehr 2013, Rolls 2014b). It can be measured by how much one would pay for the good, which might be a food, or how hard one would work to obtain the food. Stimuli with high reward value are rated as subjectively pleasant, and there is often a linear relation between the activation of the orbitofrontal cortex and the pleasantness of the stimulus (Chapter 4).

A.2 Learning theory terms

Instrumental reinforcers are stimuli that, if their occurrence, termination, or omission is made contingent upon the making of an action, alter the probability of the future emission of that action (Gray 1975, Mackintosh 1983, Dickinson 1980, Lieberman 2000, Mazur 2012, Rolls 2014b). Rewards and punishers are instrumental reinforcing stimuli. The notion of an action here is that an arbitrary action, e.g. turning right vs turning left, will be performed in order to obtain the reward or avoid the punisher, so that there is no pre-wired connection between the response and the reinforcer. Some stimuli are **primary (unlearned) reinforcers** (e.g., the taste of food if the animal is hungry, or pain); while others may become reinforcing by learning, because of their association with such primary reinforcers, thereby becoming '**secondary reinforcers**'. This type of learning may thus be called '**stimulus–reinforcer association learning**', and occurs via a stimulus–stimulus associative learning process.

A **positive reinforcer** (such as food) increases the probability of emission of an action on which it is contingent, the process is termed **positive reinforcement**, and the outcome is a **reward** (such as food).

A **negative reinforcer** (such as a painful stimulus) increases the probability of emission of an action that causes the negative reinforcer to be omitted (as in **active avoidance**) or terminated (as in **escape**), and the procedure is termed **negative reinforcement**.

Punishment refers to procedures in which the probability of an action is decreased. Punishment thus describes procedures in which an action decreases in probability if it is followed by a painful stimulus, as in **passive avoidance**. Punishment can also be used to refer to a procedure involving the omission or termination of a reward (**'extinction'** and **'time out'** respectively), both of which decrease the probability of responses (Gray 1975, Mackintosh 1983, Dickinson 1980, Lieberman 2000, Mazur 2012, Rolls 2014b).

A **punisher** when delivered acts instrumentally to decrease the probability of actions on which it is contingent, or when not delivered (escaped from or avoided) acts as a negative reinforcer in that it then increases the probability of the action on which its non-delivery is contingent. Note that my definition of a punisher, which is similar to that of an aversive stimulus, is of a stimulus or event that can either decrease the probability of actions on which it is contingent, or increase the probability of actions on which its non-delivery is contingent. The term **punishment** is restricted to situations where the probability of an action is being decreased.

Emotions are states elicited by instrumental reinforcers, where the states have the set of functions described in Chapter 3. My argument is that an affectively positive or 'appetitive' stimulus (which produces a state of pleasure) acts operationally as a **reward**, which when delivered acts instrumentally as a positive reinforcer, or when not delivered (omitted or terminated) acts to decrease the probability of responses on which it is contingent. Conversely I argue that an affectively negative or aversive stimulus (which produces an unpleasant state) acts operationally as a **punisher**, which when delivered acts instrumentally to decrease the probability of actions on which it is contingent, or when not delivered (escaped from or avoided) acts as a negative reinforcer in that it then increases the probability of the action on which its non-delivery is contingent[16].

Classical conditioning or **Pavlovian conditioning**. When a **conditioned stimulus (CS)** (such as a tone) is paired with a primary reinforcer or **unconditioned stimulus (US)** (such as a painful stimulus), then there are opportunities for a number of types of association to be formed. Some of these involve 'classical conditioning' or 'Pavlovian conditioning', in which no action is performed that affects the contingency between the conditioned stimulus and the unconditioned stimulus. Typically an **unconditioned response (UR)**, for example an alteration of heart rate, is produced by the US, and will come to be elicited by the CS as a **conditioned response (CR)**. These responses are typically autonomic (such as the heart beating faster), or endocrine (for example the release of adrenaline (epinephrine in American usage) by the adrenal gland). In addition, the organism may learn to perform an instrumental response with the skeletal muscles in order to alter the probability that the primary reinforcer will be obtained. In our example, the experimenter might alter the contingencies so that when the tone sounded, if the organism performed a response such as pressing a lever, then the painful stimulus could be avoided. In the instrumental learning situation there are still

[16] Note that my definition of a punisher, which is similar to that of an aversive stimulus, is of a stimulus or event that can either decrease the probability of actions on which it is contingent, or increase the probability of actions on which its non-delivery is contingent. The term punishment is restricted to situations where the probability of an action is being decreased.

opportunities for many classically conditioned responses, including emotional states such as fear, to occur. The associative processes involved in classical conditioning, and the influences that these processes may have on instrumental performance, are described in Section 4.6.2.

Motivated behaviour occurs when an animal will perform an instrumental (i.e. arbitrary operant) response to obtain a reward or to escape from or avoid a punisher. If this criterion of an arbitrary operant responsc is not met, and only a fixed response can be performed, then the term **drive** can be used to describe the state of the animal when it will work to obtain or escape from the stimulus.

Long-term potentiation (LTP) is the increase in synaptic strength that can occur during learning. It is typically associative, depending on conjunctive presynaptic activity and postsynaptic depolarization.

Long-term depression (LTP) is the decrease in synaptic strength that can occur during learning. It is typically associative, occurring when the presynaptic activity is low and the postsynaptic depolarization is high (heterosynaptic long-term depression), or when the presynaptic activity is high, and the postsynaptic activity is only moderate (homosynaptic long-term depression).

References

Abdallah CG, Adams TG, Kelmendi B, Esterlis I, Sanacora G, & Krystal JH (2016). Ketamine's mechanism of action: A path to rapid-acting antidepressants. *Depress Anxiety* 33: 689–97.

Abrams DI (2018). The therapeutic effects of cannabis and cannabinoids: An update from the national academies of sciences, engineering and medicine report. *Eur J Intern Med* 49: 7–11.

Adams JE (1976). Naloxone reversal of analgesia produced by brain stimulation in the human. *Pain* 2: 161–166.

Adolphs R (2003). Cognitive neuroscience of human social behavior. *Nature Reviews Neuroscience* 4: 165–178.

Adolphs R, Tranel D, Damasio H, & Damasio AR (1994). Impaired recognition of emotion in facial expressions following bilateral damage to the human amygdala. *Nature* 372: 669–672.

Adolphs R, Tranel D, & Baron-Cohen S (2002). Amygdala damage impairs recognition of social emotions from facial expressions. *Journal of Cognitive Neuroscience* 14: 1–11.

Adolphs R, Gosselin F, Buchanan TW, Tranel D, Schyns P, & Damasio AR (2005). A mechanism for impaired fear recognition after amygdala damage. *Nature* 433: 68–72.

Aggelopoulos NC & Rolls ET (2005). Natural scene perception: inferior temporal cortex neurons encode the positions of different objects in the scene. *European Journal of Neuroscience* 22: 2903–2916.

Aggelopoulos NC, Franco L, & Rolls ET (2005). Object perception in natural scenes: encoding by inferior temporal cortex simultaneously recorded neurons. *Journal of Neurophysiology* 93: 1342–1357.

Aggleton JP, editor (2000). *The Amygdala, A Functional Analysis*. Oxford University Press, Oxford, 2nd edn.

Aiello LC & Wheeler P (1995). The expensive-tissue hypothesis: the brain and the digestive system in human and primate evolution. *Current Anthropology* 36: 199–221.

Akil H, Mayer DJ, & Liebeskind JC (1976). Antagonism of stimulation-produced analgesia by naloxone, a narcotic antagonist. *Science* 191: 961–962.

Aleksandrova LR, Phillips AG, & Wang YT (2017). Antidepressant effects of ketamine and the roles of ampa glutamate receptors and other mechanisms beyond nmda receptor antagonism. *J Psychiatry Neurosci* 42: 222–229.

Alexander RD (1979). *Darwinism and Human Affairs*. University of Washington Press, Seattle.

Amaral DG (2003). The amygdala, social behavior, and danger detection. *Annals of the New York Academy of Sciences* 1000: 337–347.

Amaral DG & Price JL (1984). Amygdalo-cortical projections in the monkey (Macaca fascicularis). *Journal of Comparative Neurology* 230: 465–496.

Amaral DG, Price JL, Pitkanen A, & Carmichael ST (1992). Anatomical organization of the primate amygdaloid complex. In Aggleton JP, editor, *The Amygdala*, chap. 1, 1–66. Wiley-Liss, New York.

Amsel A (1962). Frustrative non-reward in partial reinforcement and discrimination learning: some recent history and a theoretical extension. *Psychological Review* 69: 306–328.

Anderson AK, Christoff K, Stappen I, Panitz D, Ghahremani DG, Glover G, Gabrieli JD, & Sobel N (2003). Dissociated neural representations of intensity and valence in human olfaction. *Nature Neuroscience* 6: 196–202.

Anderson IM, Haddad PM, & Scott J (2012). Bipolar disorder. *BMJ* 345: e8508.

Anderson JR (1996). ACT: a simple theory of complex cognition. *American Psychologist* 51: 355–365.

Aou S, Oomura Y, Lenard L, Nishino H, Inokuchi A, Minami T, & Misaki H (1984). Behavioral significance of monkey hypothalamic glucose-sensitive neurons. *Brain Research* 302: 69–74.

Argiolas A & Melis MR (2013). Neuropeptides and central control of sexual behavior from the past to the present: A review. *Progress in Neurobiology* doi: 10.1016/j.pneurobio.2013.06.006.

Aron AR, Robbins TW, & Poldrack RA (2014). Inhibition and the right inferior frontal cortex: one decade on. *Trends in Cognitive Sciences* 18: 177–85.

Auger SD & Maguire EA (2013). Assessing the mechanism of response in the retrosplenial cortex of good and poor navigators. *Cortex* 49: 2904–2913.

Baars BJ (1988). *A Cognitive Theory of Consciousness*. Cambridge University Press, New York.

Baker RR & Bellis MA (1995). *Human Sperm Competition: Copulation, Competition and Infidelity*. Chapman and Hall, London.

Baker RR & Shackelford TK (2017). A comparison of paternity data and relative testes size as measures of level of sperm competition in the hominoidea. *Am J Phys Anthropol* .

Balleine BW & Dickinson A (1998). The role of incentive learning in instrumental outcome revaluation by sensory-specific satiety. *Animal Learning and Behavior* 26: 46–59.

Bar-On R (1997). *The Emotional Intelligence Inventory (EQ-i): Technical Manual*. MultiHealth Systems, Toronto.

Barbaro N & Shackelford TK (2015). Book review: Nether no more: Bringing genital evolution to the forefront. *Evolutionary Psychology* 13: 262–265.

Barbas H (1988). Anatomic organization of basoventral and mediodorsal visual recipient prefrontal regions in the rhesus monkey. *Journal of Comparative Neurology* 276: 313–342.

Barbas H (1993). Organization of cortical afferent input to the orbitofrontal area in the rhesus monkey. *Neuroscience* 56: 841–864.

Barbas H (1995). Anatomic basis of cognitive–emotional interactions in the primate prefrontal cortex. *Neuroscience and Biobehavioral Reviews* 19: 499–510.

Barbas H (2007). Specialized elements of orbitofrontal cortex in primates. *Annals of the New York Academy of Sciences* 1121: 10–32.

Barbas H & Pandya DN (1989). Architecture and intrinsic connections of the prefrontal cortex in the rhesus monkey. *Journal of Comparative Neurology* 286: 353–375.

Barbas H, Zikopoulos B, & Timbie C (2011). Sensory pathways and emotional context for action in primate prefrontal cortex. *Biological Psychiatry* 69: 1133–1139.

Barrett L, Dunbar R, & Lycett J (2002). *Human Evolutionary Psychology*. Palgrave, Basingstoke.

Barsh GS & Schwartz MW (2002). Genetic approaches to studying energy balence: perception and integration. *Nature Reviews Genetics* 3: 589–600.

Barsh GS, Farooqi IS, & O'Rahilly S (2000). Genetics of body weight regulation. *Nature* 404: 644–651.

Barson JR, Karatayev O, Chang GQ, Johnson DF, Bocarsly ME, Hoebel BG, & Leibowitz SF (2009). Positive relationship between dietary fat, ethanol intake, triglycerides, and hypothalamic peptides: counteraction by lipid-lowering drugs. *Alcohol* 43: 433–441.

Bateman AJ (1948). Intra-sexual selection in drosophila. *Heredity (Edinb)* 2: 349–68.

Bateson P (1983). *Mate Choice*. Cambridge University Press, Cambridge.

Baum MJ, Everitt BJ, Herbert J, & Keverne EB (1977). Hormonal basis of proceptivity and receptivity in female primates. *Archives of Sexual Behavior* 6: 173–192.

Baylis LL & Gaffan D (1991). Amygdalectomy and ventromedial prefrontal ablation produce similar deficits in food choice and in simple object discrimination learning for an unseen reward. *Experimental Brain Research* 86: 617–622.

Baylis LL & Rolls ET (1991). Responses of neurons in the primate taste cortex to glutamate. *Physiology and Behavior* 49: 973–979.

Baylis LL, Rolls ET, & Baylis GC (1994). Afferent connections of the orbitofrontal cortex taste area of the primate. *Neuroscience* 64: 801–812.

Beauchamp GK & Yamazaki K (2003). Chemical signalling in mice. *Biochemical Society Transactions* 31: 147–151.

Beaver JD, Lawrence AD, Ditzhuijzen Jv, Davis MH, Woods A, & Calder AJ (2006). Individual differences in reward drive predict neural responses to images of food. *Journal of Neuroscience* 26: 5160–5166.

Bechara A, Damasio AR, Damasio H, & Anderson SW (1994). Insensitivity to future consequences following damage to human prefrontal cortex. *Cognition* 50: 7–15.

Bechara A, Tranel D, Damasio H, & Damasio AR (1996). Failure to respond autonomically to anticipated future outcomes following damage to prefrontal cortex. *Cerebral Cortex* 6: 215–225.

Bechara A, Damasio H, Tranel D, & Damasio AR (1997). Deciding advantageously before knowing the advantageous strategy. *Science* 275: 1293–1295.

Bechara A, Damasio H, Tranel D, & Damasio AR (2005). The Iowa Gambling Task and the somatic marker hypothesis: some questions and answers. *Trends in Cognitive Sciences* 9: 159–162.

Beck AT (1979). *Cognitive Therapy of Depression*. Guilford Press.

Beck AT (2008). The evolution of the cognitive model of depression and its neurobiological correlates. *American Journal of Psychiatry* 165: 969–977.

Becker NB, Jesus SN, Joao K, Viseu JN, & Martins RIS (2017). Depression and sleep quality in older adults: a meta-analysis. *Psychol Health Med* 22: 889–895.

Beckstead RM & Norgren R (1979). An autoradiographic examination of the central distribution of the trigeminal, facial, glossopharyngeal, and vagal nerves in the monkey. *Journal of Comparative Neurology* 184: 455–472.

Beckstead RM, Morse JR, & Norgren R (1980). The nucleus of the solitary tract in the monkey: projections to the thalamus and brainstem nuclei. *Journal of Comparative Neurology* 190: 259–282.

Beluzzi JD, Grant N, Garsky V, Sarantakis D, Wise CD, & Stein L (1976). Analgesia induced in vivo by central administration of enkephalin in rat. *Nature* 260: 625–626.

Ben-Ze'ev A (2000). *The Subtlety of Emotions*. MIT Press, Cambridge, MA.

Benes FM & Subburaj S (2016). *Circuitry-specific hypermetabolism in the hippocampus of bipolar patients*, book section 7, 70–89. Cambridge University Press, Cambridge, 3rd edn.

Berglund A & Rosenqvist G (2001). Male pipefish prefer ornamented females. *Animal Behaviour* 61: 345–350.

Berlin H & Rolls ET (2004). Time perception, impulsivity, emotionality, and personality in self-harming borderline personality disorder patients. *Journal of Personality Disorders* 18: 358–378.

Berlin H, Rolls ET, & Kischka U (2004). Impulsivity, time perception, emotion, and reinforcement sensitivity in patients with orbitofrontal cortex lesions. *Brain* 127: 1108–1126.

Berlin H, Rolls ET, & Iversen SD (2005). Borderline Personality Disorder, impulsivity, and the orbitofrontal cortex. *American Journal of Psychiatry* 58: 234–245.

Bermpohl F, Kahnt T, Dalanay U, Hagele C, Sajonz B, Wegner T, Stoy M, Adli M, Kruger S, Wrase J, Strohle A, Bauer M, & Heinz A (2010). Altered representation of expected value in the orbitofrontal cortex in mania. *Human Brain Mapping* 31: 958–969.

Berner LA, Bocarsly ME, Hoebel BG, & Avena NM (2011). Pharmacological interventions for binge eating: lessons from animal models, current treatments, and future directions. *Current Pharmaceutical Design* 17: 1180–1187.

Berntson GG, Norman GJ, Bechara A, Bruss J, Tranel D, & Cacioppo JT (2011). The insula and evaluative processes. *Psychological Science* 22: 80–66.

Berridge KC (1996). Food reward: brain substrates of wanting and liking. *Neuroscience and Biobehavioral Reviews* 20: 1–25.

Berridge KC & Robinson TE (1998). What is the role of dopamine in reward: hedonic impact, reward learning, or incentive salience? *Brain Research Reviews* 28: 309–369.

Berridge KC, Robinson TE, & Aldridge JW (2009). Dissecting components of reward: 'liking', 'wanting', and learning. *Current Opinion in Pharmacology* 9: 65–73.

Bertram BCR (1975). Social factors influencing reproduction in wild lions. *Journal of Zoology* 177: 463–482.

Betzig LL (1986). *Despotism and Differential Reproduction.* Aldine, New York.

Bhattacharya A, Derecki NC, Lovenberg TW, & Drevets WC (2016). Role of neuro-immunological factors in the pathophysiology of mood disorders. *Psychopharmacology (Berl)* 233: 1623–36.

Birkhead T (2000). *Promiscuity.* Faber and Faber, London.

Birkhead TR, Chaline N, Biggins JD, Burke T, & Pizzari T (2004). Nontransitivity of paternity in a bird. *Evolution* 58: 416–420.

Bjorklund A & Lindvall O (1986). Catecholaminergic brainstem regulatory systems. In Mountcastle VB, Bloom FE, & Geiger SR, editors, *Handbook of Physiology: The Nervous System*, vol. 4, Intrinsic systems of the Brain, 155–236. American Psychological Society, Bethesda.

Blaney PH (1986). Affect and memory: a review. *Psychological Bulletin* 99: 229–246.

Blaustein JD & Erskine MS (2002). Feminine sexual behavior. In Pfaff DW, Arnold AP, Etgen AM, Fahrbach SE, & Rubin RT, editors, *Hormones, Brain and Behavior*, vol. 1, chap. 2, 139–214. Academic Press, San Diego, CA.

Bliss-Moreau E, Moadab G, Bauman MD, & Amaral DG (2013). The impact of early amygdala damage on juvenile rhesus macaque social behavior. *J Cogn Neurosci* 25: 2124–40.

Block N (1995). On a confusion about a function of consciousness. *Behavioral and Brain Sciences* 18: 22–47.

Blood AJ & Zatorre RJ (2001). Intensely pleasureable responses to music correlate with activity of brain regions implicated in reward and emotion. *Proceedings of the National Academy of Sciences USA* 98: 11818–11823.

Blood AJ, Zatorre RJ, Bermudez P, & Evans AC (1999). Emotional responses to pleasant and unpleasant music correlate with activity in paralimbic brain regions. *Nature Neuroscience* 2: 382–387.

Blumberg J & Kreiman G (2010). How cortical neurons help us see: visual recognition in the human brain. *The Journal of Clinical Investigation* 120: 3054–3063.

Boden MA, editor (1996). *The Philosophy of Artificial Life.* Oxford University Press, Oxford.

Booth DA (1985). Food-conditioned eating preferences and aversions with interoceptive elements: learned appetites and satieties. *Annals of the New York Academy of Sciences* 443: 22–37.

Booth MCA & Rolls ET (1998). View-invariant representations of familiar objects by neurons in the inferior temporal visual cortex. *Cerebral Cortex* 8: 510–523.

Bosch OJ & Young LJ (2017). Oxytocin and social relationships: From attachment to bond disruption. *Curr Top Behav Neurosci* .

Bostan AC, Dum RP, & Strick PL (2018). Functional anatomy of basal ganglia circuits with the cerebral cortex and the cerebellum. *Prog Neurol Surg* 33: 50–61.

Bowlby J (1969). *Attachment and Loss: Volume 1 Attachment.* Hogarth Press, London.

Bowlby J (1973). *Attachment and Loss: Volume 2 Separation.* Hogarth Press, London.

Bowlby J (1980). *Attachment and Loss: Volume 3 Loss.* Hogarth Press, London.

Bowles S & Gintis H (2005). Prosocial emotions. In Blume LE & Durlauf SN, editors, *The Economy as an Evolving Complex System III.* Santa Fe Institute, Santa Fe, NM.

Boyd R, Gintis H, Bowles S, & Richerson PJ (2003). The evolution of altruistic punishment. *Proceedings of the National Academy of Sciences USA* 100: 3531–3535.

Brodersen KH, Wiech K, Lomakina EI, Lin CS, Buhmann JM, Bingel U, Ploner M, Stephan KE, & Tracey I (2012). Decoding the perception of pain from fmri using multivariate pattern analysis. *Neuroimage* 63: 1162–1170.

Bromberg-Martin ES & Hikosaka O (2011). Lateral habenula neurons signal errors in the prediction of reward information. *Nat Neurosci* 14: 1209–16.

Bromberg-Martin ES, Matsumoto M, & Hikosaka O (2010). Dopamine in motivational control: rewarding, aversive, and alerting. *Neuron* 68: 815–834.

Brothers L & Ring B (1993). Mesial temporal neurons in the macaque monkey with responses selective for aspects of social stimuli. *Behavioural Brain Research* 57: 53–61.

Brunel N & Wang XJ (2001). Effects of neuromodulation in a cortical network model of object working memory dominated by recurrent inhibition. *Journal of Computational Neuroscience* 11: 63–85.

Bubb EJ, Kinnavane L, & Aggleton JP (2017). Hippocampal - diencephalic - cingulate networks for memory and emotion: An anatomical guide. *Brain Neurosci Adv* 1.

Buot A & Yelnik J (2012). Functional anatomy of the basal ganglia: limbic aspects. *Revue Neurologique (Paris)* 168: 569–575.

Burch RL & Gallup GG (2006). *The psychobiology of human semen*, book section 8, 141–172. Cambridge University Press, Cambridge.

Bush G, Luu P, & Posner MI (2000). Cognitive and emotional influences in anterior cingulate cortex. *Trends in Cognitive Sciences* 4: 215–222.

Bush G, Vogt BA, Holmes J, Dales AM, Greve D, Jenike MA, & Rosen BR (2002). Dorsal anterior cingulate cortex: a role in reward-based decision making. *Proceedings of the National Academy of Sciences USA* 99: 523–528.

Buss DM (1989). Sex differences in human mate preferences: evolutionary hypotheses tested in 37 cultures. *Behavioural and Brain Sciences* 12: 1–14.

Buss DM (2015). *Evolutionary Psychology: The New Science of the Mind.* Pearson, Boston, MA, 5th edn.

Buss DM (2016). *Evolution of Desire. Strategies of Human Mating.* Basic Books, New York, NY, revised and updated edn.

Buss DM & Schmitt DP (1993). Sexual strategies theory: an evolutionary perspective on human mating. *Psychological Review* 100: 204–232.

Buss DM, Abbott M, Angeleitner A, Asherian A, Biaggio A, Blancovillasenor A, Bruchonschweitzer M, Chu H, Czapinski J, DeRaad B, Ekehammar B, Ellohamy N, Fioravanti M, Georgas J, Gjerde P, Guttman R, Hazan F, Iwawaki S, Janakiramaiah N, Khosroshani F, Kreitler S, Lachenicht L, Lee M, Liik K, Little B, Mika S, Moadelshahid M, Moane G, Montero M, Mundycastle AC, Niit T, Nsenduluka E, Pienkowski R, Pirttila-Backman AM, Deleon JP, Rousseau J, Runco MA, Safir MP, Samuels C, Sanitioso R, Serpell R, Smid N, Spencer C, Tadinac M, Todorova EN, Troland K, Vandenbrande L, Van Heck G, Vanlangenhove L, & Yang KS (1990). International preferences in selecting mates: a study of 37 cultures. *Journal of Cross-Cultural Psychology* 21: 5–47.

Butter CM (1969). Perseveration in extinction and in discrimination reversal tasks following selective prefrontal ablations in Macaca mulatta. *Physiology and Behavior* 4: 163–171.

Butter CM & Snyder DR (1972). Alterations in aversive and aggressive behaviors following orbitofrontal lesions in rhesus monkeys. *Acta Neurobiologica Experimentalis* 32: 525–565.

Butter CM, McDonald JA, & Snyder DR (1969). Orality, preference behavior, and reinforcement value of non-food objects in monkeys with orbital frontal lesions. *Science* 164: 1306–1307.

Butter CM, Snyder DR, & McDonald JA (1970). Effects of orbitofrontal lesions on aversive and aggressive behaviors in rhesus monkeys. *Journal of Comparative Physiology and Psychology* 72: 132–144.

Caan W, Perrett DI, & Rolls ET (1984). Responses of striatal neurons in the behaving monkey. 2. Visual processing in the caudal neostriatum. *Brain Research* 290: 53–65.

Cabanac M (1971). Physiological role of pleasure. *Science* 173: 1103–1107.

Cabanac M & Duclaux R (1970). Specificity of internal signals in producing satiety for taste stimuli. *Nature* 227: 966–967.

Cabanac M & Fantino M (1977). Origin of olfacto-gustatory alliesthesia: Intestinal sensitivity to carbohydrate concentration? *Physiology and Behavior* 10: 1039–1045.

Cai X & Padoa-Schioppa C (2012). Neuronal encoding of subjective value in dorsal and ventral anterior cingulate cortex. *Journal of Neuroscience* 32: 3791–3808.

Calder AJ, Keane J, Manes F, Antoun N, & Young AW (2000). Impaired recognition and experience of disgust following brain injury. *Nature Neuroscience* 3: 1077–1078.

Camille N, Tsuchida A, & Fellows LK (2011). Double dissociation of stimulus-value and action-value learning in humans with orbitofrontal or anterior cingulate cortex damage. *Journal of Neuroscience* 31: 15048–15052.

Canli T, Zhao Z, Desmond JE, Kang E, Gross J, & Gabrieli JD (2001). An fMRI study of personality influences on brain reactivity to emotional stimuli. *Behavioral Neuroscience* 115: 33–42.

Canli T, Sivers H, Whitfield SL, Gotlib IH, & Gabrieli JD (2002). Amygdala response to happy faces as a function of extraversion. *Science* 296: 2191.

Cannistraro PA & Rauch SL (2003). Neural circuitry of anxiety: evidence from structural and functional neuroimaging studies. *Psychopharmacology Bulletin* 37: 8–25.

Cardinal N & Everitt BJ (2004). Neural and psychological mechanisms underlying appetitive learning: links to drug addiction. *Current Opinion in Neurobiology* 14: 156–162.

Cardinal RN, Parkinson JA, Hall J, & Everitt BJ (2002). Emotion and motivation: the role of the amygdala, ventral striatum, and prefrontal cortex. *Neuroscience and Biobehavioral Reviews* 26: 321–352.

Carlson NR & Birkett MA (2017). *Physiology of Behavior.* Pearson, Boston, 12th edn.

Carmichael ST & Price JL (1994). Architectonic subdivision of the orbital and medial prefrontal cortex in the macaque monkey. *Journal of Comparative Neurology* 346: 366–402.

Carmichael ST & Price JL (1995a). Limbic connections of the orbital and medial prefrontal cortex in macaque monkeys. *Journal of Comparative Neurology* 363: 615–641.

Carmichael ST & Price JL (1995b). Sensory and premotor connections of the orbital and medial prefrontal cortex of macaque monkeys. *Journal of Comparative Neurology* 363: 642–664.

Carmichael ST, Clugnet MC, & Price JL (1994). Central olfactory connections in the macaque monkey. *Journal of Comparative Neurology* 346: 403–434.

Carruthers P (1996). *Language, Thought and Consciousness.* Cambridge University Press, Cambridge.

Carruthers P (2000). *Phenomenal Consciousness.* Cambridge University Press, Cambridge.

Carter CS (1998). Neuroendocrine perpectives on social attachment and love. *Psychoneuroendocrinology* 23: 779–818.

Carter CS (2017). Oxytocin and human evolution. *Curr Top Behav Neurosci* .

Cavanna AE & Trimble MR (2006). The precuneus: a review of its functional anatomy and behavioural correlates. *Brain* 129: 564–583.

Celada P, Puig MV, Armagos-Bosch M, Adell A, & Artigas F (2004). The therapeutic role of 5-HT_{1A} and 5-HT_{2A} receptors in depression. *Journal of Psychiatry and Neuroscience* 29: 252–265.

Chalmers DJ (1996). *The Conscious Mind.* Oxford University Press, Oxford.

Chandrashekar J, Hoon MA, Ryba NJ, & Zuker CS (2006). The receptors and cells for mammalian taste. *Nature* 444: 288–294.

Chau BK, Sallet J, Papageorgiou GK, Noonan MP, Bell AH, Walton ME, & Rushworth MF (2015). Contrasting roles for orbitofrontal cortex and amygdala in credit assignment and learning in macaques. *Neuron* 87: 1106–1118.

Chaudhari N & Roper SD (2010). The cell biology of taste. *Journal of Cell Biology* 190: 285–296.

Chaudhari N, Landin AM, & Roper S (2000). A metabolic glutamate receptor variant functions as a taste receptor. *Nature Neuroscience* 3: 113–119.

Cheng W, Rolls ET, Qiu J, Liu W, Tang Y, Huang CC, Wang X, Zhang J, Lin W, Zheng L, Pu J, Tsai SJ, Yang AC, Lin CP, Wang F, Xie P, & Feng J (2016). Medial reward and lateral non-reward orbitofrontal cortex circuits change in opposite directions in depression. *Brain* 139: 3296–3309.

Cheng W, Rolls ET, Qiu J, Xie X, Lyu W, Li Y, Huang CC, Yang AC, Tsai SJ, Lyu F, Zhuang K, Lin CP, Xie P, & Feng J (2018a). Functional connectivity of the human amygdala in health and in depression. *Social, Cognitive, and Affective Neuroscience* doi: 10.1093/scan/nsy032.

Cheng W, Rolls ET, Qiu J, Xie X, Wei D, Huang CC, Yang AC, Tsai SJ, Li Q, Meng J, Lin CP, Xie P, & Feng J (2018b). Increased functional connectivity of the posterior cingulate cortex with the lateral orbitofrontal cortex in depression. *Translational Psychiatry* 8: 90.

Cheng W, Rolls ET, Qiu J, Yang D, Ruan H, Wei D, Zhao L, Meng J, Xie P, & Feng J (2018c). Functional connectivity of the precuneus in unmedicated patients with depression. *Biological Psychiatry: Cognitive Neuroscience and Neuroimaging* in revision.

Cheng W, Rolls ET, Ruan H, & Feng J (2018d). Brain mechanisms that mediate the relationship between depressive problems and sleep quality. *JAMA Psychiatry* in press.

Chevalier-Skolnikoff S (1973). Facial expression of emotion in non-human primates. In Ekman P, editor, *Darwin and Facial Expression*, 11–89. Academic Press, New York.

Childress AR, Mozley PD, McElgin W, Fitzgerald J, Reivich M, & O'Brien CP (1999). Limbic activation during cue-induced cocaine craving. *American Journal of Psychiatry* 156: 11–18.

Cho YK, Li CS, & Smith DV (2002). Gustatory projections from the nucleus of the solitary tract to the parabrachial nuclei in the hamster. *Chemical Senses* 27: 81–90.

Churchland PS & Winkielman P (2012). Modulating social behavior with oxytocin: how does it work? What does it mean? *Hormones and Behavior* 61: 392–399.

Clutton-Brock TH & Albon SD (1979). The roaring of red deer and the evolution of honest advertisement. *Behaviour* 69: 145–170.

Cooper JR, Bloom FE, & Roth RH (2003). *The Biochemical Basis of Neuropharmacology.* Oxford University Press, Oxford, 8th edn.

Corbetta M & Shulman GL (2002). Control of goal-directed and stimulus-driven attention in the brain. *Nature Reviews Neuroscience* 3: 201–215.

Cornell CE, Rodin J, & Weingarten H (1989). Stimulus-induced eating when satiated. *Physiology and Behavior* 45: 695–704.

Corr PJ & McNaughton N (2012). Neuroscience and approach/avoidance personality traits: a two stage (valuation-motivation) approach. *Neuroscience and Biobehavioural Reviews* 36: 2339–2254.

Corrado GS, Sugrue LP, Seung HS, & Newsome WT (2005). Linear-nonlinear-Poisson models of primate choice dynamics. *Journal of the Experimental Analysis of Behavior* 84: 581–617.

Cosmides I & Tooby J (1999). Evolutionary psychology. In Wilson R & Keil F, editors, *MIT Encyclopedia of the Cognitive Sciences*, 295–298. MIT Press, Cambridge, MA.

Cowley JJ & Brooksbank BWL (1991). Human exposure to putative pheromones and changes in aspects of social behaviour. *Journal of Steroid Biochemistry and Molecular Biology* 39: 647–659.

Craig AD (2009). How do you feel–now? The anterior insula and human awareness. *Nature Reviews Neuroscience* 10: 59–70.

Craig AD (2011). Significance of the insula for the evolution of human awareness of feelings from the body. *Annals of the New York Academy of Sciences* 1225: 72–82.

Craig AD, Chen K, Bandy D, & Reiman EM (2000). Thermosensory activation of insular cortex. *Nature Neuroscience* 3: 184–190.

Crews FT & Boettiger CA (2009). Impulsivity, frontal lobes and risk for addiction. *Pharmacology Biochemistry and Behavior* 93: 237–247.

Crick FHC & Koch C (1990). Towards a neurobiological theory of consciousness. *Seminars in the Neurosciences* 2: 263–275.

Critchley HD & Harrison NA (2013). Visceral influences on brain and behavior. *Neuron* 77: 624–638.

Critchley HD & Rolls ET (1996a). Responses of primate taste cortex neurons to the astringent tastant tannic acid. *Chemical Senses* 21: 135–145.

Critchley HD & Rolls ET (1996b). Olfactory neuronal responses in the primate orbitofrontal cortex: analysis in an olfactory discrimination task. *Journal of Neurophysiology* 75: 1659–1672.

Critchley HD & Rolls ET (1996c). Hunger and satiety modify the responses of olfactory and visual neurons in the primate orbitofrontal cortex. *Journal of Neurophysiology* 75: 1673–1686.

Croxson PL, Walton ME, O'Reilly JX, Behrens TE, & Rushworth MF (2009). Effort-based cost-benefit valuation and the human brain. *Journal of Neuroscience* 29: 4531–4541.

Cummings DE & Schwartz MW (2003). Genetics and pathophysiology of human obesity. *Annual Reviews of Medicine* 54: 453–471.

Cunningham MR, Roberts AR, Barbee AP, & Druen PB (1995). Their ideas of beauty are, on the whole, the same as ours: consistency and variability in the cross-cultural perception of female physical attractiveness. *Journal of Personality and Social Psychology* 68: 261–279.

Dahlström A & Fuxe K (1965). Evidence for the existence of monoamine-containing neurons in the central nervous system: demonstration of monoamines in the cell bodies of brain stem neurons. *Acta Physiologia Scandinavica* 62: 1–55.

Dai D, Li QC, Zhu QB, Hu SH, Balesar R, Swaab D, & Bao AM (2017). Direct involvement of androgen receptor in oxytocin gene expression: Possible relevance for mood disorders. *Neuropsychopharmacology* 42: 2064–2071.

Damasio A, Damasio H, & Tranel D (2013). Persistence of feelings and sentience after bilateral damage of the insula. *Cerebral Cortex* 23: 833–846.

Damasio AR (1994). *Descartes' Error: Emotion, Reason, and the Human Brain*. Grosset/Putnam, New York.

Damasio AR (1996). The somatic marker hypothesis and the possible functions of the prefrontal cortex [and discussion]. *Philosophical Transactions of the Royal Society of London. Series B: Biological Sciences* 351: 1413–1420.

Damasio AR (2003). *Looking for Spinoza*. Heinemann, London.

Damasio AR, Grabowski TJ, Bechara A, Damasio H, Ponto LLB, Parvizi J, & Hichwa RD (2000). Subcortical and cortical brain activity during the feeling of self-generated emotions. *Nature Neuroscience* 3: 1049–1056.

Damasio H, Grabowski T, Frank R, Galaburda AM, & Damasio AR (1994). The return of Phineas Gage: clues about the brain from the skull of a famous patient. *Science* 264: 1102–1105.

Darwin C (1859). *The Origin of Species*. John Murray [reprinted (1982) by Penguin Books Ltd], London.

Darwin C (1871). *The Descent of Man, and Selection in Relation to Sex*. John Murray [reprinted (1981) by Princeton University Press], London.

Darwin C (1872). *The Expression of the Emotions in Man and Animals*. University of Chicago Press. [reprinted (1998) (3rd edn) ed. P. Ekman. Harper Collins], Glasgow.

Davis M (2006). Neural systems involved in fear and anxiety measured with fear-potentiated startle. *American Psychologist* 61: 741–756.

Davis M (2011). NMDA receptors and fear extinction: implications for cognitive behavioral therapy. *Dialogues in Clinical Neuroscience* 13: 463–474.

Davis M, Antoniadis EA, Amaral DG, & Winslow JT (2008). Acoustic startle reflex in rhesus monkeys: a review. *Reviews in Neuroscience* 19: 171–185.

Dawkins MS (1986a). *Unravelling Animal Behaviour*. Longman, Harlow, 1st edn.

Dawkins MS (1995). *Unravelling Animal Behaviour*. Longman, Harlow, 2nd edn.

Dawkins R (1976). *The Selfish Gene*. Oxford University Press, Oxford.

Dawkins R (1982). *The Extended Phenotype*. Freeman, Oxford.

Dawkins R (1986b). *The Blind Watchmaker*. Longman, Harlow.

Dawkins R (1989). *The Selfish Gene*. Oxford University Press, Oxford, 2nd edn.

Dayan P & Abbott LF (2001). *Theoretical Neuroscience*. MIT Press, Cambridge, MA.

de Araujo IE, Ferreira JG, Tellez LA, Ren X, & Yeckel CW (2012). The gut-brain dopamine axis: a regulatory system for caloric intake. *Physiol Behav* 106: 394–9.

De Araujo IET & Rolls ET (2004). Representation in the human brain of food texture and oral fat. *Journal of Neuroscience* 24: 3086–3093.

De Araujo IET, Rolls ET, & Stringer SM (2001). A view model which accounts for the response properties of hippocampal primate spatial view cells and rat place cells. *Hippocampus* 11: 699–706.

De Araujo IET, Kringelbach ML, Rolls ET, & Hobden P (2003a). Representation of umami taste in the human brain. *Journal of Neurophysiology* 90: 313–319.

De Araujo IET, Kringelbach ML, Rolls ET, & McGlone F (2003b). Human cortical responses to water in the mouth, and the effects of thirst. *Journal of Neurophysiology* 90: 1865–1876.

De Araujo IET, Rolls ET, Kringelbach ML, McGlone F, & Phillips N (2003c). Taste-olfactory convergence, and the representation of the pleasantness of flavour in the human brain. *European Journal of Neuroscience* 18: 2059–2068.

De Araujo IET, Rolls ET, Velazco MI, Margot C, & Cayeux I (2005). Cognitive modulation of olfactory processing. *Neuron* 46: 671–679.

De Gelder B, Vroomen J, Pourtois G, & Weiskrantz L (1999). Non-conscious recognition of affect in the absence of striate cortex. *NeuroReport* 10: 3759–3763.

Debiec J, LeDoux JE, & Nader K (2002). Cellular and systems reconsolidation in the hippocampus. *Neuron* 36: 527–538.

Debiec J, Doyere V, Nader K, & LeDoux JE (2006). Directly reactivated, but not indirectly reactivated, memories undergo reconsolidation in the amygdala. *Proceedings of the National Academy of Sciences USA* 103: 3428–3433.

Deco G & Kringelbach ML (2014). Great expectations: using whole-brain computational connectomics for understanding neuropsychiatric disorders. *Neuron* 84: 892–905.

Deco G & Rolls ET (2003). Attention and working memory: a dynamical model of neuronal activity in the prefrontal cortex. *European Journal of Neuroscience* 18: 2374–2390.

Deco G & Rolls ET (2004). A neurodynamical cortical model of visual attention and invariant object recognition. *Vision Research* 44: 621–644.

Deco G & Rolls ET (2005a). Synaptic and spiking dynamics underlying reward reversal in the orbitofrontal cortex. *Cerebral Cortex* 15: 15–30.

Deco G & Rolls ET (2005b). Neurodynamics of biased competition and cooperation for attention: a model with spiking neurons. *Journal of Neurophysiology* 94: 295–313.

Deco G & Rolls ET (2006). A neurophysiological model of decision-making and Weber's law. *European Journal of Neuroscience* 24: 901–916.

Deco G, Rolls ET, & Romo R (2009). Stochastic dynamics as a principle of brain function. *Progress in Neurobiology* 88: 1–16.

Deco G, Rolls ET, Albantakis L, & Romo R (2013). Brain mechanisms for perceptual and reward-related decision-making. *Progress in Neurobiology* 103: 194–213.

Dehaene S & Naccache L (2001). Towards a cognitive neuroscience of consciousness: basic evidence and a workspace framework. *Cognition* 79: 1–37.

Dehaene S, Changeux JP, Naccache L, Sackur J, & Sergent C (2006). Conscious, preconscious, and subliminal processing: a testable taxonomy. *Trends in Cognitive Sciences* 10: 204–211.

Dehaene S, Charles L, King JR, & Marti S (2014). Toward a computational theory of conscious processing. *Curr Opin Neurobiol* 25: 76–84.

Dehaene S, Lau H, & Kouider S (2017). What is consciousness, and could machines have it? *Science* 358: 486–492.

Delgado MR, Jou RL, & Phelps EA (2011). Neural systems underlying aversive conditioning in humans with primary and secondary reinforcers. *Frontiers in Neuroscience* 5: 71.

DeLong M & Wichmann T (2010). Changing views of basal ganglia circuits and circuit disorders. *Clinical EEG and Neuroscience* 41: 61–67.

Deng WL, Rolls ET, Ji X, Robbins TW, Banaschewski T, Bokde A, Bromberg U, Buechel C, Desrivieres S, Conrod P, Flor H, Frouin V, Gallinat J, Garavan H, Gowland P, Heinz A, Ittermann B, Martinot JL, Lemaitre H, Nees F, Papadopoulos Orfanos D, Poustka L, Smolka MN, Walter H, Whelan R, Schumann G, Feng J, & the Imagen consortium (2017). Separate neural systems for behavioral change and for emotional responses to failure during behavioral inhibition. *Human Brain Mapping* doi: 10.1002/hbm.23607.

Dennett DC (1991). *Consciousness Explained.* Penguin, London.

Derbyshire SWG, Vogt BA, & Jones AKP (1998). Pain and Stroop interference tasks activate separate processing modules in anterior cingulate cortex. *Experimental Brain Research* 118: 52–60.

Desimone R & Duncan J (1995). Neural mechanisms of selective visual attention. *Annual Review of Neuroscience* 18: 193–222.

DeVries AC, DeVries MB, Taymans SE, & Carter CS (1996). The effects of stress on social preferences are sexually dimorphic in prairie voles. *Proceedings of the National Academy of Science USA* 93: 11980–11984.

Di Lorenzo PM (1990). Corticofugal influence on taste responses in the parabrachial pons of the rat. *Brain Research* 530: 73–84.

Di Marzo V & Matias I (2005). Endocannabinoid control of food intake and energy balance. *Nature Neuroscience* 8: 585–590.

Diamond J (1997). *Why is Sex Fun?* Weidenfeld and Nicholson, London.

Dickinson A (1980). *Contemporary Animal Learning Theory*. Cambridge University Press, Cambridge.

Dickinson A (1994). Instrumental conditioning. In Mackintosh NJ, editor, *Animal Learning and Cognition*, 45–80. Academic Press, San Diego.

Disner SG, Beevers CG, Haigh EA, & Beck AT (2011). Neural mechanisms of the cognitive model of depression. *Nat Rev Neurosci* 12: 467–77.

Douglas RJ, Markram H, & Martin KAC (2004). Neocortex. In Shepherd GM, editor, *The Synaptic Organization of the Brain*, chap. 12, 499–558. Oxford University Press, Oxford, 5th edn.

Downar J, Blumberger DM, Rizvi SJ, Daskalakis ZJ, Kennedy H, & Giacobbe P (2018). Targeting the neural subtypes of depression .

Doyere V, Debiec J, Monfils MH, Schafe GE, & LeDoux JE (2007). Synapse-specific reconsolidation of distinct fear memories in the lateral amygdala. *Nature Neuroscience* 10: 414–416.

Drevets WC (2007). Orbitofrontal cortex function and structure in depression. *Annals of the New York Academy of Sciences* 1121: 499–527.

Drysdale AT, Grosenick L, Downar J, Dunlop K, Mansouri F, Meng Y, Fetcho RN, Zebley B, Oathes DJ, Etkin A, Schatzberg AF, Sudheimer K, Keller J, Mayberg HS, Gunning FM, Alexopoulos GS, Fox MD, Pascual-Leone A, Voss HU, Casey BJ, Dubin MJ, & Liston C (2017). Resting-state connectivity biomarkers define neurophysiological subtypes of depression. *Nat Med* 23: 28–38.

Dulac C & Kimchi T (2007). Neural mechanisms underlying sex-specific behaviors in vertebrates. *Current Opinion in Neurobiology* 17: 675–683.

Dulac C & Torello AT (2003). Molecular detection of pheromone signals in mammals: from genes to behaviour. *Nature Reviews Neuroscience* 4: 551–562.

Duman RS & Aghajanian GK (2012). Synaptic dysfunction in depression: potential therapeutic targets. *Science* 338: 68–72.

Dunbar R (1993). Co-evolution of neocortex size, group size and language in humans. *Behavioural and Brain Sciences* 16: 681–735.

Dunbar R (1996). *Grooming, Gossip, and the Evolution of Language*. Faber and Faber, London.

Edward DA, Stockley P, & Hosken DJ (2015). Sexual conflict and sperm competition. *Cold Spring Harbor perspectives in biology* 7: a017707.

Eisenberger NI & Lieberman MD (2004). Why rejection hurts: a common neural alarm system for physical and social pain. *Trends in Cognitive Neuroscience* 8: 294–300.

Ekman P (1992). An argument for basic emotions. *Cognition and Emotion* 6: 169–200.

Ekman P (2003). *Emotions Revealed: Understanding Faces and Feelings*. Weidenfeld and Nicolson, London.

Engelhardt A, Pfeifer JB, Heistermann M, Niemitz C, Van Hoof JARAM, & Jodges JK (2004). Assessment of females' reproductive status by male longtailed macques, Macaca fascicularis, under natural conditions. *Animal Behaviour* 67: 915–924.

Eshel N & Roiser JP (2010). Reward and punishment processing in depression. *Biological Psychiatry* 68: 118–124.

Eslinger P & Damasio A (1985). Severe disturbance of higher cognition after bilateral frontal lobe ablation: patient EVR. *Neurology* 35: 1731–1741.

Everitt BJ (1990). Sexual motivation: a neural and behavioural analysis of the mechanisms underlying appetitive and copulatory responses of male rats. *Neuroscience and Biobehavioral Reviews* 14: 217–232.

Everitt BJ & Robbins TW (1992). Amygdala-ventral striatal interactions and reward-related processes. In Aggleton JP, editor, *The Amygdala*, chap. 15, 401–429. Wiley, Chichester.

Everitt BJ & Robbins TW (2013). From the ventral to the dorsal striatum: Devolving views of their roles in drug addiction. *Neuroscience and Biobehavioural Reviews* 37: 1946–1954.

Everitt BJ, Cador M, & Robbins TW (1989). Interactions between the amygdala and ventral striatum in stimulus–reward association: studies using a second order schedule of sexual reinforcement. *Neuroscience* 30: 63–75.

Everitt BJ, Belin D, Economidou D, Pelloux Y, Dalley JW, & Robbins TW (2008). Review. neural mechanisms underlying the vulnerability to develop compulsive drug-seeking habits and addiction. *Philosopjical Transactions of the Royal Society London B Biological Sciences* 363: 3125–3135.

Eysenck HJ & Eysenck SBG (1985). *Personality and Individual Differences: a Natural Science Approach*. Plenum, New York.

Faisal A, Selen L, & Wolpert D (2008). Noise in the nervous system. *Nature Reviews Neuroscience* 9: 292–303.

Farb DH & Ratner MH (2014). Targeting the modulation of neural circuitry for the treatment of anxiety disorders. *Pharmacol Rev* 66: 1002–32.

Farooqi IS & O'Rahilly S (2017). *The Genetics of Obesity in Humans*. South Dartmouth (MA).

Farrow TF, Zheng Y, Wilkinson ID, Spence SA, Deakin JF, Tarrier N, Griffiths PD, & Woodruff PW (2001). Investigating the functional anatomy of empathy and forgiveness. *NeuroReport* 12: 2433–2438.

Feffer K, Fettes P, Giacobbe P, Daskalakis ZJ, Blumberger DM, & Downar J (2018). 1hz rtms of the right orbitofrontal cortex for major depression: Safety, tolerability and clinical outcomes. *Eur Neuropsychopharmacol* 28: 109–117.

Feinstein JS, Adolphs R, Damasio A, & Tranel D (2011). The human amygdala and the induction and experience of fear. *Current Biology* 21: 34–38.

Fellows LK (2007). The role of orbitofrontal cortex in decision making: a component process account. *Annalls of the New York Academy of Sciences* 1121: 421–430.

Fellows LK (2011). Orbitofrontal contributions to value-based decision making: evidence from humans with frontal lobe damage. *Annals of the New York Academy of Sciences* 1239: 51–58.

Fellows LK & Farah MJ (2003). Ventromedial frontal cortex mediates affective shifting in humans: evidence from a reversal learning paradigm. *Brain* 126: 1830–1837.

Ferguson JN, Aldag JM, Insel TR, & Young LJ (2001). Oxytocin in the medial amygdala is essential for social recognition in the mouse. *Journal of Neuroscience* 21: 8278–8285.

Fiorillo CD, Tobler PN, & Schultz W (2003). Discrete coding of reward probability and uncertainty by dopamine neurons. *Science* 299: 1898–1902.

Firman RC, Gasparini C, Manier MK, & Pizzari T (2017). Postmating female control: 20 years of cryptic female choice. *Trends Ecol Evol* 32: 368–382.

Fisher RA (1930). *The Genetical Theory of Natural Selection.* Clarendon Press, Oxford.

Fisher RA (1958). *The Genetical Theory of Natural Selection.* Dover, New York, 2nd edn.

Flint J & Kendler KS (2014). The genetics of major depression. *Neuron* 81: 1214.

Fodor JA (1994). *The Elm and the Expert: Mentalese and its Semantics.* MIT Press, Cambridge, MA.

Forgeard MJ, Haigh EA, Beck AT, Davidson RJ, Henn FA, Maier SF, Mayberg HS, & Seligman ME (2011). Beyond depression: Towards a process-based approach to research, diagnosis, and treatment. *Clinical Psychology (New York)* 18: 275–299.

Fox C, Wolff H, & Baker J (1970). Measurement of intra-vaginal and intra-uterine pressures during human coitus by radio-telemetry. *Journal of Reproduction and Fertility* 22: 243–51.

Francis S, Rolls ET, Bowtell R, McGlone F, O'Doherty J, Browning A, Clare S, & Smith E (1999). The representation of pleasant touch in the brain and its relationship with taste and olfactory areas. *NeuroReport* 10: 453–459.

Franco L, Rolls ET, Aggelopoulos NC, & Treves A (2004). The use of decoding to analyze the contribution to the information of the correlations between the firing of simultaneously recorded neurons. *Experimental Brain Research* 155: 370–384.

Freeman WJ & Watts JW (1950). *Psychosurgery in the Treatment of Mental Disorders and Intractable Pain.* Thomas, Springfield, IL, 2nd edn.

Freese JL & Amaral DG (2009). Neuroanatomy of the primate amygdala. In Whalen PJ & Phelps EA, editors, *The Human Amygdala*, chap. 1, 3–42. Guilford, New York.

Freton M, Lemogne C, Bergouignan L, Delaveau P, Lehericy S, & Fossati P (2014). The eye of the self: precuneus volume and visual perspective during autobiographical memory retrieval. *Brain Struct Funct* 219: 959–68.

Frey S, Kostopoulos P, & Petrides M (2000). Orbitofrontal involvement in the processing of unpleasant auditory information. *European Journal of Neuroscience* 12: 3709–3712.

Fries P (2005). A mechanism for cognitive dynamics: neuronal communication through neuronal coherence. *Trends in Cognitive Sciences* 9: 474–480.

Fries P (2009). Neuronal gamma-band synchronization as a fundamental process in cortical computation. *Annual Reviews of Neuroscience* 32: 209–224.

Frijda NH (1986). *The Emotions.* Cambridge University Press, Cambridge.

Frith U & Frith CD (2003). Development and neurophysiology of mentalizing. *Philosophical Transactions of the Royal Society London B* 358: 459–473.

Fujisawa TX & Cook ND (2011). The perception of harmonic triads: an fMRI study. *Brain Imaging Behav* 5: 109–125.

Fulton JF (1951). *Frontal Lobotomy and Affective Behavior. A Neurophysiological Analysis.* W. W. Norton, New York.

Fuster JM (2008). *The Prefrontal Cortex.* Academic Press, London, 4th edn.

Gabbott PL, Warner TA, Jays PR, & Bacon SJ (2003). Areal and synaptic interconnectivity of prelimbic (area 32), infralimbic (area 25) and insular cortices in the rat. *Brain Research* 993: 59–71.

Gaffan D, Saunders RC, Gaffan EA, Harrison S, Shields C, & Owen MJ (1984). Effects of fornix section upon associative memory in monkeys: role of the hippocampus in learned action. *Quarterly Journal of Experimental Psychology* 36B: 173–221.

Gallagher HL & Frith CD (2003). Functional imaging of 'theory of mind'. *Trends in Cogntive Neuroscience* 7: 77–83.

Gallagher M & Holland PC (1992). Understanding the function of the central nucleus: is simple conditioning enough? In Aggleton JP, editor, *The Amygdala: Neurobiological Aspects of Emotion, Memory, and Mental Dysfunction*, 307–321. Wiley-Liss, New York.

Gallagher M & Holland PC (1994). The amygdala complex: multiple roles in associative learning and attention. *Proceedings of the National Academy of Sciences USA* 91: 11771–11776.

Gallo M, Gamiz F, Perez-Garcia M, Del Moral RG, & Rolls ET (2014). Taste and olfactory status in a gourmand with a right amygdala lesion. *Neurocase: The neural Basis of Cognition* 20: 421–433.

Gangestad SW & Simpson JA (2000). The evolution of human mating: trade-offs and strategic pluralism. *Behavioural and Brain Sciences* 23: 573–644.

Gangestad SW & Thornhill R (1999). Individual differences in developmental precision and fluctuating asymmetry: a model and its implications. *Journal of Evolutionary Biology* 12: 402–416.
Garrison J, Erdeniz B, & Done J (2013). Prediction error in reinforcement learning: a meta-analysis of neuroimaging studies. *Neurosci Biobehav Rev* 37: 1297–310.
Gazzaniga MS (1988). Brain modularity: towards a philosophy of conscious experience. In Marcel AJ & Bisiach E, editors, *Consciousness in Contemporary Science*, chap. 10, 218–238. Oxford University Press, Oxford.
Gazzaniga MS (1995). Consciousness and the cerebral hemispheres. In Gazzaniga MS, editor, *The Cognitive Neurosciences*, chap. 92, 1392–1400. MIT Press, Cambridge, MA.
Gazzaniga MS & LeDoux J (1978). *The Integrated Mind.* Plenum, New York.
Ge T, Feng J, Grabenhorst F, & Rolls ET (2012). Componential Granger causality, and its application to identifying the source and mechanisms of the top-down biased activation that controls attention to affective vs sensory processing. *Neuroimage* 59: 1846–1858.
Gennaro RJ (2004). *Higher Order Theories of Consciousness.* John Benjamins, Amsterdam.
Georges-François P, Rolls ET, & Robertson RG (1999). Spatial view cells in the primate hippocampus: allocentric view not head direction or eye position or place. *Cerebral Cortex* 9: 197–212.
Georgiadis JR & Kringelbach ML (2012). The human sexual response cycle: brain imaging evidence linking sex to other pleasures. *Progress in Neurobiology* 98: 49–81.
Georgiadis JR, Kortekaas R, Kuipers R, Nieuwenburg A, Pruim J, Reinders AA, & Holstege G (2006). Regional cerebral blood flow changes associated with clitorally induced orgasm in healthy women. *European Journal of Neuroscience* 24: 3305–3316.
Gerfen CR & Surmeier DJ (2011). Modulation of striatal projection systems by dopamine. *Annual Reviews of Neuroscience* 34: 441–466.
Ghasemi M, Phillips C, Fahimi A, McNerney MW, & Salehi A (2017). Mechanisms of action and clinical efficacy of nmda receptor modulators in mood disorders. *Neurosci Biobehav Rev* 80: 555–572.
Ghashghaei HT & Barbas H (2002). Pathways for emotion: interactions of prefrontal and anterior temporal pathways in the amygdala of the rhesus monkey. *Neuroscience* 115: 1261–1279.
Gilbert SJ & Burgess PW (2008). Executive function. *Curr Biol* 18: R110–4.
Gilson M, Moreno-Bote R, Ponce-Alvarez A, Ritter P, & Deco G (2016). Estimation of directed effective connectivity from fmri functional connectivity hints at asymmetries in the cortical connectome. *PLoS Computational Biology* 12: e1004762.
Gintis H (2003). The hitchhiker's guide to altruism: genes, culture, and the internalization of norms. *Journal of Theoretical Biology* 220: 407–418.
Gintis H (2007). A framework for the unification of the behavioral sciences. *Behavioral and Brain Sciences* 30: 1–16.
Gintis H (2011). Gene-culture coevolution and the nature of human sociality. *Philosophical Transactions of the Royal Society London B Biological Sciences* 366: 878–888.
Giza BK & Scott TR (1983). Blood glucose selectively affects taste-evoked activity in rat nucleus tractus solitarius. *Physiology and Behaviour* 31: 643–650.
Giza BK & Scott TR (1987a). Intravenous insulin infusions in rats decrease gustatory-evoked responses to sugars. *American Journal of Physiology* 252: R994–R1002.
Giza BK & Scott TR (1987b). Blood glucose level affects perceived sweetness intensity in rats. *Physiology and Behaviour* 41: 459–464.
Giza BK, Scott TR, & Vanderweele DA (1992). Administration of satiety factors and gustatory responsiveness in the nucleus tractus solitarius of the rat. *Brain Research Bulletin* 28: 637–639.
Giza BK, Deems RO, Vanderweele DA, & Scott TR (1993). Pancreatic glucagon suppresses gustatory responsiveness to glucose. *American Journal of Physiology* 265: R1231–7.
Glascher J, Adolphs R, Damasio H, Bechara A, Rudrauf D, Calamia M, Paul LK, & Tranel D (2012). Lesion mapping of cognitive control and value-based decision making in the prefrontal cortex. *Proceedings of the National Academy of Sciences U S A* 109: 14681–14686.
Gleen JF & Erickson RP (1976). Gastric modulation of gustatory afferent activity. *Physiology and Behaviour* 16: 561–568.
Glimcher P (2004). *Decisions, Uncertainty, and the Brain.* MIT Press, Cambridge, MA.
Glimcher P (2005). Indeterminacy in brain and behavior. *Annual Review of Psychology* 56: 25–56.
Glimcher P (2011a). *Foundations of Neuroeconomic Analysis.* Oxford University Press, Oxford.
Glimcher PW (2011b). Understanding dopamine and reinforcement learning: the dopamine reward prediction error hypothesis. *Proceedings of the National Academy of Sciences U S A* 108 Suppl 3: 15647–15654.
Glimcher PW & Fehr E (2013). *Neuroeconomics: Decision-Making and the Brain.* Academic Press, New York, 2nd edn.
Goetz AT & Shackelford TK (2009). Sexual conflict in humans: Evolutionary consequences of asymmetric parental investment and paternity uncertainty. *Animal Biology* 59: 449–456.
Gold JI & Shadlen MN (2007). The neural basis of decision making. *Annual Review of Neuroscience* 30: 535–574.

Gold PW (2015). The organization of the stress system and its dysregulation in depressive illness. *Molecular Psychiatry* 20: 32–47.

Goldbach M, Loh M, Deco G, & Garcia-Ojalvo J (2008). Neurodynamical amplification of perceptual signals via system-size resonance. *Physica D* 237: 316–323.

Goldman PS & Nauta WJH (1977). An intricately patterned prefronto-caudate projection in the rhesus monkey. *Journal of Comparative Neurology* 171: 369–386.

Goldman-Rakic PS (1996). The prefrontal landscape: implications of functional architecture for understanding human mentation and the central executive. *Philosophical Transactions of the Royal Society B* 351: 1445–1453.

Goleman D (1995). *Emotional Intelligence*. Bantam, New York.

Goodale MA (2004). Perceiving the world and grasping it: dissociations between conscious and unconscious visual processing. In Gazzaniga MS, editor, *The Cognitive Neurosciences III*, 1159–1172. MIT Press, Cambridge, MA.

Goodglass H & Kaplan E (1979). Assessment of cognitive deficit in brain-injured patient. In Gazzaniga MS, editor, *Handbook of Behavioural Neurobiology*, vol. 2, Neuropsychology, 3–22. Plenum, New York.

Gothard KM, Battaglia FP, Erickson CA, Spitler KM, & Amaral DG (2007). Neural responses to facial expression and face identity in the monkey amygdala. *Journal of Neurophysiology* 97: 1671–1683.

Gothard KM, Mosher CP, Zimmerman PE, Putnam PT, Morrow JK, & Fuglevand AJ (2018). New perspectives on the neurophysiology of primate amygdala emerging from the study of naturalistic social behaviors. *Wiley Interdiscip Rev Cogn Sci* 9.

Gotlib IH & Hammen CL (2009). *Handbook of Depression*. Guilford Press, New York.

Gottfried JA, O'Doherty J, & Dolan RJ (2003). Encoding predictive reward value in human amygdala and orbitofrontal cortex. *Science* 301: 1104–1107.

Grabenhorst F & Rolls ET (2008). Selective attention to affective value alters how the brain processes taste stimuli. *European Journal of Neuroscience* 27: 723–729.

Grabenhorst F & Rolls ET (2009). Different representations of relative and absolute subjective value in the human brain. *Neuroimage* 48: 258–268.

Grabenhorst F & Rolls ET (2010). Attentional modulation of affective vs sensory processing: functional connectivity and a top down biased activation theory of selective attention. *Journal of Neurophysiology* 104: 1649–1660.

Grabenhorst F & Rolls ET (2011). Value, pleasure, and choice systems in the ventral prefrontal cortex. *Trends in Cognitive Sciences* 15: 56–67.

Grabenhorst F, Rolls ET, Margot C, da Silva M, & Velazco MI (2007). How pleasant and unpleasant stimuli combine in the brain: odor combinations. *Journal of Neuroscience* 27: 13532–13540.

Grabenhorst F, Rolls ET, & Bilderbeck A (2008a). How cognition modulates affective responses to taste and flavor: top-down influences on the orbitofrontal and pregenual cingulate cortices. *Cerebral Cortex* 18: 1549–1559.

Grabenhorst F, Rolls ET, & Parris BA (2008b). From affective value to decision-making in the prefrontal cortex. *European Journal of Neuroscience* 28: 1930–1939.

Grabenhorst F, D'Souza A, Parris BA, Rolls ET, & Passingham RE (2010a). A common neural scale for the subjective value of different primary rewards. *Neuroimage* 51: 1265–1274.

Grabenhorst F, Rolls ET, Parris BA, & D'Souza A (2010b). How the brain represents the reward value of fat in the mouth. *Cerebral Cortex* 20: 1082–1091.

Grabenhorst F, Hernadi I, & Schultz W (2012). Prediction of economic choice by primate amygdala neurons. *Proceedings of the National Academy of Sciences U S A* 109: 18950–18955.

Gray JA (1970). The psychophysiological basis of introversion-extraversion. *Behaviour Research and Therapy* 8: 249–266.

Gray JA (1975). *Elements of a Two-Process Theory of Learning*. Academic Press, London.

Gray JA (1981). Anxiety as a paradigm case of emotion. *British Medical Bulletin* 37: 193–197.

Gray JA (1987). *The Psychology of Fear and Stress*. Cambridge University Press, Cambridge, 2nd edn.

Guyenet SJ & Schwartz MW (2012). Clinical review: Regulation of food intake, energy balance, and body fat mass: implications for the pathogenesis and treatment of obesity. *Journal of Clinical Endocrinology and Metabolism* 97: 745–755.

Haber SN (2016). Corticostriatal circuitry. *Dialogues Clin Neurosci* 18: 7–21.

Hahn AC & Perrett DI (2014). Neural and behavioral responses to attractiveness in adult and infant faces. *Neurosci Biobehav Rev* 46 Pt 4: 591–603.

Haid D, Widmayer P, Voigt A, Chaudhari N, Boehm U, & Breer H (2013). Gustatory sensory cells express a receptor responsive to protein breakdown products (GPR92). *Histochemistry and Cell Biology* 140: 137–145.

Hajnal A, Takenouchi K, & Norgren R (1999). Effect of intraduodenal lipid on parabrachial gustatory coding in awake rats. *Journal of Neuroscience* 19: 7182–7190.

Hamani C, Mayberg H, Snyder B, Giacobbe P, Kennedy S, & Lozano AM (2009). Deep brain stimulation of the subcallosal cingulate gyrus for depression: anatomical location of active contacts in clinical responders and a suggested guideline for targeting. *Journal of Neurosurgery* 111: 1209–1215.

Hamani C, Mayberg H, Stone S, Laxton A, Haber S, & Lozano AM (2011). The subcallosal cingulate gyrus in the context of major depression. *Biological Psychiatry* 69: 301–308.

Hamann S & Canli T (2004). Individual differnces in emotion processing. *Current Opinion in Neurobiology* 14: 233–238.
Hamilton JP, Chen MC, & Gotlib IH (2013). Neural systems approaches to understanding major depressive disorder: an intrinsic functional organization perspective. *Neurobiology of Disease* 52: 4–11.
Hamilton WD (1964). The genetical evolution of social behaviour. *Journal of Theoretical Biology* 7: 1–52.
Hamilton WD (1996). *Narrow Roads of Gene Land.* W. H. Freeman, New York.
Hamilton WD & Zuk M (1982). Heritable true fitness and bright birds: a role for parasites. *Science* 218: 384–387.
Hampton AN & O'Doherty JP (2007). Decoding the neural substrates of reward-related decision making with functional MRI. *Proceedings of the National Academy of Sciences USA* 104: 1377–1382.
Hampton RR (2001). Rhesus monkeys know when they can remember. *Proceedings of the National Academy of Sciences of the USA* 98: 5539–5362.
Harlow CM (1986). *Learning to Love: The Selected Papers of HF Harlow.* Praeger, New York.
Harlow HF & Stagner R (1933). Psychology of feelings and emotion. *Psychological Review* 40: 84–194.
Harlow JM (1848). Passage of an iron rod though the head. *Boston Medical and Surgical Journal* 39: 389–393.
Harmer CJ & Cowen PJ (2013). 'it's the way that you look at it'–a cognitive neuropsychological account of ssri action in depression. *Philosophical Transactions of the Royal Society of London B Biological Sciences* 368: 20120407.
Harrison NA, Gray MA, Gianaros PJ, & Critchley HD (2010). The embodiment of emotional feelings in the brain. *Journal of Neuroscience* 30: 12878–12884.
Hassanpour MS, Simmons WK, Feinstein JS, Luo Q, Lapidus RC, Bodurka J, Paulus MP, & Khalsa SS (2018). The insular cortex dynamically maps changes in cardiorespiratory interoception. *Neuropsychopharmacology* 43: 426–434.
Hasselmo ME, Rolls ET, & Baylis GC (1989a). The role of expression and identity in the face-selective responses of neurons in the temporal visual cortex of the monkey. *Behavioural Brain Research* 32: 203–218.
Hasselmo ME, Rolls ET, Baylis GC, & Nalwa V (1989b). Object-centered encoding by face-selective neurons in the cortex in the superior temporal sulcus of the monkey. *Experimental Brain Research* 75: 417–429.
Hauser MD (1996). *The Evolution of Communication.* MIT Press, Cambridge, MA.
Hayden BY, Pearson JM, & Platt ML (2011). Neuronal basis of sequential foraging decisions in a patchy environment. *Nature Neuroscience* 14: 933–939.
Haynes JD & Rees G (2005a). Predicting the orientation of invisible stimuli from activity in human primary visual cortex. *Nature Neuroscience* 8: 686–691.
Haynes JD & Rees G (2005b). Predicting the stream of consciousness from activity in human visual cortex. *Current Biology* 15: 1301–1307.
Haynes JD & Rees G (2006). Decoding mental states from brain activity in humans. *Nature Reviews Neuroscience* 7: 523–534.
Haynes JD, Sakai K, Rees G, Gilbert S, Frith C, & Passingham RE (2007). Reading hidden intentions in the human brain. *Current Biology* 17: 323–328.
Hebb DO (1949). *The Organization of Behavior: a Neuropsychological Theory.* Wiley, New York.
Heberlein AS, Padon AA, Gillihan SJ, Farah MJ, & Fellows LK (2008). Ventromedial frontal lobe plays a critical role in facial emotion recognition. *Journal of Cognitive Neuroscience* 20: 721–733.
Heistermann M, Ziegler T, van Schaik CP, Launhardt K, Winkler P, & Hodges JK (2001). Loss of oestrus, concealed ovulation and paternity confusion in free-ranging Hanuman langurs. *Proceedings of the Royal Society of London B* 268: 2445–2451.
Heitmann BL, Westerterp KR, Loos RJ, Sorensen TI, O'Dea K, Mc Lean P, Jensen TK, Eisenmann J, Speakman JR, Simpson SJ, Reed DR, & Westerterp-Plantenga MS (2012). Obesity: lessons from evolution and the environment. *Obesity Reviews* 13: 910–922.
Henningsson S, Hovey D, Vass K, Walum H, Sandnabba K, Santtila P, Jern P, & Westberg L (2017). A missense polymorphism in the putative pheromone receptor gene vn1r1 is associated with sociosexual behavior. *Translational psychiatry* 7: e1102.
Hertz JA, Krogh A, & Palmer RG (1991). *Introduction to the Theory of Neural Computation.* Addison-Wesley, Wokingham, UK.
Heyes C (2008). Beast machines? Questions of animal consciousness. In Weiskrantz L & Davies M, editors, *Frontiers of Consciousness*, chap. 9, 259–274. Oxford University Press, Oxford.
Hilton NZ, Harris GT, & Rice ME (2015). The step-father effect in child abuse: Comparing discriminative parental solicitude and antisociality. *Psychology of Violence* 5: 8.
Hines M (2010). Sex-related variation in human behavior and the brain. *Trends in Cognitive Sciences* 14: 448–456.
Hines M, Constantinescu M, & Spencer D (2015). Early androgen exposure and human gender development. *Biol Sex Differ* 6: 3.
Hoge EA, Ivkovic A, & Fricchione GL (2012). Generalized anxiety disorder: diagnosis and treatment. *BMJ* 345: e7500.
Holland PC & Gallagher M (1999). Amygdala circuitry in attentional and representational processes. *Trends in Cognitive Sciences* 3: 65–73.

Hölscher C, Jacob W, & Mallot HA (2003). Reward modulates neuronal activity in the hippocampus of the rat. *Behavioural Brain Research* 142: 181–191.

Holtzheimer PE, Husain MM, Lisanby SH, Taylor SF, Whitworth LA, McClintock S, Slavin KV, Berman J, McKhann GM, Patil PG, Rittberg BR, Abosch A, Pandurangi AK, Holloway KL, Lam RW, Honey CR, Neimat JS, Henderson JM, DeBattista C, Rothschild AJ, Pilitsis JG, Espinoza RT, Petrides G, Mogilner AY, Matthews K, Peichel D, Gross RE, Hamani C, Lozano AM, & Mayberg HS (2017). Subcallosal cingulate deep brain stimulation for treatment-resistant depression: a multisite, randomised, sham-controlled trial. *Lancet Psychiatry* 4: 839–849.

Hopfield JJ (1982). Neural networks and physical systems with emergent collective computational abilities. *Proceedings of the National Academy of Sciences USA* 79: 2554–2558.

Hornak J, Rolls ET, & Wade D (1996). Face and voice expression identification in patients with emotional and behavioural changes following ventral frontal lobe damage. *Neuropsychologia* 34: 247–261.

Hornak J, Bramham J, Rolls ET, Morris RG, O'Doherty J, Bullock PR, & Polkey CE (2003). Changes in emotion after circumscribed surgical lesions of the orbitofrontal and cingulate cortices. *Brain* 126: 1691–1712.

Hornak J, O'Doherty J, Bramham J, Rolls ET, Morris RG, Bullock PR, & Polkey CE (2004). Reward-related reversal learning after surgical excisions in orbitofrontal and dorsolateral prefrontal cortex in humans. *Journal of Cognitive Neuroscience* 16: 463–478.

Horvath TL (2005). The hardship of obesity: a soft-wired hypothalamus. *Nature Neuroscience* 8: 561–565.

Hughes J (1975). Isolation of an endogenous compound from the brain with pharmacological properties similar to morphine. *Brain Research* 88: 293–308.

Hughes J, Smith TW, Kosterlitz HW, Fothergill LA, Morgan BA, & Morris HR (1975). Identification of two related pentapeptides from the brain with potent opiate antagonist activity. *Nature* 258: 577–579.

Hull EM, Meisel RL, & Sachs BD (2002). Male sexual behavior. In Pfaff DW, Arnold AP, Etgen AM, Fahrbach SE, & Rubin RT, editors, *Hormones, Brain and Behavior*, vol. 1, chap. 1, 3–137. Academic Press, San Diego, CA.

Humphrey NK (1980). Nature's psychologists. In Josephson BD & Ramachandran VS, editors, *Consciousness and the Physical World*, 57–80. Pergamon, Oxford.

Humphrey NK (1986). *The Inner Eye*. Faber, London.

Hunt JN (1980). A possible relation between the regulation of gastric emptying and food intake. *American Journal of Physiology* 239: G1–G4.

Hunt JN & Stubbs DF (1975). The volume and energy content of meals as determinants of gastric emptying. *Journal of Physiology* 245: 209–225.

Iadarola ND, Niciu MJ, Richards EM, Vande Voort JL, Ballard ED, Lundin NB, Nugent AC, Machado-Vieira R, & Zarate J C A (2015). Ketamine and other n-methyl-d-aspartate receptor antagonists in the treatment of depression: a perspective review. *Therapetic Advances in Chronic Disease* 6: 97–114.

Ide JS, Nedic S, Wong KF, Strey SL, Lawson EA, Dickerson BC, Wald LL, La Camera G, & Mujica-Parodi LR (2018). Oxytocin attenuates trust as a subset of more general reinforcement learning, with altered reward circuit functional connectivity in males. *Neuroimage* 174: 35–43.

Ikeda K (1909). On a new seasoning. *Journal of the Tokyo Chemistry Society* 30: 820–836.

Imamura K, Mataga N, & Mori K (1992). Coding of odor molecules by mitral/tufted cells in rabbit olfactory bulb. I. Aliphatic compounds. *Journal of Neurophysiology* 68: 1986–2002.

Insabato A, Pannunzi M, Rolls ET, & Deco G (2010). Confidence-related decision-making. *Journal of Neurophysiology* 104: 539–547.

Ishizu T & Zeki S (2011). Toward a brain-based theory of beauty. *PLoS ONE* 6: e21852.

Ishizu T & Zeki S (2013). The brain's specialized systems for aesthetic and perceptual judgment. *European Journal of Neuroscience* 37: 1413–14120.

Iversen LL, Iversen SD, Bloom FE, & Roth RH, editors (2009). *Introduction to Neuropharmacology*. Oxford University Press, Oxford.

Iversen SD & Mishkin M (1970). Perseverative interference in monkey following selective lesions of the inferior prefrontal convexity. *Experimental Brain Research* 11: 376–386.

Jackendoff R (2002). *Foundations of Language*. Oxford University Press, Oxford.

Jacobsen CF (1936). The functions of the frontal association areas in monkeys. *Comparative Psychology Monographs* 13: 1–60.

James W (1884). What is an emotion? *Mind* 9: 188–205.

Jenni DA & Collier G (1972). Polyandry in the American jacana. *The Auk* 89: 743–765.

Johansen-Berg H, Gutman DA, Behrens TE, Matthews PM, Rushworth MF, Katz E, Lozano AM, & Mayberg HS (2008). Anatomical connectivity of the subgenual cingulate region targeted with deep brain stimulation for treatment-resistant depression. *Cerebral Cortex* 18: 1374–1383.

Johnson SC, Baxter LC, Wilder LS, Pipe JG, Heiserman JE, & Prigatano GP (2002). Neural correlates of self-reflection. *Brain* 125: 1808–14.

Johnson-Laird PN (1988). *The Computer and the Mind: An Introduction to Cognitive Science*. Harvard University Press, Cambridge, MA.

Johnston VS, Hagel R, Franklin M, Fink B, & Grammer K (2001). Male facial attractiveness: evidence for hormone-mediated adaptive design. *Evolution and Human Behaviour* 22: 251–267.

Johnstone S & Rolls ET (1990). Delay, discriminatory, and modality specific neurons in striatum and pallidum during short-term memory tasks. *Brain Research* 522: 147–151.

Jones B & Mishkin M (1972). Limbic lesions and the problem of stimulus–reinforcement associations. *Experimental Neurology* 36: 362–377.

Jones EG & Powell TPS (1970). An anatomical study of converging sensory pathways within the cerebral cortex of the monkey. *Brain* 93: 793–820.

Jouandet M & Gazzaniga MS (1979). The frontal lobes. In Gazzaniga MS, editor, *Handbook of Behavioural Neurobiology*, vol. 2, Neuropsychology, 25–59. Plenum, New York.

Julian JB, Keinath AT, Frazzetta G, & Epstein RA (2018). Human entorhinal cortex represents visual space using a boundary-anchored grid. *Nat Neurosci* 21: 191–194.

Jurgens U (2002). Neural pathways underlying vocal control. *Neuroscience and Biobehavioral Reviews* 26: 235–258.

Kacelnik A & Brito e Abreu F (1998). Risky choice and Weber's Law. *Journal of Theoretical Biology* 194: 289–298.

Kadohisa M, Rolls ET, & Verhagen JV (2004). Orbitofrontal cortex neuronal representation of temperature and capsaicin in the mouth. *Neuroscience* 127: 207–221.

Kadohisa M, Rolls ET, & Verhagen JV (2005a). The primate amygdala: neuronal representations of the viscosity, fat texture, grittiness and taste of foods. *Neuroscience* 132: 33–48.

Kadohisa M, Rolls ET, & Verhagen JV (2005b). Neuronal representations of stimuli in the mouth: the primate insular taste cortex, orbitofrontal cortex, and amygdala. *Chemical Senses* 30: 401–419.

Kagel JH, Battalio RC, & Green L (1995). *Economic Choice Theory: An Experimental Analysis of Animal Behaviour.* Cambridge University Press, Cambridge.

Kapoor E, Collazo-Clavell ML, & Faubion SS (2017). Weight gain in women at midlife: A concise review of the pathophysiology and strategies for management. *Mayo Clin Proc* 92: 1552–1558.

Kappeler PM & van Schaik CP (2004). Sexual selection in primates: review and selective preview. In Kappeler PM & van Schaik CP, editors, *Sexual Selection in Primates*, chap. 1, 3–23. Cambridge University Press, Cambridge.

Katz LD (2000). Emotion, representation, and consciousness. *Behavioral and Brain Sciences* 23: 204–205.

Kawamura Y & Kare MR, editors (1992). *Umami: a Basic Taste.* Dekker, New York.

Kemp JM & Powell TPS (1970). The cortico-striate projections in the monkey. *Brain* 93: 525–546.

Kennedy DP & Adolphs R (2011). Reprint of: Impaired fixation to eyes following amygdala damage arises from abnormal bottom-up attention. *Neuropsychologia* 49: 589–595.

Kennerley SW & Wallis JD (2009). Encoding of reward and space during a working memory task in the orbitofrontal cortex and anterior cingulate sulcus. *Journal of Neurophysiology* 102: 3352–3364.

Kennerley SW, Walton ME, Behrens TE, Buckley MJ, & Rushworth MF (2006). Optimal decision making and the anterior cingulate cortex. *Nature Neuroscience* 9: 940–947.

Kennerley SW, Behrens TE, & Wallis JD (2011). Double dissociation of value computations in orbitofrontal and anterior cingulate neurons. *Nature Neuroscience* 14: 1581–1589.

Kennis M, Rademaker AR, & Geuze E (2013). Neural correlates of personality: an integrative review. *Neuroscience and Biobehavioural Reviews* 37: 73–95.

Kesner RP & Rolls ET (2015). A computational theory of hippocampal function, and tests of the theory: New developments. *Neuroscience and Biobehavioral Reviews* 48: 92–147.

Keverne EB (1995). Neurochemical changes accompanying the reproductive process; their significance for maternal care in primates and other mammals. In Pryce CR, Martin RD, & Skuse D, editors, *Motherhood in Human and Nonhuman Primates*, 69–77. Karger, Basel.

Keverne EB, Nevison CM, & Martel FL (1997). Early learning and the social bond. *Annals of the New York Academy of Science* 807: 329–339.

Killcross S & Coutureau E (2003). Coordination of actions and habits in the medial prefrontal cortex of rats. *Cerebral Cortex* 13: 400–408.

Kim HF, Ghazizadeh A, & Hikosaka O (2015). Dopamine neurons encoding long-term memory of object value for habitual behavior. *Cell* 163: 1165–1175.

Kim KS, Seeley RJ, & Sandoval DA (2018). Signalling from the periphery to the brain that regulates energy homeostasis. *Nat Rev Neurosci* 19: 185–196.

Kircher TT, Senior C, Phillips ML, Benson PJ, Bullmore ET, Brammer M, Simmons A, Williams SC, Bartels M, & David AS (2000). Towards a functional neuroanatomy of self processing: effects of faces and words. *Brain Res Cogn Brain Res* 10: 133–44.

Kircher TT, Brammer M, Bullmore E, Simmons A, Bartels M, & David AS (2002). The neural correlates of intentional and incidental self processing. *Neuropsychologia* 40: 683–92.

Kluver H & Bucy PC (1939). Preliminary analysis of functions of the temporal lobe in monkeys. *Archives of Neurology and Psychiatry* 42: 979–1000.

Kobayashi S (2012). Organization of neural systems for aversive information processing: pain, error, and punishment. *Frontiers in Neuroscience* 6: 136.

Kobayashi Y & Amaral DG (2003). Macaque monkey retrosplenial cortex: Ii. cortical afferents. *J Comp Neurol* 466: 48–79.

Kobayashi Y & Amaral DG (2007). Macaque monkey retrosplenial cortex: Iii. cortical efferents. *J Comp Neurol* 502: 810–33.

Kolb B & Whishaw IQ (2015). *Fundamentals of Human Neuropsychology*. Macmillan, New York, 7th edn.

Kolling N, Wittmann MK, Behrens TE, Boorman ED, Mars RB, & Rushworth MF (2016). Value, search, persistence and model updating in anterior cingulate cortex. *Nat Neurosci* 19: 1280–5.

Koob GF & Le Moal M (1997). Drug abuse: hedonic homeostatic dysregulation. *Science* 278: 52–58.

Koob GF & Volkow ND (2016). Neurobiology of addiction: a neurocircuitry analysis. *Lancet Psychiatry* 3: 760–73.

Kosar E, Grill HJ, & Norgren R (1986). Gustatory cortex in the rat. II. Thalamocortical projections. *Brain Research* 379: 342–352.

Koski L & Paus T (2000). Functional connectivity of anterior cingulate cortex within human frontal lobe: a brain mapping meta-analysis. *Experimental Brain Research* 133: 55–65.

Krebs JR, Davies NB, & West WA (2012). *An Introduction to Behavioural Ecology*. Wiley-Blackwell, Oxford, 4th edn.

Kringelbach ML & Rolls ET (2003). Neural correlates of rapid reversal learning in a simple model of human social interaction. *Neuroimage* 20: 1371–1383.

Kringelbach ML & Rolls ET (2004). The functional neuroanatomy of the human orbitofrontal cortex: evidence from neuroimaging and neuropsychology. *Progress in Neurobiology* 72: 341–372.

Kringelbach ML, O'Doherty J, Rolls ET, & Andrews C (2003). Activation of the human orbitofrontal cortex to a liquid food stimulus is correlated with its subjective pleasantness. *Cerebral Cortex* 13: 1064–1071.

Kroes MC, Schiller D, LeDoux JE, & Phelps EA (2016). Translational approaches targeting reconsolidation. *Curr Top Behav Neurosci* 28: 197–230.

Krolak-Salmon P, Henaff MA, Isnard J, Tallon-Baudry C, Guenot M, Vighetto A, Bertrand O, & Mauguiere F (2003). An attention modulated response to disgust in human ventral anterior insula. *Annals of Neurology* 53: 446–453.

Krug R, Plihal W, Fehm HL, & Born J (2000). Selective influence of the menstrual cycle on perception of stimuli with reproductive significance: an event-related potential study. *Psychophysiology* 37: 111–122.

Kuehner C (2017). Why is depression more common among women than among men? *Lancet Psychiatry* 4: 146–158.

Kuhar MJ, Pert CB, & Snyder SH (1973). Regional distribution of opiate receptor binding in monkey and human brain. *Nature* 245: 447–450.

Kumar V, Croxson PL, & Simonyan K (2016). Structural organization of the laryngeal motor cortical network and its implication for evolution of speech production. *J Neurosci* 36: 4170–81.

Kunz G & Leyendecker G (2002). Uterine peristaltic activity during the menstrual cycle: characterization, regulation, function and dysfunction. *Reproductive biomedicine online* 4: 5–9.

Kupferman I (2000). Reward: Wanted - a better definition. *Behavioral and Brain Sciences* 23: 208.

Laland KN & Brown GR (2002). *Sense and Nonsense. Evolutionary Perspectives on Human Behaviour*. Oxford University Press, Oxford.

Lally N, Nugent AC, Luckenbaugh DA, Niciu MJ, Roiser JP, & Zarate J C A (2015). Neural correlates of change in major depressive disorder anhedonia following open-label ketamine. *Journal of Psychopharmacology* 29: 596–607.

Lane RD, Fink GR, Chau PML, & Dolan RJ (1997a). Neural activation during selective attention to subjective emotional responses. *Neuroreport* 8: 3969–3972.

Lane RD, Reiman EM, Ahern GL, Schwartz GE, & Davidson RJ (1997b). Neuroanatomical correlates of happiness, sadness, and disgust. *American Journal of Psychiatry* 154: 926–933.

Lane RD, Reiman EM, Bradley MM, Lang PJ, Ahern GL, Davidson RJ, & Schwartz GE (1997c). Neuroanatomical correlates of pleasant and unpleasant emotion. *Neuropsychologia* 35: 1437–1444.

Lane RD, Reiman E, Axelrod B, Yun LS, Holmes AH, & Schwartz G (1998). Neural correlates of levels of emotional awareness. Evidence of an interaction between emotion and attention in the anterior cingulate cortex. *Journal of Cognitive Neuroscience* 10: 525–535.

Lange C (1885). The emotions. In Dunlap E, editor, *The Emotions*. Williams and Wilkins, Baltimore, 1922nd edn.

Langlois JH, Roggman LA, Casey RJ, & Ritter JM (1987). Infant preferences for attractive faces: Rudiments of a stereotype? *Developmental Psychology* 23: 363–369.

Langlois JH, Roggman LA, & Reiser-Danner LA (1990). Infants' differential social responses to attractive and unattractive faces. *Developmental Psychology* 29: 153–159.

Langlois JH, Ritter JM, Roggman LA, & Vaughn LS (1991). Facial diversity and infant preferences for attractive faces. *Developmental Psychology* 27: 79–84.

Langlois JH, Kalakanis L, Rubenstein AJ, Larson A, Hallam M, & Smoot M (2000). Maxims or myths of beauty? A meta-analytic and theoretical review. *Psychological Bulletin* 126: 390–423.

Lau H & Rosenthal D (2011). Empirical support for higher-order theories of conscious awareness. *Trends in Cognitive Sciences* 15: 365–373.

Lau HC, Rogers RD, & Passingham RE (2006). On measuring the perceived onsets of spontaneous actions. *Journal of Neuroscience* 26: 7265–7271.

Laxton AW, Neimat JS, Davis KD, Womelsdorf T, Hutchison WD, Dostrovsky JO, Hamani C, Mayberg HS, & Lozano AM (2013). Neuronal coding of implicit emotion categories in the subcallosal cortex in patients with depression. *Biological Psychiatry* 74: 714–719.

LeDoux JE (1992). Emotion and the amygdala. In Aggleton JP, editor, *The Amygdala*, chap. 12, 339–351. Wiley-Liss, New York.

LeDoux JE (1995). Emotion: clues from the brain. *Annual Review of Psychology* 46: 209–235.

LeDoux JE (1996). *The Emotional Brain*. Simon and Schuster, New York.

LeDoux JE (2008). Emotional coloration of consciousness: how feelings come about. In Weiskrantz L & Davies M, editors, *Frontiers of Consciousness*, 69–130. Oxford University Press, Oxford.

LeDoux JE (2012). Rethinking the emotional brain. *Neuron* 73: 653–676.

LeDoux JE & Brown R (2017). A higher-order theory of emotional consciousness. *Proc Natl Acad Sci U S A* 114: E2016–E2025.

LeDoux JE & Daw ND (2018). Surviving threats: neural circuit and computational implications of a new taxonomy of defensive behaviour. *Nat Rev Neurosci* 19: 269–282.

LeDoux JE & Pine DS (2016). Using neuroscience to help understand fear and anxiety: A two-system framework. *Am J Psychiatry* 173: 1083–1093.

LeDoux JE, Brown R, Pine DS, & Hofmann SG (2018). Know thyself: Well-being and subjective experience. *Cerebrum https://www.dana.org/Cerebrum* .

Leech R & Sharp DJ (2014). The role of the posterior cingulate cortex in cognition and disease. *Brain* 137: 12–32.

Leonard CM, Rolls ET, Wilson FAW, & Baylis GC (1985). Neurons in the amygdala of the monkey with responses selective for faces. *Behavioural Brain Research* 15: 159–176.

Li CS & Cho YK (2006). Efferent projection from the bed nucleus of the stria terminalis suppresses activity of taste-responsive neurons in the hamster parabrachial nuclei. *American Journal of Physiology Regul Integr Comp Physiol* 291: R914–R926.

Li CS, Cho YK, & Smith DV (2002). Taste responses of neurons in the hamster solitary nucleus are modulated by the central nucleus of the amygdala. *Journal of Neurophysiology* 88: 2979–2992.

Lieberman DA, editor (2000). *Learning: Behavior and Cognition*. Wadsworth, Belmont, CA.

Liebeskind JC & Paul LA (1977). Psychological and physiological mechanisms of pain. *Annual Review of Psychology* 88: 41–60.

Liebeskind JC, Giesler GJ, & Urca G (1985). Evidence pertaining to an endogenous mechanism of pain inhibition in the central nervous system. In Zotterman Y, editor, *Sensory Functions of the Skin*. Pergamon, Oxford.

Lim MM, Wang Z, Olazabal DE, Ren X, Terwilliger EF, & Young LJ (2004). Enhanced partner preference in a promiscuous species by manipulating the expression of a single gene. *Nature* 429: 754–757.

Lin W, Ogura T, & Kinnamon SC (2003). Responses to di-sodium guanosine 5′-monophosphate and monosodium L-glutamate in taste receptor cells of rat fungiform papillae. *Journal of Neurophysiology* 89: 1434–1439.

Liu Z, Ma N, Rolls ET, Wei D, Zhang J, Chen Q, Meng J, Qiu J, & Feng J (2018). Integrating multi-modal data to explore the neural, genetic and behavioral correlates of happiness .

Loh M, Rolls ET, & Deco G (2007a). A dynamical systems hypothesis of schizophrenia. *PLoS Computational Biology* 3: e228. doi:10.1371/journal.pcbi.0030228.

Loh M, Rolls ET, & Deco G (2007b). Statistical fluctuations in attractor networks related to schizophrenia. *Pharmacopsychiatry* 40: S78–84.

Longtin A (1993). Stochastic resonance in neuron models. *Journal of Statistical Physics* 70: 309–327.

Loonen AJ & Ivanova SA (2016). Circuits regulating pleasure and happiness: the evolution of the amygdalar-hippocampal-habenular connectivity in vertebrates. *Front Neurosci* 10: 539.

Lovlie H, Gillingham MAF, Worley K, Pizzari T, & Richardson DS (2013). Cryptic female choice favours sperm from major histocompatibility complex-dissimilar males. *Proceedings of the Royal Society B* 280: 20131296.

Lozano AM, Giacobbe P, Hamani C, Rizvi SJ, Kennedy SH, Kolivakis TT, Debonnel G, Sadikot AF, Lam RW, Howard AK, Ilcewicz-Klimek M, Honey CR, & Mayberg HS (2012). A multicenter pilot study of subcallosal cingulate area deep brain stimulation for treatment-resistant depression. *Journal of Neurosurgery* 116: 315–322.

Lujan JL, Chaturvedi A, Choi KS, Holtzheimer PE, Gross RE, Mayberg HS, & McIntyre CC (2013). Tractography-activation models applied to subcallosal cingulate deep brain stimulation. *Brain Stimulation* 6: 737–739.

Luk CH & Wallis JD (2009). Dynamic encoding of responses and outcomes by neurons in medial prefrontal cortex. *Journal of Neuroscience* 29: 7526–7539.

Luk CH & Wallis JD (2013). Choice coding in frontal cortex during stimulus-guided or action-guided decision-making. *Journal of Neuroscience* 33: 1864–1871.

Lundy J R F & Norgren R (2004). Activity in the hypothalamus, amygdala, and cortex generates bilateral and convergent modulation of pontine gustatory neurons. *Journal of Neurophysiology* 91: 1143–1157.

Luo Q, Ge T, Grabenhorst F, Feng J, & Rolls ET (2013). Attention-dependent modulation of cortical taste circuits revealed by Granger causality with signal-dependent noise. *PLoS Computational Biology* 9: e1003265.

Lycan WG (1997). Consciousness as internal monitoring. In Block N, Flanagan O, & Guzeldere G, editors, *The Nature of Consciousness: Philosophical Debates*, 755–771. MIT Press, Cambridge, MA.

Ma Y (2015). Neuropsychological mechanism underlying antidepressant effect: a systematic meta-analysis. *Molecular Psychiatry* 20: 311–319.

Mackey S & Petrides M (2010). Quantitative demonstration of comparable architectonic areas within the ventromedial and lateral orbital frontal cortex in the human and the macaque monkey brains. *European Journal of Neuroscience* 32: 1940–1950.

Mackintosh NJ (1983). *Conditioning and Associative Learning*. Oxford University Press, Oxford.

Malsburg Cvd (1990). A neural architecture for the representation of scenes. In McGaugh JL, Weinberger NM, & Lynch G, editors, *Brain Organization and Memory: Cells, Systems and Circuits*, chap. 19, 356–372. Oxford University Press, New York.

Maltbie EA, Kaundinya GS, & Howell LL (2017). Ketamine and pharmacological imaging: use of functional magnetic resonance imaging to evaluate mechanisms of action. *Behav Pharmacol* 28: 610–622.

Matrix (2013). Economic analysis of workplace mental health promotion and mental disorder prevention programmes and of their potential contribution to eu health, social and economic policy objectives. *Executive Agency for Health and Consumers, Specific Request EAHC/2011/Health/19 for the Implementation of Framework Contract EAHC/2010/Health/01 /Lot 2* .

Matsumoto K, Suzuki W, & Tanaka K (2003). Neuronal correlates of goal-based motor selection in the prefrontal cortex. *Science* 301: 229–232.

Matsumoto M & Hikosaka O (2009a). Two types of dopamine neuron distinctly convey positive and negative motivational signals. *Nature* 459: 837–841.

Matsumoto M & Hikosaka O (2009b). Representation of negative motivational value in the primate lateral habenula. *Nat Neurosci* 12: 77–84.

Matsumoto M, Matsumoto K, Abe H, & Tanaka K (2007). Medial prefrontal selectivity signalling prediction errors of action values. *Nature Neuroscience* 10: 647–656.

Matthews G & Gilliland K (1999). The personality theories of H.J.Eysenck and J.A.Gray: a comparative review. *Personality and Individual Differences* 26: 583–626.

Matthews G, Zeidner M, & Roberts RD (2002). *Emotional Intelligence: Science and Myth*. MIT Press, Cambridge, MA.

Mayberg HS (2003). Positron emission tomography imaging in depression: a neural systems perspective. *Neuroimaging Clinics of North America* 13: 805–815.

Maynard Smith J (1982). *Evolution and the Theory of Games*. Cambridge University Press, Cambridge.

Maynard Smith J (1984). Game theory and the evolution of behaviour. *Behavioral and Brain Sciences* 7: 95–125.

Maynard Smith J & Harper D (2003). *Animal Signals*. Oxford University Press, Oxford.

Mayr E (1961). Cause and effect in biology. *Science* 134: 1501–1506.

Mazur JE (2012). *Learning and Behavior*. Pearson, Boston, MA, 7th edn.

McCabe C & Rolls ET (2007). Umami: a delicious flavor formed by convergence of taste and olfactory pathways in the human brain. *European Journal of Neuroscience* 25: 1855–1864.

McCabe C, Rolls ET, Bilderbeck A, & McGlone F (2008). Cognitive influences on the affective representation of touch and the sight of touch in the human brain. *Social, Cognitive and Affective Neuroscience* 3: 97–108.

McClure SM, Laibson DI, Loewenstein G, & Cohen JD (2004). Separate neural systems value immediate and delayed monetary rewards. *Science* 306: 503–507.

McEwen BS, Gray JD, & Nasca C (2015). 60 years of neuroendocrinology: Redefining neuroendocrinology: stress, sex and cognitive and emotional regulation. *J Endocrinol* 226: T67–83.

McLeod P, Plunkett K, & Rolls ET (1998). *Introduction to Connectionist Modelling of Cognitive Processes*. Oxford University Press, Oxford.

McQuaid RJ, McInnis OA, Abizaid A, & Anisman H (2014). Making room for oxytocin in understanding depression. *Neurosci Biobehav Rev* 45: 305–22.

Meehan TP, Bressler SL, Tang W, Astafiev SV, Sylvester CM, Shulman GL, & Corbetta M (2017). Top-down cortical interactions in visuospatial attention. *Brain Struct Funct* 222: 3127–3145.

Melzack R & Wall PD (1996). *The Challenge of Pain*. Penguin, Harmondsworth, UK.

Menon V & Uddin LQ (2010). Saliency, switching, attention and control: a network model of insula function. *Brain Structure and Function* 214: 655–667.

Mesulam MM & Mufson EJ (1982a). Insula of the Old World monkey. I: Architectonics in the insulo-orbito-temporal component of the paralimbic brain. *Journal of Comparative Neurology* 212: 1–22.

Mesulam MM & Mufson EJ (1982b). Insula of the Old World monkey. III. Efferent cortical output and comments on function. *Journal of Comparative Neurology* 212: 38–52.

Micevych PE & Meisel RL (2017). Integrating neural circuits controlling female sexual behavior. *Front Syst Neurosci* 11: 42.

Millar R (1952). Forces observed during coitus in thoroughbreds. *Australian Veterinary Journal* 28: 127–128.

Millenson JR (1967). *Principles of Behavioral Analysis*. MacMillan, New York.

Miller GA (1956). The magic number seven, plus or minus two: some limits on our capacity for the processing of information. *Psychological Review* 63: 81–93.

Miller GF (2000). *The Mating Mind*. Heinemann, London.

Milner A (2008). Conscious and unconscious visual processing in the human brain. In Weiskrantz L & Davies M, editors, *Frontiers of Consciousness*, chap. 5, 169–214. Oxford University Press, Oxford.

Milner AD & Goodale MA (1995). *The Visual Brain in Action*. Oxford University Press, Oxford.

Milton AL, Lee JL, Butler VJ, Gardner R, & Everitt BJ (2008). Intra-amygdala and systemic antagonism of NMDA receptors prevents the reconsolidation of drug-associated memory and impairs subsequently both novel and previously acquired drug-seeking behaviors. *Journal of Neuroscience* 28: 8230–8237.

Moller AP & Thornhill R (1998). Male parental care, differential parental investment by females and sexual selection. *Animal Behaviour* 55: 1507–1515.

Mombaerts P (2006). Axonal wiring in the mouse olfactory system. *Annual Review of Cell and Developmental Biology* 22: 713–737.

Moniz E (1936). *Tentatives Opératoires dans le Traitment de Certaines Psychoses*. Masson, Paris.

Montague PR, King-Casas B, & Cohen JD (2006). Imaging valuation models in human choice. *Annual Review of Neuroscience* 29: 417–448.

Moors A, Ellsworth PC, Scherer, & Frijda NH (2013). Appraisal theories of emotion: state of the art and future development. *Emotion Review* 5: 119–124.

Mora F, Mogenson GJ, & Rolls ET (1977). Activity of neurones in the region of the substantia nigra during feeding. *Brain Research* 133: 267–276.

Morecraft RJ & Tanji J (2009). Cingulofrontal interactions and the cingulate motor areas. In Vogt B, editor, *Cingulate Neurobiology and Disease*, chap. 5, 113–144. Oxford University Press, Oxford.

Morecraft RJ, Geula C, & Mesulam MM (1992). Cytoarchitecture and neural afferents of orbitofrontal cortex in the brain of the monkey. *Journal of Comparative Neurology* 323: 341–358.

Morecraft RJ, McNeal DW, Stilwell-Morecraft KS, Gedney M, Ge J, Schroeder CM, & van Hoesen GW (2007). Amygdala interconnections with the cingulate motor cortex in the rhesus monkey. *J Comp Neurol* 500: 134–65.

Mori K & Sakano H (2011). How is the olfactory map formed and interpreted in the mammalian brain? *Annual Reviews of Neuroscience* 34: 467–499.

Mori K, Mataga N, & Imamura K (1992). Differential specificities of single mitral cells in rabbit olfactory bulb for a homologous series of fatty acid odor molecules. *Journal of Neurophysiology* 67: 786–789.

Mori K, Nagao H, & Yoshihara Y (1999). The olfactory bulb: coding and processing of odor molecule information. *Science* 286: 711–715.

Morris JA, Jordan CL, & Breedlove MS (2004). Sexual differentiation of the vertebrate nervous system. *Nature Neuroscience* 7: 1034–1039.

Morrison SE, Saez A, Lau B, & Salzman CD (2011). Different time courses for learning-related changes in amygdala and orbitofrontal cortex. *Neuron* 71: 1127–40.

Morrot G, Brochet F, & Dubourdieu D (2001). The color of odors. *Brain and Language* 79: 309–320.

Motta-Mena NV & Puts DA (2017). Endocrinology of human female sexuality, mating, and reproductive behavior. *Horm Behav* 91: 19–35.

Mufson EJ & Mesulam MM (1982). Insula of the Old World monkey II: Afferent cortical input and comments on the claustrum. *Journal of Comparative Neurology* 212: 23–37.

Munzberg H & Myers MG (2005). Molecular and anatomical determinants of central leptin resistance. *Nature Neuroscience* 8: 566–570.

Murray EA & Izquierdo A (2007). Orbitofrontal cortex and amygdala contributions to affect and action in primates. *Annals of the New York Academy of Sciences* 1121: 273–296.

Nagai Y, Critchley HD, Featherstone E, Trimble MR, & Dolan RJ (2004). Activity in ventromedial prefrontal cortex covaries with sympathetic skin conductance level: a physiological account of a "default mode" of brain function. *Neuroimage* 22: 243–251.

Nakazawa K, Quirk MC, Chitwood RA, Watanabe M, Yeckel MF, Sun LD, Kato A, Carr CA, Johnston D, Wilson MA, & Tonegawa S (2002). Requirement for hippocampal CA3 NMDA receptors in associative memory recall. *Science* 297: 211–218.

Nakazawa K, Sun LD, Quirk MC, Rondi-Reig L, Wilson MA, & Tonegawa S (2003). Hippocampal CA3 NMDA receptors are crucial for memory acquisition of one-time experience. *Neuron* 38: 305–315.

Nakazawa K, McHugh TJ, Wilson MA, & Tonegawa S (2004). NMDA receptors, place cells and hippocampal spatial memory. *Nature Reviews Neuroscience* 5: 361–372.

Nemeroff CB (2003). The role of GABA in the pathophysiology and treatment of anxiety disorders. *Psychopharmacology Bulletin* 37: 133–146.

Nesse RM (2000). Is depression an adaptation? *Archives of General Psychiatry* 57: 14–20.

Nesse RM & Lloyd AT (1992). The evolution of psychodynamic mechanisms. In Barkow JH, Cosmides L, & Tooby J, editors, *The Adapted Mind*, 601–624. Oxford University Press, New York.

Niki H & Watanabe M (1979). Prefrontal and cingulate unit activity during timing behavior in the monkey. *Brain Research* 171: 213–224.

Nishijo H, Ono T, & Nishino H (1988). Single neuron responses in amygdala of alert monkey during complex sensory stimulation with affective significance. *Journal of Neuroscience* 8: 3570–3583.

Norgren R (1974). Gustatory afferents to ventral forebrain. *Brain Research* 81: 285–295.

Norgren R (1976). Taste pathways to hypothalamus and amygdala. *Journal of Comparative Neurology* 166: 17–30.

Norgren R (1990). Gustatory system. In Paxinos G, editor, *The Human Nervous System*, 845–861. Academic Press, San Diego.

Norgren R & Leonard CM (1971). Taste pathways in rat brainstem. *Science* 173: 1136–1139.

Norgren R & Leonard CM (1973). Ascending central gustatory pathways. *Journal of Comparative Neurology* 150: 217–238.

Nugent AC, Milham MP, Bain EE, Mah L, Cannon DM, Marrett S, Zarate CA, Pine DS, Price JL, & Drevets WC (2006). Cortical abnormalities in bipolar disorder investigated with mri and voxel-based morphometry. *Neuroimage* 30: 485–497.

Nusslock R, Young CB, & Damme KS (2014). Elevated reward-related neural activation as a unique biological marker of bipolar disorder: assessment and treatment implications. *Behaviour Research and Therapy* 62: 74–87.

Nutt DJ, Lingford-Hughes A, Erritzoe D, & Stokes PR (2015). The dopamine theory of addiction: 40 years of highs and lows. *Nat Rev Neurosci* 16: 305–12.

Oatley K & Jenkins JM (1996). *Understanding Emotions*. Blackwell, Oxford.

Oatley K, Keltner D, & Jenkins JM (2018). *Understanding Emotions*. Wiley-Blackwell, Hoboken, NJ, 4th edn.

O'Doherty J, Rolls ET, Francis S, Bowtell R, McGlone F, Kobal G, Renner B, & Ahne G (2000). Sensory-specific satiety related olfactory activation of the human orbitofrontal cortex. *NeuroReport* 11: 893–897.

O'Doherty J, Kringelbach ML, Rolls ET, Hornak J, & Andrews C (2001a). Abstract reward and punishment representations in the human orbitofrontal cortex. *Nature Neuroscience* 4: 95–102.

O'Doherty J, Rolls ET, Francis S, Bowtell R, & McGlone F (2001b). The representation of pleasant and aversive taste in the human brain. *Journal of Neurophysiology* 85: 1315–1321.

O'Doherty J, Winston J, Critchley HD, Perrett DI, Burt DM, & Dolan RJ (2003). Beauty in a smile: the role of the medial orbitofrontal cortex in facial attractiveness. *Neuropsychologia* 41: 147–155.

Ongur D & Price JL (2000). The organisation of networks within the orbital and medial prefrontal cortex of rats, monkeys and humans. *Cerebral Cortex* 10: 206–219.

Ongur D, Ferry AT, & Price JL (2003). Architectonic subdivision of the human orbital and medial prefrontal cortex. *Journal of Comparative Neurology* 460: 425–449.

Ono T & Nishijo H (1992). Neurophysiological basis of the Kluver–Bucy syndrome: responses of monkey amygdaloid neurons to biologically significant objects. In Aggleton JP, editor, *The Amygdala*, chap. 6, 167–190. Wiley-Liss, New York.

Ono T, Nishino H, Sasaki K, Fukuda M, & Muramoto K (1980). Role of the lateral hypothalamus and amygdala in feeding behavior. *Brain Research Bulletin* 5, Suppl.: 143–149.

Ono T, Tamura R, Nishijo H, Nakamura K, & Tabuchi E (1989). Contribution of amygdala and LH neurons to the visual information processing of food and non-food in the monkey. *Physiology and Behavior* 45: 411–421.

O'Rahilly S (2009). Human genetics illuminates the paths to metabolic disease. *Nature* 462: 307–314.

Orban GA (2011). The extraction of 3D shape in the visual system of human and nonhuman primates. *Annual Reviews of Neuroscience* 34: 361–388.

Oring LW (1986). Avian polyandry. In Johnston RF, editor, *Current Ornithology*, vol. 3, 309–351. Plenum, New York.

Overath P, Sturm T, & Rammensee HG (2014). Of volatiles and peptides: in search for mhc-dependent olfactory signals in social communication. *Cell Mol Life Sci* 71: 2429–42.

Padoa-Schioppa C (2011). Neurobiology of economic choice: a good-based model. *Annual Review of Neuroscience* 34: 333–359.

Padoa-Schioppa C & Assad JA (2006). Neurons in the orbitofrontal cortex encode economic value. *Nature* 441: 223–226.

Palomero-Gallagher N & Zilles K (2004). Isocortex. In Paxinos G, editor, *The Rat Nervous System*, 729–757. Elsevier Academic Press, San Diego.

Panksepp J (1998). *Affective Neuroscience: The Foundations of Human and Animal Emotions*. Oxford University Press, New York.

Panksepp J (2011). The basic emotional circuits of mammalian brains: Do animals have affective lives? *Neuroscience and Biobehavioral Reviews* 35: 1791–1804.

Panksepp J, Nelson E, & Bekkedal M (1997). Brain systems for the mediation of social separation-distress and social reward. *Annals of the New York Academy of Sciences* 807: 78–100.

Parker GA & Pizzari T (2015). *Sexual selection: the logical imperative*, 119–163. Springer.

Passingham REP & Wise SP (2012). *The Neurobiology of the Prefrontal Cortex*. Oxford University Press, Oxford.

Paton JJ, Belova MA, Morrison SE, & Salzman CD (2006). The primate amygdala represents the positive and negative value of visual stimuli during learning. *Nature* 439: 865–870.

Pearce JM (2008). *Animal Learning and Cognition*. Psychology Press, Hove, Sussex, 3rd edn.

Penton-Voak IS, Perrett DI, Castles DL, Kobayashi T, Burt DM, Murray LK, & Minamisawa R (1999). Menstrual cycle alters faces preference. *Nature* 399: 741–742.

Percheron G, Yelnik J, & François C (1984a). A Golgi analysis of the primate globus pallidus. III. Spatial organization of the striato-pallidal complex. *Journal of Comparative Neurology* 227: 214–227.

Percheron G, Yelnik J, & François C (1984b). The primate striato-pallido-nigral system: an integrative system for cortical information. In McKenzie JS, Kemm RE, & Wilcox LN, editors, *The Basal Ganglia: Structure and Function*, 87–105. Plenum, New York.

Percheron G, Yelnik J, François C, Fenelon G, & Talbi B (1994). Informational neurology of the basal ganglia related system. *Revue Neurologique (Paris)* 150: 614–626.

Perl ER & Kruger L (1996). Nociception and pain: evolution of concepts and observations. In Kruger L, editor, *Pain and Touch*, chap. 4, 180–211. Academic Press, San Diego.

Perrett DI, Rolls ET, & Caan W (1982). Visual neurons responsive to faces in the monkey temporal cortex. *Experimental Brain Research* 47: 329–342.

Perrett DI, Smith PAJ, Potter DD, Mistlin AJ, Head AS, Milner D, & Jeeves MA (1985). Visual cells in temporal cortex sensitive to face view and gaze direction. *Proceedings of the Royal Society of London, Series B* 223: 293–317.

Pessoa L & Adolphs R (2010). Emotion processing and the amygdala: from a 'low road' to 'many roads' of evaluating biological significance. *Nature Reviews Neuroscience* 11: 773–783.

Pessoa L & Padmala S (2005). Quantitative prediction of perceptual decisions during near-threshold fear detection. *Proceedings of the National Academy of Sciences USA* 102: 5612–5617.

Petrides M (1996). Specialized systems for the processing of mnemonic information within the primate frontal cortex. *Philosophical Transactions of the Royal Society of London B* 351: 1455–1462.

Petrides M (2007). The orbitofrontal cortex: novelty, deviation from expectation, and memory. *Annals of the New York Academy of Sciences* 1121: 33–53.

Petrides M & Pandya DN (1988). Association fiber pathways to the frontal cortex from the superior temporal region in the rhesus monkey. *Journal of Comparative Neurology* 273: 52–66.

Petrides M, Tomaiuolo F, Yeterian EH, & Pandya DN (2012). The prefrontal cortex: comparative architectonic organization in the human and the macaque monkey brains. *Cortex* 48: 46–57.

Pfaff DW & Baum MJ (2018). Hormone-dependent medial preoptic/lumbar spinal cord/autonomic coordination supporting male sexual behaviors. *Mol Cell Endocrinol* 467: 21–30.

Pfaff DW, Gagnidze K, & Hunter RG (2018). Molecular endocrinology of female reproductive behavior. *Mol Cell Endocrinol* 467: 14–20.

Phelps E, O'Connor KJ, Gatenby JC, Gore JC, Grillon C, & Davis M (2001). Activation of the left amygdala to a cognitive representation of fear. *Nature Neuroscience* 4: 437–441.

Phelps EA (2004). Human emotion and memory: interactions of the amygdala and hippocampal complex. *Current Opinion in Neurobiology* 14: 198–202.

Phelps EA (2006). Emotion and cognition: insights from studies of the human amygdala. *Annual Review of Psychology* 57: 27–53.

Phelps EA & LeDoux JE (2005). Contributions of the amygdala to emotion processing: from animal models to human behavior. *Neuron* 48: 175–187.

Phillips AG, Mora F, & Rolls ET (1981). Intra-cerebral self-administration of amphetamine by rhesus monkeys. *Neuroscience Letters* 24: 81–86.

Phillips AG, Pfaus JG, & Blaha CD (1991). Dopamine and motivated behavior: insights provided by in vivo analysis. In Willner P & Scheel-Kruger J, editors, *The Mesolimbic Dopamine System: From Motivation to Action*, chap. 8, 199–224. Wiley, New York.

Phillips AG, Vacca G, & Ahn S (2008). A top-down perspective on dopamine, motivation and memory. *Pharmacol Biochem Behav* 90: 236–49.

Phillips ML (2004). Facial processing deficits and social dysfunction: how are they related? *Brain* 127: 1691–1692.

Phillips ML, Drevets WC, Rauch SL, & Lane R (2003). Neurobiology of emotion perception II: Implications for major psychiatric disorders. *Biological Psychiatry* 54: 515–528.

Phillips ML, Williams LM, Heining M, Herba CM, Russell T, Andrew C, Bullmore ET, Brammer MJ, Williams SC, Morgan M, Young AW, & Gray JA (2004). Differential neural responses to overt and covert presentations of facial expressions of fear and disgust. *Neuroimage* 21: 1484–1496.

Piguet O (2011). Eating disturbance in behavioural-variant frontotemporal dementia. *Journal of Molecuar Neuroscience* 45: 589–593.

Pitkanen A, Kelly JL, & Amaral DG (2002). Projections from the lateral, basal, and accessory basal nuclei of the amygdala to the entorhinal cortex in the macaque monkey. *Hippocampus* 12: 186–205.

Pizzari T, Cornwallis CK, Lovlie H, Jakobsson S, & Birkhead TR (2003). Sophisticated sperm allocation in male fowl. *Nature* 426: 70–74.

Preuss TM (1995). Do rats have prefrontal cortex? The Rose-Woolsey-Akert program reconsidered. *Journal of Cognitive Neuroscience* 7: 1–24.

Preuss TM & Goldman-Rakic PS (1989). Connections of the ventral granular frontal cortex of macaques with perisylvian premotor and somatosensory areas: anatomical evidence for somatic representation in primate frontal association cortex. *Journal of Comparative Neurology* 282: 293–316.

Price J (2006). Connections of orbital cortex. In Zald DH & Rauch SL, editors, *The Orbitofrontal Cortex*, chap. 3, 39–55. Oxford University Press, Oxford.

Price JL & Drevets WC (2012). Neural circuits underlying the pathophysiology of mood disorders. *Trends in Cognitive Science* 16: 61–71.

Price JL, Carmichael ST, Carnes KM, Clugnet MC, & Kuroda M (1991). Olfactory input to the prefrontal cortex. In Davis JL & Eichenbaum H, editors, *Olfaction: A Model System for Computational Neuroscience*, 101–120. MIT Press, Cambridge, MA.

Pritchard TC, Hamilton RB, & Norgren R (1989). Neural coding of gustatory information in the thalamus of Macaca mulatta. *Journal of Neurophysiology* 61: 1–14.

Proulx CD, Hikosaka O, & Malinow R (2014). Reward processing by the lateral habenula in normal and depressive behaviors. *Nat Neurosci* 17: 1146–52.

Pryce CR, Azzinnari D, Spinelli S, Seifritz E, Tegethoff M, & Meinlschmidt G (2011). Helplessness: a systematic translational review of theory and evidence for its relevance to understanding and treating depression. *Pharmacol Ther* 132: 242–267.

Puts D (2015). Human sexual selection. *Current Opinion in Psychology* 7: 28–32.

Rachlin H (1989). *Judgement, Decision, and Choice: A Cognitive/Behavioural Synthesis*. Freeman, New York.

Rada P, Mark GP, & Hoebel BG (1998). Dopamine in the nucleus accumbens released by hypothalamic stimulation-escape behavior. *Brain Research* 782: 228–234.

Rahman S, Sahakian BJ, Hodges JR, Rogers RD, & Robbins TW (1999). Specific cognitive deficits in mild frontal variant frontotemporal dementia. *Brain* 122: 1469–1493.

Rantala MJ, Luoto S, Krams I, & Karlsson H (2018). Depression subtyping based on evolutionary psychiatry: Proximate mechanisms and ultimate functions. *Brain Behav Immun* 69: 603–617.

Rascovsky K, Hodges JR, & al (2011). Sensitivity of revised diagnostic criteria for the behavioural variant of frontotemporal dementia. *Brain* 134: 2456–2477.

Ratcliff R & Rouder JF (1998). Modeling response times for two-choice decisions. *Psychological Science* 9: 347–356.

Ratcliff R, Zandt TV, & McKoon G (1999). Connectionist and diffusion models of reaction time. *Psychological Reviews* 106: 261–300.

Rawlins JN, Winocur G, & Gray JA (1983). The hippocampus, collateral behavior, and timing. *Behavioral Neuroscience* 97: 857–872.

Reddy WM (2001). *The Navigation of Feeling: A Framework for the History of Emotions*. Cambridge University Press, Cambridge.

Reisenzein R (1983). The Schachter theory of emotion: two decades later. *Psychological Bulletin* 94: 239–264.

Rempel-Clower NL & Barbas H (1998). Topographic organization of connections between the hypothalamus and prefrontal cortex in the rhesus monkey. *Journal of Comparative Neurology* 398: 393–419.

Riani M & Simonotto E (1994). Stochastic resonance in the perceptual interpretation of ambiguous figures: A neural network model. *Physical Review Letters* 72: 3120–3123.

Ridley M (1993a). *The Red Queen: Sex and the Evolution of Human Nature*. Penguin, London.

Ridley M (1993b). *Evolution*. Blackwell, Oxford.

Ridley M (1996). *The Origins of Virtue*. Viking, London.

Ridley M (2003). *Nature via Nurture*. Harper, London.

Robbins TW, Gillan CM, Smith DG, de Wit S, & Ersche KD (2012). Neurocognitive endophenotypes of impulsivity and compulsivity: towards dimensional psychiatry. *Trends in Cognitive Sciences* 16: 81–91.

Robertson RG, Rolls ET, & Georges-François P (1998). Spatial view cells in the primate hippocampus: Effects of removal of view details. *Journal of Neurophysiology* 79: 1145–1156.

Robinson MD, Watkins ER, & Harmon-Jones E (2013). *Handbook of Cognition and Emotion*. Guilford, New York.

Rodin J (1976). The role of perception of internal and external signals in the regulation of feeding in overweight and non-obese individuals. *Dahlem Konferenzen, Life Sciences Research Report* 2: 265–281.

Rolls BJ (2012a). Dietary strategies for weight management. *Nestle Nutrition Institute Workshop Series* 73: 37–48.

Rolls BJ & Hetherington M (1989). The role of variety in eating and body weight regulation. In Shepherd R, editor, *Handbook of the Psychophysiology of Human Eating*, chap. 3, 57–84. Wiley, Chichester.

Rolls BJ & Rolls ET (1982a). *Thirst*. Cambridge University Press, Cambridge.

Rolls BJ, Rolls ET, Rowe EA, & Sweeney K (1981a). Sensory specific satiety in man. *Physiology and Behavior* 27: 137–142.

Rolls BJ, Rowe EA, Rolls ET, Kingston B, Megson A, & Gunary R (1981b). Variety in a meal enhances food intake in man. *Physiology and Behavior* 26: 215–221.

Rolls BJ, Rowe EA, & Rolls ET (1982a). How sensory properties of foods affect human feeding behavior. *Physiology and Behavior* 29: 409–417.

Rolls BJ, Rowe EA, & Rolls ET (1982b). How flavour and appearance affect human feeding. *Proceedings of the Nutrition Society* 41: 109–117.

Rolls BJ, Van Duijenvoorde PM, & Rowe EA (1983a). Variety in the diet enhances intake in a meal and contributes to the development of obesity in the rat. *Physiology and Behavior* 31: 21–27.

Rolls BJ, Van Duijenvoorde PM, & Rolls ET (1984a). Pleasantness changes and food intake in a varied four course meal. *Appetite* 5: 337–348.

Rolls ET (1975). *The Brain and Reward.* Pergamon Press, Oxford.

Rolls ET (1981a). Processing beyond the inferior temporal visual cortex related to feeding, learning, and striatal function. In Katsuki Y, Norgren R, & Sato M, editors, *Brain Mechanisms of Sensation*, chap. 16, 241–269. Wiley, New York.

Rolls ET (1981b). Central nervous mechanisms related to feeding and appetite. *British Medical Bulletin* 37: 131–134.

Rolls ET (1981c). Responses of amygdaloid neurons in the primate. In Ben-Ari Y, editor, *The Amygdaloid Complex*, 383–393. Elsevier, Amsterdam.

Rolls ET (1986a). A theory of emotion, and its application to understanding the neural basis of emotion. In Oomura Y, editor, *Emotions. Neural and Chemical Control*, 325–344. Japan Scientific Societies Press; and Karger, Tokyo; and Basel.

Rolls ET (1986b). Neural systems involved in emotion in primates. In Plutchik R & Kellerman H, editors, *Emotion: Theory, Research, and Experience*, vol. 3: Biological Foundations of Emotion, chap. 5, 125–143. Academic Press, New York.

Rolls ET (1989). Functions of neuronal networks in the hippocampus and neocortex in memory. In Byrne JH & Berry WO, editors, *Neural Models of Plasticity: Experimental and Theoretical Approaches*, chap. 13, 240–265. Academic Press, San Diego, CA.

Rolls ET (1990a). A theory of emotion, and its application to understanding the neural basis of emotion. *Cognition and Emotion* 4: 161–190.

Rolls ET (1990b). Theoretical and neurophysiological analysis of the functions of the primate hippocampus in memory. *Cold Spring Harbor Symposia in Quantitative Biology* 55: 995–1006.

Rolls ET (1992a). Neurophysiology and functions of the primate amygdala. In Aggleton JP, editor, *The Amygdala*, chap. 5, 143–165. Wiley-Liss, New York.

Rolls ET (1992b). Neurophysiological mechanisms underlying face processing within and beyond the temporal cortical visual areas. *Philosophical Transactions of the Royal Society* 335: 11–21.

Rolls ET (1995). A theory of emotion and consciousness, and its application to understanding the neural basis of emotion. In Gazzaniga MS, editor, *The Cognitive Neurosciences*, chap. 72, 1091–1106. MIT Press, Cambridge, MA.

Rolls ET (1996). A theory of hippocampal function in memory. *Hippocampus* 6: 601–620.

Rolls ET (1997a). Brain mechanisms of vision, memory, and consciousness. In Ito M, Miyashita Y, & Rolls E, editors, *Cognition, Computation, and Consciousness*, chap. 6, 81–120. Oxford University Press, Oxford.

Rolls ET (1997b). Consciousness in neural networks? *Neural Networks* 10: 1227–1240.

Rolls ET (1999a). *The Brain and Emotion.* Oxford University Press, Oxford.

Rolls ET (1999b). Spatial view cells and the representation of place in the primate hippocampus. *Hippocampus* 9: 467–480.

Rolls ET (1999c). The functions of the orbitofrontal cortex. *Neurocase* 5: 301–312.

Rolls ET (2000a). Précis of The Brain and Emotion. *Behavioral and Brain Sciences* 23: 177–233.

Rolls ET (2000b). The orbitofrontal cortex and reward. *Cerebral Cortex* 10: 284–294.

Rolls ET (2000c). Neurophysiology and functions of the primate amygdala, and the neural basis of emotion. In Aggleton JP, editor, *The Amygdala: Second Edition. A Functional Analysis*, chap. 13, 447–478. Oxford University Press, Oxford.

Rolls ET (2000d). Memory systems in the brain. *Annual Review of Psychology* 51: 599–630.

Rolls ET (2001). The representation of umami taste in the human and macaque cortex. *Sensory Neuron* 3: 227–242.

Rolls ET (2003). Consciousness absent and present: a neurophysiological exploration. *Progress in Brain Research* 144: 95–106.

Rolls ET (2004a). The operation of memory systems in the brain. In Feng J, editor, *Computational Neuroscience: A Comprehensive Approach*, chap. 16, 491–534. CRC Press (UK), London.

Rolls ET (2004b). The functions of the orbitofrontal cortex. *Brain and Cognition* 55: 11–29.

Rolls ET (2004c). A higher order syntactic thought (HOST) theory of consciousness. In Gennaro RJ, editor, *Higher Order Theories of Consciousness*, chap. 7, 137–172. John Benjamins, Amsterdam.

Rolls ET (2005). *Emotion Explained.* Oxford University Press, Oxford.

Rolls ET (2006a). Consciousness absent and present: a neurophysiological exploration of masking. In Ogmen H & Breitmeyer BG, editors, *The First Half Second*, chap. 6, 89–108. MIT Press, Cambridge, MA.

Rolls ET (2006b). Brain mechanisms underlying flavour and appetite. *Philosophical Transactions of the Royal Society B* 361: 1123–1136.

Rolls ET (2007a). The affective neuroscience of consciousness: higher order syntactic thoughts, dual routes to emotion and action, and consciousness. In Zelazo PD, Moscovitch M, & Thompson E, editors, *Cambridge Handbook of Consciousness*, chap. 29, 831–859. Cambridge University Press, New York.

Rolls ET (2007b). Understanding the mechanisms of food intake and obesity. *Obesity Reviews* 8: 67–72.

Rolls ET (2007c). A computational neuroscience approach to consciousness. *Neural Networks* 20: 962–982.

Rolls ET (2008a). Emotion, higher order syntactic thoughts, and consciousness. In Weiskrantz L & Davies M, editors, *Frontiers of Consciousness*, chap. 4, 131–167. Oxford University Press, Oxford.

Rolls ET (2008b). Functions of the orbitofrontal and pregenual cingulate cortex in taste, olfaction, appetite and emotion. *Acta Physiologica Hungarica* 95: 131–164.

Rolls ET (2009a). Functional neuroimaging of umami taste: what makes umami pleasant. *American Journal of Clinical Nutrition* 90: 803S–814S.

Rolls ET (2009b). The anterior and midcingulate cortices and reward. In Vogt B, editor, *Cingulate Neurobiology and Disease*, chap. 8, 191–206. Oxford University Press, Oxford.

Rolls ET (2010a). Noise in the brain, decision-making, determinism, free will, and consciousness. In Perry E, Collerton D, LeBeau F, & Ashton H, editors, *New Horizons in the Neuroscience of Consciousness*, 113–120. John Benjamins, Amsterdam.

Rolls ET (2010b). A computational theory of episodic memory formation in the hippocampus. *Behavioural Brain Research* 215: 180–196.

Rolls ET (2010c). The affective and cognitive processing of touch, oral texture, and temperature in the brain. *Neuroscience and Biobehavioral Reviews* 34: 237–245.

Rolls ET (2010d). Taste, olfactory and food texture processing in the brain and the control of appetite. In LDube, ABechara, ADagher, ADrewnowski, JLeBel, PJames, & RYYada, editors, *Obesity Prevention*, chap. 4, 41–56. Academic Press, London.

Rolls ET (2011a). Consciousness, decision-making, and neural computation. In Cutsuridis V, Hussain A, & Taylor JG, editors, *Perception-Action Cycle: Models, architecture, and hardware*, chap. 9, 287–333. Springer, Berlin.

Rolls ET (2011b). Taste, olfactory, and food texture reward processing in the brain and obesity. *International Journal of Obesity* 35: 550–561.

Rolls ET (2011c). Face neurons. In Calder AJ, Rhodes G, Johnson MH, & Haxby JV, editors, *The Oxford Handbook of Face Perception*, chap. 4, 51–75. Oxford University Press, Oxford.

Rolls ET (2011d). A neurobiological basis for affective feelings and aesthetics. In Schellekens E & Goldie P, editors, *The Aesthetic Mind: Philosophy and Psychology*, chap. 8, 116–165. Oxford University Press, Oxford.

Rolls ET (2011e). The neural representation of oral texture including fat texture. *Journal of Texture Studies* 42: 137–156.

Rolls ET (2011f). Chemosensory learning in the cortex. *Frontiers in Systems Neuroscience* 5: 78 (1–13).

Rolls ET (2012b). Glutamate, obsessive-compulsive disorder, schizophrenia, and the stability of cortical attractor neuronal networks. *Pharmacology, Biochemistry and Behavior* 100: 736–751.

Rolls ET (2012c). Taste, olfactory, and food texture reward processing in the brain and the control of appetite. *Proceedings of the Nutrition Society* 71: 488–501.

Rolls ET (2012d). *Neuroculture: On the Implications of Brain Science*. Oxford University Press, Oxford.

Rolls ET (2012e). Invariant visual object and face recognition: neural and computational bases, and a model, VisNet. *Frontiers in Computational Neuroscience* 6: 1–70.

Rolls ET (2013a). A biased activation theory of the cognitive and attentional modulation of emotion. *Frontiers in Human Neuroscience* 7: 74.

Rolls ET (2013b). On the relation between the mind and the brain: a neuroscience perspective. *Philosophia Scientiae* 17: 31–70.

Rolls ET (2013c). A quantitative theory of the functions of the hippocampal CA3 network in memory. *Frontiers in Cellular Neuroscience* 7: 98.

Rolls ET (2013d). What are emotional states, and why do we have them? *Emotion Review* 5: 241–247.

Rolls ET (2014a). Neuroculture: art, aesthetics, and the brain. *Rendiconti Lincei Scienze Fisiche e Naturali* 25: 291–307. doi:DOI:10.1007/s12210-013-0276-7.

Rolls ET (2014b). *Emotion and Decision-Making Explained*. Oxford University Press, Oxford.

Rolls ET (2014c). Emotion and decision-making explained: Précis. *Cortex* 59: 185–193.

Rolls ET (2015a). Limbic systems for emotion and for memory, but no single limbic system. *Cortex* 62: 119–157.

Rolls ET (2015b). Central neural integration of taste, smell and other sensory modalities. In Doty RL, editor, *Handbook of Olfaction and Gustation*, chap. 44, 1027–1048. Wiley, New York, 3rd edn.

Rolls ET (2015c). Taste, olfactory, and food reward value processing in the brain. *Progress in Neurobiology* 127–128: 64–90.

Rolls ET (2015d). Limbic systems for emotion and for memory, but no single limbic system. *Cortex* 62: 119–157.

Rolls ET (2015e). Neurobiological foundations of art and aesthetics. In Huston JP, Nadal M, Mora F, Agnati L, & Cela-Conde CJ, editors, *Art, Aesthetics and the Brain*, chap. 23, 453–478. Oxford University Press, Oxford.

Rolls ET (2016a). Brain processing of reward for touch, temperature, and oral texture. In Olausson H, Wessberg J, Morrison I, & McGlone F, editors, *Affective Touch and the Neurophysiology of CT Afferents*, chap. 13, 209–225. Springer, Berlin.

Rolls ET (2016b). Functions of the anterior insula in taste, autonomic, and related functions. *Brain and Cognition* 110: 4–19.

Rolls ET (2016c). *Cerebral Cortex: Principles of Operation*. Oxford University Press, Oxford.

Rolls ET (2016d). A non-reward attractor theory of depression. *Neuroscience and Biobehavioral Reviews* 68: 47–58.

Rolls ET (2016e). Reward systems in the brain and nutrition. *Annual Review of Nutrition* 36: 435–470.

Rolls ET (2017a). Neurobiological foundations of aesthetics and art. *New Ideas in Psychology* 47: 121–135.
Rolls ET (2017b). The roles of the orbitofrontal cortex via the habenula in non-reward and depression, and in the responses of serotonin and dopamine neurons. *Neuroscience and Biobehavioral Reviews* 75: 331–334.
Rolls ET (2017c). Evolution of the emotional brain. In Watanabe S, Hofman MA, & Shimizu T, editors, *Evolution of Brain, Cognition, and Emotion in Vertebrates*, chap. 12, 251–272. Springer, Tokyo.
Rolls ET (2017d). The orbitofrontal cortex and emotion in health and disease, including depression. *Neuropsychologia* doi: 10.1016/j.neuropsychologia.2017.09.021.
Rolls ET (2018). The storage and recall of memories in the hippocampo-cortical system. *Cell and Tissue Research* doi: 10.1007/s00441–017–2744–3.
Rolls ET & Baylis GC (1986). Size and contrast have only small effects on the responses to faces of neurons in the cortex of the superior temporal sulcus of the monkey. *Experimental Brain Research* 65: 38–48.
Rolls ET & Baylis LL (1994). Gustatory, olfactory and visual convergence within the primate orbitofrontal cortex. *Journal of Neuroscience* 14: 5437–5452.
Rolls ET & de Waal AWL (1985). Long-term sensory-specific satiety: evidence from an Ethiopian refugee camp. *Physiology and Behavior* 34: 1017–1020.
Rolls ET & Deco G (2002). *Computational Neuroscience of Vision*. Oxford University Press, Oxford.
Rolls ET & Deco G (2006). Attention in natural scenes: neurophysiological and computational bases. *Neural Networks* 19: 1383–1394.
Rolls ET & Deco G (2010). *The Noisy Brain: Stochastic Dynamics as a Principle of Brain Function*. Oxford University Press, Oxford.
Rolls ET & Deco G (2011a). A computational neuroscience approach to schizophrenia and its onset. *Neuroscience and Biobehavioral Reviews* 35: 1644–1653.
Rolls ET & Deco G (2011b). Prediction of decisions from noise in the brain before the evidence is provided. *Frontiers in Neuroscience* 5: 33.
Rolls ET & Deco G (2015a). A stochastic neurodynamics approach to the changes in cognition and memory in aging. *Neurobiology of Learning and Memory* 118: 150–161.
Rolls ET & Deco G (2015b). Networks for memory, perception, and decision-making, and beyond to how the syntax for language might be implemented in the brain. *Brain Research* 1621: 316–334.
Rolls ET & Deco G (2016). Non-reward neural mechanisms in the orbitofrontal cortex. *Cortex* 83: 27–38.
Rolls ET & Grabenhorst F (2008). The orbitofrontal cortex and beyond: from affect to decision-making. *Progress in Neurobiology* 86: 216–244.
Rolls ET & Johnstone S (1992). Neurophysiological analysis of striatal function. In Vallar G, Cappa S, & Wallesch C, editors, *Neuropsychological Disorders Associated with Subcortical Lesions*, chap. 3, 61–97. Oxford University Press, Oxford.
Rolls ET & Kesner RP (2006). A theory of hippocampal function, and tests of the theory. *Progress in Neurobiology* 79: 1–48.
Rolls ET & McCabe C (2007). Enhanced affective brain representations of chocolate in cravers vs non-cravers. *European Journal of Neuroscience* 26: 1067–1076.
Rolls ET & Mills WPC (2018). Non-accidental properties, metric invariance, and encoding by neurons in a model of ventral stream visual object recognition, visnet. *Neurobiology of Learning and Memory* .
Rolls ET & Rolls BJ (1977). Activity of neurones in sensory, hypothalamic and motor areas during feeding in the monkey. In Katsuki Y, Sato M, Takagi S, & Oomura Y, editors, *Food Intake and Chemical Senses*, 525–549. University of Tokyo Press, Tokyo.
Rolls ET & Rolls BJ (1982b). Brain mechanisms involved in feeding. In Barker L, editor, *Psychobiology of Human Food Selection*, chap. 3, 33–62. AVI Publishing Company, Westport, Connecticut.
Rolls ET & Rolls JH (1997). Olfactory sensory-specific satiety in humans. *Physiology and Behavior* 61: 461–473.
Rolls ET & Scott TR (2003). Central taste anatomy and neurophysiology. In Doty R, editor, *Handbook of Olfaction and Gustation*, chap. 33, 679–705. Dekker, New York, 2nd edn.
Rolls ET & Stringer SM (2000). On the design of neural networks in the brain by genetic evolution. *Progress in Neurobiology* 61: 557–579.
Rolls ET & Stringer SM (2001). A model of the interaction between mood and memory. *Network: Computation in Neural Systems* 12: 89–109.
Rolls ET & Tovee MJ (1994). Processing speed in the cerebral cortex and the neurophysiology of visual masking. *Proceedings of the Royal Society, B* 257: 9–15.
Rolls ET & Tovee MJ (1995). Sparseness of the neuronal representation of stimuli in the primate temporal visual cortex. *Journal of Neurophysiology* 73: 713–726.
Rolls ET & Treves A (1990). The relative advantages of sparse versus distributed encoding for associative neuronal networks in the brain. *Network* 1: 407–421.
Rolls ET & Treves A (1998). *Neural Networks and Brain Function*. Oxford University Press, Oxford.
Rolls ET & Treves A (2011). The neuronal encoding of information in the brain. *Progress in Neurobiology* 95: 448–490.
Rolls ET & Webb TJ (2014). Finding and recognising objects in natural scenes: complementary computations in the dorsal and ventral visual systems. *Frontiers in Computational Neuroscience* 8: 85.

Rolls ET & Williams GV (1987). Neuronal activity in the ventral striatum of the primate. In Carpenter MB & Jayamaran A, editors, *The Basal Ganglia II – Structure and Function – Current Concepts*, 349–356. Plenum, New York.

Rolls ET & Wirth S (2018). Spatial representations in the primate hippocampus, and their functions in memory and navigation .

Rolls ET & Xiang JZ (2005). Reward–spatial view representations and learning in the primate hippocampus. *Journal of Neuroscience* 25: 6167–6174.

Rolls ET & Xiang JZ (2006). Spatial view cells in the primate hippocampus, and memory recall. *Reviews in the Neurosciences* 17: 175–200.

Rolls ET, Judge SJ, & Sanghera M (1977). Activity of neurones in the inferotemporal cortex of the alert monkey. *Brain Research* 130: 229–238.

Rolls ET, Rolls BJ, & Rowe EA (1983b). Sensory-specific and motivation-specific satiety for the sight and taste of food and water in man. *Physiology and Behavior* 30: 185–192.

Rolls ET, Thorpe SJ, & Maddison SP (1983c). Responses of striatal neurons in the behaving monkey. 1. Head of the caudate nucleus. *Behavioural Brain Research* 7: 179–210.

Rolls ET, Thorpe SJ, Boytim M, Szabo I, & Perrett DI (1984b). Responses of striatal neurons in the behaving monkey. 3. Effects of iontophoretically applied dopamine on normal responsiveness. *Neuroscience* 12: 1201–1212.

Rolls ET, Baylis GC, & Leonard CM (1985). Role of low and high spatial frequencies in the face-selective responses of neurons in the cortex in the superior temporal sulcus. *Vision Research* 25: 1021–1035.

Rolls ET, Murzi E, Yaxley S, Thorpe SJ, & Simpson SJ (1986). Sensory-specific satiety: food-specific reduction in responsiveness of ventral forebrain neurons after feeding in the monkey. *Brain Research* 368: 79–86.

Rolls ET, Baylis GC, & Hasselmo ME (1987). The responses of neurons in the cortex in the superior temporal sulcus of the monkey to band-pass spatial frequency filtered faces. *Vision Research* 27: 311–326.

Rolls ET, Scott TR, Sienkiewicz ZJ, & Yaxley S (1988). The responsiveness of neurones in the frontal opercular gustatory cortex of the macaque monkey is independent of hunger. *Journal of Physiology* 397: 1–12.

Rolls ET, Miyashita Y, Cahusac PMB, Kesner RP, Niki H, Feigenbaum J, & Bach L (1989a). Hippocampal neurons in the monkey with activity related to the place in which a stimulus is shown. *Journal of Neuroscience* 9: 1835–1845.

Rolls ET, Sienkiewicz ZJ, & Yaxley S (1989b). Hunger modulates the responses to gustatory stimuli of single neurons in the caudolateral orbitofrontal cortex of the macaque monkey. *European Journal of Neuroscience* 1: 53–60.

Rolls ET, Yaxley S, & Sienkiewicz ZJ (1990). Gustatory responses of single neurons in the orbitofrontal cortex of the macaque monkey. *Journal of Neurophysiology* 64: 1055–1066.

Rolls ET, Hornak J, Wade D, & McGrath J (1994a). Emotion-related learning in patients with social and emotional changes associated with frontal lobe damage. *Journal of Neurology, Neurosurgery and Psychiatry* 57: 1518–1524.

Rolls ET, Tovee MJ, Purcell DG, Stewart AL, & Azzopardi P (1994b). The responses of neurons in the temporal cortex of primates, and face identification and detection. *Experimental Brain Research* 101: 474–484.

Rolls ET, Critchley HD, Mason R, & Wakeman EA (1996a). Orbitofrontal cortex neurons: role in olfactory and visual association learning. *Journal of Neurophysiology* 75: 1970–1981.

Rolls ET, Critchley HD, Wakeman EA, & Mason R (1996b). Responses of neurons in the primate taste cortex to the glutamate ion and to inosine 5′-monophosphate. *Physiology and Behavior* 59: 991–1000.

Rolls ET, Robertson RG, & Georges-François P (1997a). Spatial view cells in the primate hippocampus. *European Journal of Neuroscience* 9: 1789–1794.

Rolls ET, Treves A, Foster D, & Perez-Vicente C (1997b). Simulation studies of the CA3 hippocampal subfield modelled as an attractor neural network. *Neural Networks* 10: 1559–1569.

Rolls ET, Treves A, Tovee M, & Panzeri S (1997c). Information in the neuronal representation of individual stimuli in the primate temporal visual cortex. *Journal of Computational Neuroscience* 4: 309–333.

Rolls ET, Treves A, & Tovee MJ (1997d). The representational capacity of the distributed encoding of information provided by populations of neurons in the primate temporal visual cortex. *Experimental Brain Research* 114: 149–162.

Rolls ET, Critchley HD, Browning A, & Hernadi I (1998a). The neurophysiology of taste and olfaction in primates, and umami flavor. *Annals of the New York Academy of Sciences* 855: 426–437.

Rolls ET, Treves A, Robertson RG, Georges-François P, & Panzeri S (1998b). Information about spatial view in an ensemble of primate hippocampal cells. *Journal of Neurophysiology* 79: 1797–1813.

Rolls ET, Critchley HD, Browning AS, Hernadi A, & Lenard L (1999a). Responses to the sensory properties of fat of neurons in the primate orbitofrontal cortex. *Journal of Neuroscience* 19: 1532–1540.

Rolls ET, Tovee MJ, & Panzeri S (1999b). The neurophysiology of backward visual masking: information analysis. *Journal of Cognitive Neuroscience* 11: 335–346.

Rolls ET, Stringer SM, & Trappenberg TP (2002). A unified model of spatial and episodic memory. *Proceedings of The Royal Society B* 269: 1087–1093.

Rolls ET, Aggelopoulos NC, & Zheng F (2003a). The receptive fields of inferior temporal cortex neurons in natural scenes. *Journal of Neuroscience* 23: 339–348.
Rolls ET, Franco L, Aggelopoulos NC, & Reece S (2003b). An information theoretic approach to the contributions of the firing rates and the correlations between the firing of neurons. *Journal of Neurophysiology* 89: 2810–2822.
Rolls ET, Kringelbach ML, & De Araujo IET (2003c). Different representations of pleasant and unpleasant odours in the human brain. *European Journal of Neuroscience* 18: 695–703.
Rolls ET, O'Doherty J, Kringelbach ML, Francis S, Bowtell R, & McGlone F (2003d). Representations of pleasant and painful touch in the human orbitofrontal and cingulate cortices. *Cerebral Cortex* 13: 308–317.
Rolls ET, Verhagen JV, & Kadohisa M (2003e). Representations of the texture of food in the primate orbitofrontal cortex: neurons responding to viscosity, grittiness, and capsaicin. *Journal of Neurophysiology* 90: 3711–3724.
Rolls ET, Aggelopoulos NC, Franco L, & Treves A (2004). Information encoding in the inferior temporal visual cortex: contributions of the firing rates and the correlations between the firing of neurons. *Biological Cybernetics* 90: 19–32.
Rolls ET, Browning AS, Inoue K, & Hernadi S (2005a). Novel visual stimuli activate a population of neurons in the primate orbitofrontal cortex. *Neurobiology of Learning and Memory* 84: 111–123.
Rolls ET, Xiang JZ, & Franco L (2005b). Object, space and object-space representations in the primate hippocampus. *Journal of Neurophysiology* 94: 833–844.
Rolls ET, Critchley HD, Browning AS, & Inoue K (2006). Face-selective and auditory neurons in the primate orbitofrontal cortex. *Experimental Brain Research* 170: 74–87.
Rolls ET, Grabenhorst F, Margot C, da Silva M, & Velazco MI (2008a). Selective attention to affective value alters how the brain processes olfactory stimuli. *Journal of Cognitive Neuroscience* 20: 1815–1826.
Rolls ET, Grabenhorst F, & Parris B (2008b). Warm pleasant feelings in the brain. *Neuroimage* 41: 1504–1513.
Rolls ET, Loh M, & Deco G (2008c). An attractor hypothesis of obsessive-compulsive disorder. *European Journal of Neuroscience* 28: 782–793.
Rolls ET, Loh M, Deco G, & Winterer G (2008d). Computational models of schizophrenia and dopamine modulation in the prefrontal cortex. *Nature Reviews Neuroscience* 9: 696–709.
Rolls ET, McCabe C, & Redoute J (2008e). Expected value, reward outcome, and temporal difference error representations in a probabilistic decision task. *Cerebral Cortex* 18: 652–663.
Rolls ET, Grabenhorst F, & Franco L (2009). Prediction of subjective affective state from brain activations. *Journal of Neurophysiology* 101: 1294–1308.
Rolls ET, Critchley H, Verhagen JV, & Kadohisa M (2010a). The representation of information about taste and odor in the primate orbitofrontal cortex. *Chemosensory Perception* 3: 16–33.
Rolls ET, Grabenhorst F, & Deco G (2010b). Choice, difficulty, and confidence in the brain. *Neuroimage* 53: 694–706.
Rolls ET, Grabenhorst F, & Deco G (2010c). Decision-making, errors, and confidence in the brain. *Journal of Neurophysiology* 104: 2359–2374.
Rolls ET, Grabenhorst F, & Parris BA (2010d). Neural systems underlying decisions about affective odors. *Journal of Cognitive Neuroscience* 10: 1068–1082.
Rolls ET, Webb TJ, & Deco G (2012). Communication before coherence. *European Journal of Neuroscience* 36: 2689–2709.
Rolls ET, Dempere-Marco L, & Deco G (2013). Holding multiple items in short term memory: a neural mechanism. *PLoS One* 8: e61078.
Rolls ET, Joliot M, & Tzourio-Mazoyer N (2015). Implementation of a new parcellation of the orbitofrontal cortex in the automated anatomical labeling atlas. *Neuroimage* 122: 1–5.
Rolls ET, Cheng W, Gilson M, Qiu J, Hu Z, Li Y, Huang CC, Yang AC, Tsai SJ, Zhang X, Zhuang K, Lin CP, Deco G, Xie P, & Feng J (2018a). Effective connectivity in depression. *Biological Psychiatry: Cognitive Neuroscience and Neuroimaging* 3: 187–197.
Rolls ET, Cheng W, Qiu J, Zhou C, Zhang J, Lyu W, Ruan H, Wei D, Huang CC, Yang AC, Tsai SJ, Cheng K, Meng J, Lin CP, Xie P, & Feng J (2018b). Functional connectivity of the anterior cingulate cortex in depression and in health. *Cerebral Cortex* .
Rolls ET, Mills T, Norton A, Lazidis A, & Norton IT (2018c). Neuronal encoding of fat using the coefficient of sliding friction .
Rosati AG (2017). *The Evolution of Primate Executive Function: From Response Control to Strategic Decision-Making*, vol. 3, book section 23, 423–437. Elsevier, Amsterdam, 2nd edn. doi:http://dx.doi.org/10.1016/B978-0-12-804042-3.00093-2.
Rosenkilde CE (1979). Functional heterogeneity of the prefrontal cortex in the monkey: a review. *Behavioral and Neural Biology* 25: 301–345.
Rosenkilde CE, Bauer RH, & Fuster JM (1981). Single unit activity in ventral prefrontal cortex in behaving monkeys. *Brain Research* 209: 375–394.
Rosenthal D (1990). A theory of consciousness. *ZIF Report 40/1990. Zentrum für Interdisziplinaire Forschung, Bielefeld* 40. Reprinted in Block, N., Flanagan, O. and Guzeldere, G. (eds.) (1997) *The Nature of Consciousness: Philosophical Debates*. MIT Press, Cambridge MA, pp. 729–853.

Rosenthal DM (1986). Two concepts of consciousness. *Philosophical Studies* 49: 329–359.
Rosenthal DM (1993). Thinking that one thinks. In Davies M & Humphreys GW, editors, *Consciousness*, chap. 10, 197–223. Blackwell, Oxford.
Rosenthal DM (2004). Varieties of higher order theory. In Gennaro RJ, editor, *Higher Order Theories of Consciousness*, 17–44. John Benjamins, Amsterdam.
Rosenthal DM (2005). *Consciousness and Mind*. Oxford University Press, Oxford.
Rosenthal DM (2012). Higher-order awareness, misrepresentation, and function. *Philosophical Transactions of the Royal Society B: Biological Sciences* 367: 1424–1438.
Royet JP, Zald D, Versace R, Costes N, Lavenne F, Koenig O, Gervais R, Routtenberg A, Gardner EI, & Huang YH (2000). Emotional responses to pleasant and unpleasant olfactory, visual, and auditory stimuli: a positron emission tomography study. *Journal of Neuroscience* 20: 7752–7759.
Rudebeck PH & Murray EA (2011). Dissociable effects of subtotal lesions within the macaque orbital prefrontal cortex on reward-guided behavior. *Journal of Neuroscience* 31: 10569–10578.
Rudebeck PH & Murray EA (2014). The orbitofrontal oracle: cortical mechanisms for the prediction and evaluation of specific behavioral outcomes. *Neuron* 84: 1143–56.
Rudebeck PH, Behrens TE, Kennerley SW, Baxter MG, Buckley MJ, Walton ME, & Rushworth MF (2008). Frontal cortex subregions play distinct roles in choices between actions and stimuli. *Journal of Neuroscience* 28: 13775–13785.
Rudebeck PH, Saunders RC, Lundgren DA, & Murray EA (2017). Specialized representations of value in the orbital and ventrolateral prefrontal cortex: Desirability versus availability of outcomes. *Neuron* 95: 1208–1220 e5.
Rumelhart DE, Hinton GE, & Williams RJ (1986). Learning internal representations by error propagation. In Rumelhart DE, McClelland JL, & the PDP Research Group, editors, *Parallel Distributed Processing: Explorations in the Microstructure of Cognition*, vol. 1, chap. 8, 318–362. MIT Press, Cambridge, MA.
Rupp HA & Wallen K (2009). Sex-specific content preferences for visual sexual stimuli. *Archives in Sexual Behavior* 38: 417–426.
Rushworth MF, Noonan MP, Boorman ED, Walton ME, & Behrens TE (2011). Frontal cortex and reward-guided learning and decision-making. *Neuron* 70: 1054–1069.
Rushworth MF, Kolling N, Sallet J, & Mars RB (2012). Valuation and decision-making in frontal cortex: one or many serial or parallel systems? *Current Opinion in Neurobiology* 22: 946–955.
Rushworth MFS, Hadland KA, Paus T, & Sipila PK (2002). Role of the human medial frontal cortex in task-switching: a combined fMRI and TMS study. *Journal of Neurophysiology* 87: 2577–2592.
Rushworth MFS, Walton ME, Kennerley SW, & Bannerman DM (2004). Action sets and decisions in the medial frontal cortex. *Trends in Cognitive Sciences* 8: 410–417.
Rushworth MFS, Buckley MJ, Behrens TE, Walton ME, & Bannerman DM (2007). Functional organization of the medial frontal cortex. *Current Opinion in Neurobiology* 17: 220–227.
Rusting C & Larsen R (1998). Personality and cognitive processing of affective information. *Personality and Social Psychology Bulletin* 24: 200–213.
Rutishauser U, Tudusciuc O, Neumann D, Mamelak AN, Heller AC, Ross IB, Philpott L, Sutherling WW, & Adolphs R (2011). Single-unit responses selective for whole faces in the human amygdala. *Current Biology* 21: 1654–1660.
Rutishauser U, Mamelak AN, & Adolphs R (2015). The primate amygdala in social perception - insights from electrophysiological recordings and stimulation. *Trends Neurosci* 38: 295–306.
Rylander G (1948). Personality analysis before and after frontal lobotomy. *Association for Research into Nervous and Mental Disorders* 27 (The Frontal Lobes): 691–705.
Saez RA, Saez A, Paton JJ, Lau B, & Salzman CD (2017). Distinct roles for the amygdala and orbitofrontal cortex in representing the relative amount of expected reward. *Neuron* 95: 70–77 e3.
Saint-Cyr JA, Ungerleider LG, & Desimone R (1990). Organization of visual cortical inputs to the striatum and subsequent outputs to the pallido-nigral complex in the monkey. *Journal of Comparative Neurology* 298: 129–156.
Saleem KS, Kondo H, & Price JL (2008). Complementary circuits connecting the orbital and medial prefrontal networks with the temporal, insular, and opercular cortex in the macaque monkey. *Journal of Comparative Neurology* 506: 659–693.
Saleem KS, Miller B, & Price JL (2014). Subdivisions and connectional networks of the lateral prefrontal cortex in the macaque monkey. *Journal of Comparative Neurology* 522: 1641–1690.
Sandman N, Merikanto I, Maattanen H, Valli K, Kronholm E, Laatikainen T, Partonen T, & Paunio T (2016). Winter is coming: nightmares and sleep problems during seasonal affective disorder. *J Sleep Res* 25: 612–619.
Sanfey AG, Rilling JK, Aronson JA, Nystrom LE, & Cohen JD (2003). The neural basis of economic decision-making in the ultimatum game. *Science* 300: 1755–1758.
Sanghera MK, Rolls ET, & Roper-Hall A (1979). Visual responses of neurons in the dorsolateral amygdala of the alert monkey. *Experimental Neurology* 63: 610–626.
Savic I (2014). *Pheromone Processing in Relation to Sex and Sexual Orientation*, book section 18. Frontiers in Neuroscience. CRC Press, Boca Raton (FL).

Schachter S (1971). Importance of cognitive control in obesity. *American Psychologist* 26: 129–144.

Schachter S & Singer J (1962). Cognitive, social and physiological determinants of emotional state. *Psychological Review* 69: 378–399.

Scherer K (2009). The dynamic architecture of emotion: Evidence for the component process model. *Cognition and Emotion* 23: 1307–1351.

Schiller D, Monfils MH, Raio CM, Johnson DC, LeDoux JE, & Phelps EA (2010). Preventing the return of fear in humans using reconsolidation update mechanisms. *Nature* 463: 49–53.

Schilthuizen M (2015). *Nature's Nether Regions: What the Sex Lives of Bugs, Birds, and Beasts Tell Us about Evolution, Biodiversity, and Ourselves.* Penguin, New York.

Schirmer A, Zysset S, Kotz SA, & von Cramon YD (2004). Gender differences in the activation of inferior frontal cortex during emotional speech perception. *Neuroimage* 21: 1114–1123.

Schoenbaum G & Eichenbaum H (1995). Information encoding in the rodent prefrontal cortex. I. Single-neuron activity in orbitofrontal cortex compared with that in pyriform cortex. *Journal of Neurophysiology* 74: 733–750.

Schoenbaum G, Roesch MR, Stalnaker TA, & Takahashi YK (2009). A new perspective on the role of the orbitofrontal cortex in adaptive behaviour. *Nature Reviews Neuroscience* 10: 885–892.

Schultz W (2013). Updating dopamine reward signals. *Current Opinion in Neurobiology* 23: 229–238.

Schultz W (2016a). Dopamine reward prediction-error signalling: a two-component response. *Nat Rev Neurosci* 17: 183–95.

Schultz W (2016b). Reward functions of the basal ganglia. *J Neural Transm (Vienna)* 123: 679–693.

Schultz W, Romo R, Ljunberg T, Mirenowicz J, Hollerman JR, & Dickinson A (1995). Reward-related signals carried by dopamine neurons. In Houk JC, Davis JL, & Beiser DG, editors, *Models of Information Processing in the Basal Ganglia*, chap. 12, 233–248. MIT Press, Cambridge, MA.

Schwartz MW & Porte D (2005). Diabetes, obesity, and the brain. *Science* 307: 375–379.

Scott SK, Young AW, Calder AJ, Hellawell DJ, Aggleton JP, & Johnson M (1997). Impaired auditory recognition of fear and anger following bilateral amygdala lesions. *Nature* 385: 254–257.

Scott TR (2011). Learning through the taste system. *Frontiers in Systems Neuroscience* 5: 87.

Scott TR & Giza BK (1987). A measure of taste intensity discrimination in the rat through conditioned taste aversions. *Physiology and Behaviour* 41: 315–320.

Scott TR & Giza BK (1992). Gustatory control of ingestion. In Booth DA, editor, *The Neurophysiology of Ingestion.* Manchester University Press, Manchester.

Scott TR & Small DM (2009). The role of the parabrachial nucleus in taste processing and feeding. *Annals of the New York Academy of Sciences* 1170: 372–377.

Scott TR, Yaxley S, Sienkiewicz ZJ, & Rolls ET (1986). Gustatory responses in the frontal opercular cortex of the alert cynomolgus monkey. *Journal of Neurophysiology* 56: 876–890.

Scott TR, Karadi Z, Oomura Y, Nishino H, Plata-Salaman CR, Lenard L, Giza BK, & Aou S (1993). Gustatory neural coding in the amygdala of the alert monkey. *Journal of Neurophysiology* 69: 1810–1820.

Scott TR, Yan J, & Rolls ET (1995). Brain mechanisms of satiety and taste in macaques. *Neurobiology* 3: 281–292.

Seleman LD & Goldman-Rakic PS (1985). Longitudinal topography and interdigitation of corticostriatal projections in the rhesus monkey. *Journal of Neuroscience* 5: 776–794.

Seligman ME (1970). On the generality of the laws of learning. *Psychological Review* 77: 406–418.

Seligman ME (1978). Learned helplessness as a model of depression. Comment and integration. *Journal of Abnormal Psychology* 87: 165–179.

Seltzer B & Pandya DN (1989). Frontal lobe connections of the superior temporal sulcus in the rhesus monkey. *Journal of Comparative Neurology* 281: 97–113.

Shackelford TK & Goetz AT (2007). Adaptation to sperm competition in humans. *Current Directions in Psychological Science* 16: 47–50.

Shackelford TK, Le Blanc GL, Weekes-Shackelford VA, Bleske-Rechek AL, Euler HA, & Hoier S (2002). Psychological adaptation to human sperm competition. *Evolution and Human Behaviour* 23: 123–138.

Shang Y, Claridge-Chang A, Sjulson L, Pypaert M, & Miesenböck G (2007). Excitatory local circuits and their implications for olfactory processing in the fly antennal lobe. *Cell* 128: 601–612.

Shen X, Tokoglu F, Papademetris X, & Constable RT (2013). Groupwise whole-brain parcellation from resting-state fmri data for network node identification. *Neuroimage* 82: 403–15.

Shima K & Tanji J (1998). Role for cingulate motor area cells in voluntary movement selection based on reward. *Science* 13: 1335–1338.

Shimura T & Shimokochi M (1990). Involvement of the lateral mesencephalic tegmentum in copulatory behavior of male rats: neuron activity in freely moving animals. *Neuroscience Research* 9: 173–183.

Simmen-Tulberg B & Moller AP (1993). The relationship between concealed ovulation and mating systems in anthropoid primates: a phylogenetic analysis. *American Naturalist* 141: 1–25.

Simmons JM, Minamimoto T, Murray EA, & Richmond BJ (2010). Selective ablations reveal that orbital and lateral prefrontal cortex play different roles in estimating predicted reward value. *Journal of Neuroscience* 30: 15878–15887.

Simmons LW, Firman RC, Rhodes G, & Peters M (2004). Human sperm competition: testis size, sperm production and rate of extra-pair copulations. *Animal Behaviour* 68: 297–302.

Singer P (1981). *The Expanding Circle: Ethics and Sociobiology*. Oxford University Press, Oxford.

Singer T, Seymour B, O'Doherty J, Kaube H, Dolan RJ, & Frith CD (2004). Empathy for pain involves the affective but not sensory components of pain. *Science* 303: 1157–1162.

Singer W (1999). Neuronal synchrony: A versatile code for the definition of relations? *Neuron* 24: 49–65.

Singh D & Bronstad MP (2001). Female body odour is a potential cue to ovulation. *Proceedings of the Royal Society of London B* 268: 797–801.

Singh D & Young RK (1995). Body weight, waist-to-hip ratio, breasts and hips: role in judgements of female attractiveness and desirability for relationships. *Ethology and Sociobiology* 16: 483–507.

Singh D, Meyer W, Zambarano RJ, & Hurlbert DF (1998). Frequency and timing of coital orgasm in women desirous of becoming pregnant. *Archives of Sexual Behaviour* 27: 15–29.

Small DM & Scott TR (2009). Symposium overview: What happens to the pontine processing? Repercussions of interspecies differences in pontine taste representation for tasting and feeding. *Annals of the New York Academy of Science* 1170: 343–346.

Small DM, Zald DH, Jones-Gotman M, Zatorre RJ, Petrides M, & Evans AC (1999). Human cortical gustatory areas: a review of functional neuroimaing data. *NeuroReport* 8: 3913–3917.

Small DM, Bender G, Veldhuizen MG, Rudenga K, Nachtigal D, & Felsted J (2007). The role of the human orbitofrontal cortex in taste and flavor processing. *Annals of the New York Academy of Sciences* 1121: 136–151.

Smerieri A, Rolls ET, & Feng J (2010). Decision time, slow inhibition, and theta rhythm. *Journal of Neuroscience* 30: 14173–14181.

Snyder SH (2004). Opiate receptors and beyond: 30 years of neural signaling research. *Neuropharmacology* 47 Suppl 1: 274–85.

Soares JC & Young AH (2016). *Bipolar Disorder: basic mechanisms and therapeutic implications*. Cambridge University Press, Cambridge, 3rd edn.

Sobel N, Prabhakaran V, Hartley CA, Desmond JE, Glover GH, Sullivan EV, & Gabrieli JD (1999). Blind smell: brain activation induced by an undetected air-borne chemical. *Brain* 122: 209–217.

Spiridon M, Fischl B, & Kanwisher N (2006). Location and spatial profile of category-specific regions in human extrastriate cortex. *Human Brain Mapping* 27: 77–89.

Squire LR, Stark CEL, & Clark RE (2004). The medial temporal lobe. *Annual Review of Neuroscience* 27: 279–306.

Stalnaker TA, Cooch NK, & Schoenbaum G (2015). What the orbitofrontal cortex does not do. *Nat Neurosci* 18: 620–7.

Stefanacci L, Suzuki WA, & Amaral DG (1996). Organization of connections between the amygdaloid complex and the perirhinal and parahippocampal cortices in macaque monkeys. *Journal of Comparative Neurology* 375: 552–582.

Stephan KE, Weiskopf N, Drysdale PM, Robinson PA, & Friston KJ (2007). Comparing hemodynamic models with DCM. *Neuroimage* 38: 387–401.

Stephenson-Jones M, Yu K, Ahrens S, Tucciarone JM, van Huijstee AN, Mejia LA, Penzo MA, Tai LH, Wilbrecht L, & Li B (2016). A basal ganglia circuit for evaluating action outcomes. *Nature* 539: 289–293.

Stocks NG (2000). Suprathreshold stochastic resonance in multilevel threshold systems. *Physical Review Letters* 84: 2310–2313.

Stowers L & Kuo TH (2015). Mammalian pheromones: emerging properties and mechanisms of detection. *Curr Opin Neurobiol* 34: 103–9.

Strongman KT (2003). *The Psychology of Emotion*. Wiley, New York, 5th edn.

Sugiura M, Watanabe J, Maeda Y, Matsue Y, Fukuda H, & Kawashima R (2005). Cortical mechanisms of visual self-recognition. *Neuroimage* 24: 143–9.

Sugrue LP, Corrado GS, & Newsome WT (2005). Choosing the greater of two goods: neural currencies for valuation and decision making. *Nature Reviews Neuroscience* 6: 363–375.

Suleiman AB, Galvan A, Harden KP, & Dahl RE (2017). Becoming a sexual being: The 'elephant in the room' of adolescent brain development. *Dev Cogn Neurosci* 25: 209–220.

Suzuki WA & Amaral DG (1994). Perirhinal and parahippocampal cortices of the macaque monkey – cortical afferents. *Journal of Comparative Neurology* 350: 497–533.

Swaddle JP & Reierson GW (2002). Testosterone increases perceived dominance but not attractiveness in human males. *Proceedings of the Royal Society of London B* 269: 2285–2289.

Swann AC (2009). Impulsivity in mania. *Current Psychiatry Reports* 11: 481–487.

Tabuchi E, Mulder AB, & Wiener SI (2003). Reward value invariant place responses and reward site associated activity in hippocampal neurons of behaving rats. *Hippocampus* 13: 117–132.

Tanaka D (1973). Effects of selective prefrontal decortication on escape behavior in the monkey. *Brain Research* 53: 161–173.

Terenius L & Johansson B (2010). The opioid systems–panacea and nemesis. *Biochemical and Biophysical Research Communications* 396: 140–142.

Tessman I (1995). Human altruism as a courtship display. *Oikos* 74: 157–158.
Thibaut F (2017). Anxiety disorders: a review of current literature. *Dialogues Clin Neurosci* 19: 87–88.
Thomas DM, Bouchard C, Church T, Slentz C, Kraus WE, Redman LM, Martin CK, Silva AM, Vossen M, Westerterp K, & Heymsfield SB (2012). Why do individuals not lose more weight from an exercise intervention at a defined dose? An energy balance analysis. *Obesity Reviews* 13: 835–847.
Thornhill R & Gangestad SW (2015). *The functional design and phylogeny of womenâ^s sexuality*, 149–184. Springer.
Thornhill R & Gangstad SW (1999). The scent of symmetry: a human sex pheromone that signals fitness? *Evolution and Human Behaviour* 20: 175–201.
Thornhill R & Grammer K (1999). The body and face of woman: one ornament that signals quality? *Evolution and Human Behaviour* 20: 105–120.
Thornhill R, Gangestad SW, & Comer R (1995). Human female orgasm and mate fluctuating asymmetry. *Animal Behaviour* 50: 1601–1615.
Thorpe SJ, Maddison S, & Rolls ET (1979). Single unit activity in the orbitofrontal cortex of the behaving monkey. *Neuroscience Letters* S3: S77.
Thorpe SJ, Rolls ET, & Maddison S (1983). Neuronal activity in the orbitofrontal cortex of the behaving monkey. *Experimental Brain Research* 49: 93–115.
Tiihonen J, Kuikka J, Kupila J, Partanen K, Vainio P, Airaksinen J, Eronen M, Hallikainen T, Paanila J, Kinnunen I, & Huttunen J (1994). Increase in cerebral blood flow of right prefrontal cortex in man during orgasm. *Neuroscience Letters* 170: 241–243.
Tinbergen N (1951). *The Study of Instinct.* Oxford University Press, Oxford.
Tinbergen N (1963). On aims and methods of ethology. *Zeitschrift fur Tierpsychologie* 20: 410–433.
Tomkins SS (1995). *Exploring Affect: The Selected Writings of Sylvan S. Tomkins.* Cambridge University Press, New York.
Tonegawa S, Nakazawa K, & Wilson MA (2003). Genetic neuroscience of mammalian learning and memory. *Philosophical Transactions of the Royal Society of London B Biological Sciences* 358: 787–795.
Tovee MJ & Rolls ET (1992). Oscillatory activity is not evident in the primate temporal visual cortex with static stimuli. *Neuroreport* 3: 369–372.
Tovee MJ & Rolls ET (1995). Information encoding in short firing rate epochs by single neurons in the primate temporal visual cortex. *Visual Cognition* 2: 35–58.
Tovee MJ, Rolls ET, Treves A, & Bellis RP (1993). Information encoding and the responses of single neurons in the primate temporal visual cortex. *Journal of Neurophysiology* 70: 640–654.
Tovee MJ, Rolls ET, & Azzopardi P (1994). Translation invariance and the responses of neurons in the temporal visual cortical areas of primates. *Journal of Neurophysiology* 72: 1049–1060.
Tranel D, Bechara A, & Denburg NL (2002). Asymmetric functional roles of right and left ventromedial prefrontal cortices in social conduct, decision-making and emotional processing. *Cortex* 38: 589–612.
Trappenberg TP, Rolls ET, & Stringer SM (2002). Effective size of receptive fields of inferior temporal visual cortex neurons in natural scenes. In Dietterich TG, Becker S, & Gharamani Z, editors, *Advances in Neural Information Processing Systems*, vol. 14, 293–300. MIT Press, Cambridge, MA.
Tremblay L & Schultz W (1999). Relative reward preference in primate orbitofrontal cortex. *Nature* 398: 704–708.
Treves A & Rolls ET (1991). What determines the capacity of autoassociative memories in the brain? *Network* 2: 371–397.
Treves A & Rolls ET (1992). Computational constraints suggest the need for two distinct input systems to the hippocampal CA3 network. *Hippocampus* 2: 189–199.
Treves A & Rolls ET (1994). A computational analysis of the role of the hippocampus in memory. *Hippocampus* 4: 374–391.
Treves A, Panzeri S, Rolls ET, Booth M, & Wakeman EA (1999). Firing rate distributions and efficiency of information transmission of inferior temporal cortex neurons to natural visual stimuli. *Neural Computation* 11: 601–631.
Trivers R (1971). The evolution of reciprocal altruism. *Quarterly Review of Biology* 46: 35–57.
Trivers R (1974). Parent-offspring conflict. *American Zoologist* 14: 249–264.
Trivers RL (1985). *Social Evolution.* Benjamin, Cummings, CA.
Troisi A & Carosi M (1998). Female orgasm rate increases with male dominance in Japanese macaque. *Animal Behaviour* 56: 1261–1266.
Trull TJ & Widiger TA (2013). Dimensional models of personality: the five-factor model and the dsm-5. *Dialogues Clin Neurosci* 15: 135–46.
Tsao DY & Livingstone MS (2008). Mechanisms of face perception. *Annual Reviews of Neuroscience* 31: 411–437.
Udry JR & Eckland BK (1984). Benefits of being attractive: differential pay-offs for men and women. *Psychological Reports* 54: 47–56.
Ullsperger M & von Cramon DY (2001). Subprocesses of performance monitoring: a dissociation of error processing and response competition revealed by event-related fMRI and ERPs. *Neuroimage* 14: 1387–1401.

Ungerstedt U (1971). Adipsia and aphagia after 6-hydroxydopamine induced degeneration of the nigrostriatal dopamine system. *Acta Physiologia Scandinavica* 81 (Suppl. 367): 95–122.

Valenstein ES (1974). *Brain Control. A Critical Examination of Brain Stimulation and Psychosurgery*. Wiley, New York.

Van Hoesen GW (1981). The differential distribution, diversity and sprouting of cortical projections to the amygdala in the rhesus monkey. In Ben-Ari Y, editor, *The Amygdaloid Complex*, 77–90. Elsevier, Amsterdam.

Van Hoesen GW, Yeterian EH, & Lavizzo-Mourey R (1981). Widespread corticostriate projections from temporal cortex of the rhesus monkey. *Journal of Comparative Neurology* 199: 205–219.

van Veen V, Cohen JD, Botvinick MM, Stenger AV, & Carter CS (2001). Anterior cingulate cortex, conflict monitoring, and levels of processing. *Neuroimage* 14: 1302–1308.

vandenBerghe PL & Frost P (1986). Skin colour preferences, sexual dimorphism and sexual selection: a case for gene culture evolution. *Ethnic and Racial Studies* 9: 87–113.

Veening JG, de Jong TR, Waldinger MD, Korte SM, & Olivier B (2015). The role of oxytocin in male and female reproductive behavior. *Eur J Pharmacol* 753: 209–28.

Verhagen JV, Rolls ET, & Kadohisa M (2003). Neurons in the primate orbitofrontal cortex respond to fat texture independently of viscosity. *Journal of Neurophysiology* 90: 1514–1525.

Verhagen JV, Kadohisa M, & Rolls ET (2004). The primate insular taste cortex: neuronal representations of the viscosity, fat texture, grittiness, and the taste of foods in the mouth. *Journal of Neurophysiology* 92: 1685–1699.

Voellm BA, De Araujo IET, Cowen PJ, Rolls ET, Kringelbach ML, Smith KA, Jezzard P, Heal RJ, & Matthews PM (2004). Methamphetamine activates reward circuitry in drug naive human subjects. *Neuropsychopharmacology* 29: 1715–1722.

Vogt BA, editor (2009). *Cingulate Neurobiology and Disease*. Oxford University Press, Oxford.

Vogt BA & Laureys S (2009). *The primate posterior cingulate gyrus: connections, sensorimotor orientation, gateway to limbic processing*, book section 13, 275–308. Oxford University Press, Oxford.

Vogt BA & Pandya DN (1987). Cingulate cortex of the rhesus monkey: II. Cortical afferents. *Journal of Comparative Neurology* 262: 271–289.

Vogt BA & Sikes RW (2000). The medial pain system, cingulate cortex, and parallel processing of nociceptive information. *Progress in Brain Research* 122: 223–235.

Vogt BA, Derbyshire S, & Jones AKP (1996). Pain processing in four regions of human cingulate cortex localized with co-registered PET and MR imaging. *European Journal of Neuroscience* 8: 1461–1473.

Vogt BA, Berger GR, & Derbyshire SWG (2003). Structural and functional dichotomy of human midcingulate cortex. *European Journal of Neuroscience* 18: 3134–3144.

Volkow ND, Wang GJ, Tomasi D, & Baler RD (2013). Obesity and addiction: neurobiological overlaps. *Obesity Reviews* 14: 2–18.

Waelti P, Dickinson A, & Schultz W (2001). Dopamine responses comply with basic assumptions of formal learning theory. *Nature* 412: 43–48.

Walker DM, Bell MR, Flores C, Gulley JM, Willing J, & Paul MJ (2017). Adolescence and reward: Making sense of neural and behavioral changes amid the chaos. *J Neurosci* 37: 10855–10866.

Wallis G & Rolls ET (1997). Invariant face and object recognition in the visual system. *Progress in Neurobiology* 51: 167–194.

Wallis JD & Miller EK (2003). Neuronal activity in primate dorsolateral and orbital prefrontal cortex during performance of a reward preference task. *European Journal of Neuroscience* 18: 2069–2081.

Wallrabenstein I, Gerber J, Rasche S, Croy I, Kurtenbach S, Hummel T, & Hatt H (2015). The smelling of hedione results in sex-differentiated human brain activity. *Neuroimage* 113: 365–73.

Walton ME, Bannerman DM, & Rushworth MFS (2002). The role of rat medial frontal cortex in effort-based decision making. *Journal of Neuroscience* 22: 10996–11003.

Walton ME, Bannerman DM, Alterescu K, & Rushworth MFS (2003). Functional specialization within medial frontal cortex of the anterior cingulate for evaluating effort-related decisions. *Journal of Neuroscience* 23: 6475–6479.

Walton ME, Devlin JT, & Rushworth MF (2004). Interactions between decision making and performance monitoring within prefrontal cortex. *Nature Neuroscience* 7: 1259–1265.

Wang XJ (2002). Probabilistic decision making by slow reverberation in cortical circuits. *Neuron* 36: 955–968.

Wang XJ (2008). Decision making in recurrent neuronal circuits. *Neuron* 60: 215–234.

Watson JB (1930). *Behaviorism: Revised Edition*. University of Chicago Press, Chicago.

Wedell N, Gage MJ, & Parker G (2002). Sperm competition, male prudence and sperm limited females. *Proceedings of the Royal Society of London B* 260: 245–249.

Weiner KS & Grill-Spector K (2013). Neural representations of faces and limbs neighbor in human high-level visual cortex: evidence for a new organization principle. *Psychological Research* 77: 74–97.

Weisenfeld K (1993). An introduction to stochastic resonance. *Annals of the New York Academy of Sciences* 706: 13–25.

Weiskrantz L (1956). Behavioral changes associated with ablation of the amygdaloid complex in monkeys. *Journal of Comparative and Physiological Psychology* 49: 381–391.

Weiskrantz L (1968). Emotion. In Weiskrantz L, editor, *Analysis of Behavioural Change*, 50–90. Harper and Row, New York.
Weiskrantz L (1997). *Consciousness Lost and Found*. Oxford University Press, Oxford.
Weiskrantz L (1998). *Blindsight*. Oxford University Press, Oxford, 2nd edn.
Weiskrantz L (2009). Is blindsight just degraded normal vision? *Experimental Brain Research* 192: 413–416.
Wessa M, Kanske P, & Linke J (2014). Bipolar disorder: a neural network perspective on a disorder of emotion and motivation. *Restorative Neurology and Neuroscience* 32: 51–62.
West RA & Larson CR (1995). Neurons of the anterior mesial cortex related to faciovocal activity in the awake monkey. *Journal of Neurophysiology* 74: 1856–1869.
Whalen PJ & Phelps EA (2009). *The Human Amygdala*. Guilford, New York.
Wheeler EZ & Fellows LK (2008). The human ventromedial frontal lobe is critical for learning from negative feedback. *Brain* 131: 1323–1331.
Whelan R, Conrod PJ, Poline JB, Lourdusamy A, Banaschewski T, Barker GJ, Bellgrove MA, Büchel C, Byrne M, Cummins TDR, et al. (2012). Adolescent impulsivity phenotypes characterized by distinct brain networks. *Nature Neuroscience* 15: 920–925.
Wiech K & Tracey I (2013). Pain, decisions, and actions: a motivational perspective. *Frontiers in Neuroscience* 7: 46.
Wilks DC, Besson H, Lindroos AK, & Ekelund U (2011). Objectively measured physical activity and obesity prevention in children, adolescents and adults: a systematic review of prospective studies. *Obesity Reviews* 12: 119–129.
Williams GV, Rolls ET, Leonard CM, & Stern C (1993). Neuronal responses in the ventral striatum of the behaving macaque. *Behavioural Brain Research* 55: 243–252.
Wilson FAW & Rolls ET (1990a). Neuronal responses related to the novelty and familiarity of visual stimuli in the substantia innominata, diagonal band of Broca and periventricular region of the primate. *Experimental Brain Research* 80: 104–120.
Wilson FAW & Rolls ET (1990b). Neuronal responses related to reinforcement in the primate basal forebrain. *Brain Research* 509: 213–231.
Wilson FAW & Rolls ET (1990c). Learning and memory are reflected in the responses of reinforcement-related neurons in the primate basal forebrain. *Journal of Neuroscience* 10: 1254–1267.
Wilson FAW & Rolls ET (1993). The effects of stimulus novelty and familiarity on neuronal activity in the amygdala of monkeys performing recognition memory tasks. *Experimental Brain Research* 93: 367–382.
Wilson FAW & Rolls ET (2005). The primate amygdala and reinforcement: a dissociation between rule-based and associatively-mediated memory revealed in amygdala neuronal activity. *Neuroscience* 133: 1061–1072.
Wilson RI & Nicoll RA (2002). Endocannabinoid signalling in the brain. *Science* 296: 678–682.
Winkielman P & Berridge KC (2003). What is an unconscious emotion? *Cognition and Emotion* 17: 181–211.
Winkielman P & Berridge KC (2005). Unconscious affective reactions to masked happy versus angry faces influence consumption behavior and judgments of value. *Personality and Social Psychology Bulletin* 31: 111–135.
Winslow JT & Insel TR (2004). Neuroendrocrine basis of social recognition. *Current Opinion in Neurobiology* 14: 248–253.
Wise SP (2008). Forward frontal fields: phylogeny and fundamental function. *Trends in Neuroscience* 31: 599–608.
Wyatt TD (2014). *Pheromones and Animal Behaviour*. Cambridge University Press, Cambridge, 2nd edn.
Yamaguchi S (1967). The synergistic taste effect of monosodium glutamate and disodium 5′-inosinate. *Journal of Food Science* 32: 473–478.
Yamaguchi S & Kimizuka A (1979). Psychometric studies on the taste of monosodium glutamate. In Filer LJ, Garattini S, Kare MR, Reynolds AR, & Wurtman RJ, editors, *Glutamic Acid: Advances in Biochemistry and Physiology*, 35–54. Raven Press, New York.
Yan J & Scott TR (1996). The effect of satiety on responses of gustatory neurons in the amygdala of alert cynomolgus macaques. *Brain Research* 740: 193–200.
Yaxley S, Rolls ET, Sienkiewicz ZJ, & Scott TR (1985). Satiety does not affect gustatory activity in the nucleus of the solitary tract of the alert monkey. *Brain Research* 347: 85–93.
Yaxley S, Rolls ET, & Sienkiewicz ZJ (1988). The responsiveness of neurones in the insular gustatory cortex of the macaque monkey is independent of hunger. *Physiology and Behavior* 42: 223–229.
Yaxley S, Rolls ET, & Sienkiewicz ZJ (1990). Gustatory responses of single neurons in the insula of the macaque monkey. *Journal of Neurophysiology* 63: 689–700.
Yelnik J (2002). Functional anatomy of the basal ganglia. *Movement Disorders* 17 Suppl 3: S15–S21.
Yeterian EH, Pandya DN, Tomaiuolo F, & Petrides M (2012). The cortical connectivity of the prefrontal cortex in the monkey brain. *Cortex* 48: 58–81.
Yohn CN, Gergues MM, & Samuels BA (2017). The role of 5-ht receptors in depression. *Mol Brain* 10: 28.
Young AW, Aggleton JP, Hellawell DJ, Johnson M, Broks P, & Hanley JR (1995). Face processing impairments after amygdalotomy. *Brain* 118: 15–24.
Young AW, Hellawell DJ, Van de Wal C, & Johnson M (1996). Facial expression processing after amygdalotomy. *Neuropsychologia* 34: 31–39.

Young KA, Gobrogge KL, Liu Y, & Wang Z (2011). The neurobiology of pair bonding: insights from a socially monogamous rodent. *Frontiers in Neuroendocrinology* 32: 53–69.

Young LJ & Wang Z (2004). The neurobiology of pairbonding. *Nature Neuroscience* 7: 1048–1054.

Zahavi A (1975). Mate selection: a selection for a handicap. *Journal of Theoretical Biology* 53: 205–214.

Zahavi A & Zahavi A (1997). *The Handicap Principle: A Missing Piece of Darwin's Puzzle.* Oxford University Press, Oxford.

Zald DH & Rauch SL, editors (2006). *The Orbitofrontal Cortex.* Oxford University Press, Oxford.

Zangemeister L, Grabenhorst F, & Schultz W (2016). Neural basis for economic saving strategies in human amygdala-prefrontal reward circuits. *Curr Biol* 26: 3004–3013.

Zanos P & Gould TD (2018). Mechanisms of ketamine action as an antidepressant. *Mol Psychiatry* 23: 801–811.

Zanos P, Moaddel R, Morris PJ, Georgiou P, Fischell J, Elmer GI, Alkondon M, Yuan P, Pribut HJ, Singh NS, Dossou KS, Fang Y, Huang XP, Mayo CL, Wainer IW, Albuquerque EX, Thompson SM, Thomas CJ, Zarate J C A, & Gould TD (2016). Nmdar inhibition-independent antidepressant actions of ketamine metabolites. *Nature* 533: 481–6.

Zatorre RJ, Jones-Gotman M, Evans AC, & Meyer E (1992). Functional localization of human olfactory cortex. *Nature* 360: 339–340.

Zatorre RJ, Jones-Gotman M, & Rouby C (2000). Neural mechanisms involved in odor pleasantness and intensity judgments. *NeuroReport* 11: 2711–2716.

Zhao GQ, Zhang Y, Hoon MA, Chandrashekar J, Erlenbach I, Ryba NJ, & Zucker CS (2003). The receptors for mammalian sweet and umami taste. *Cell* 115: 255–266.

Zorumski CF, Izumi Y, & Mennerick S (2016). Ketamine: Nmda receptors and beyond. *J Neurosci* 36: 11158–11164.

Index